ADOLESCENT PSYCHIATRY

DEVELOPMENTAL AND CLINICAL STUDIES

VOLUME 12

Annals of the American Society for Adolescent Psychiatry

ADOLESCENT PSYCHIATRY

DEVELOPMENTAL AND CLINICAL STUDIES

VOLUME 12

Edited by
SHERMAN C. FEINSTEIN
Coordinating Editor

Senior Editors
MAX SUGAR
AARON H. ESMAN
JOHN G. LOONEY
ALLAN Z. SCHWARTZBERG
ARTHUR D. SOROSKY

The University of Chicago Press
Chicago and London

The University of Chicago Press, Chicago 60637
The University of Chicago Press, Ltd., London

Printed in the United States of America

International Standard Book Number: 0-226-24058-4
Library of Congress Catalog Card Number: 70-147017

CONTENTS

PART II. DEVELOPMENTAL ISSUES

PART III. PSYCHOPATHOLOGICAL ASPECTS OF ADOLESCENCE

PART IV. CLINICAL INSTITUTE: PERSPECTIVES IN THE TREATMENT OF ADOLESCENTS AND YOUTH

ROBERT M. GALATZER-LEVY, Special Editor

PART V. PSYCHOTHERAPEUTIC ISSUES IN ADOLESCENT PSYCHIATRY

PART VI. COUNTERTRANSFERENCE RESPONSES TO ADOLESCENTS

PETER L. GIOVACCHINI, Special Editor

PREFACE

The United Nations General Assembly has designated 1985 International Youth Year. Among major social and cultural changes, unique in the extent of their generality, is the emergence of adolescence as an essential stage in the life cycle. The history of adolescence barely takes in this century, and yet the adolescent population and its social and cultural apparatus have become an international phenomenon.

The significance of adolescence can easily be obscured as being reactive or masked—both partially true. Clearly, however, its purpose is to gather together and consolidate the emotional structures and cognitive processes required to achieve individual mental maturity. Great flexibility is required for this psychic work, which can easily become brutalized and impoverished. The opening up of social space has resulted in several phenomena: the elimination of the need for child and adolescent labor; the lengthening of the period of education and dependency; and the establishment of adolescence as the social norm.

With the establishment of the adolescent experience have come vast problems. This now-large, sociodemographic group is marked by problematic and destructive trends. Adolescents have become a "growth industry" for commercial exploitation, leaving them notably vulnerable. Broad educational problems can only be solved by achievement of the psychic aim of adolescence—emergence of the individual into adult mental maturity—still an enigma for science and society. If the general progress of modern society and culture is to be equated with higher levels of achievement, the enormous importance of adolescence becomes apparent.

These observations by Beresford Hayward of the Organization for Economic Cooperation and Development recognize the importance of adolescence in the developing nations of the world as well as in Western society. Adolescent psychiatry is, therefore, becoming increasingly transcultural and is achieving further levels of interest throughout the world as more behavioral scientists and educators accept its influence.

The American Society for Adolescent Psychiatry is dedicated to providing a forum for the communication of information about adolescence.

The Society has joined with other sponsoring societies in Europe, North and South America, and Asia to form an International Society for Adolescent Psychiatry, a project bequeathed to ASAP by our first president, William A. Schonfeld. Truly, the 1985 International Youth Year should be a significant coming of age for the adolescent.

PART I

ADOLESCENCE: GENERAL CONSIDERATIONS

EDITORS' INTRODUCTION

The question of identity formation is of concern to adolescent psychiatrists with respect not only to their patients but to their own profession as well. The consolidation of personal identity is, as Erikson has taught us, a particular task of adolescent development, and its failure in one way or another is linked with the psychopathology of adolescence as well as representing its legacy to adult impoverishment.

But adolescent psychiatry as a fledgling discipline is also concerned with consolidating its professional identity as manifested in the formation of organized programs for clinical, educational, and research activities that will serve to promote progress in these areas. The chapters in this part, therefore, emphasize the developmental aspects of adolescent psychiatry from a wide range of perspectives: research, creativity, training, coping, parenting, and sociocultural factors—all have as a common denominator Erikson's generative motive of human development.

Clarice J. Kestenbaum focuses on diagnostic criteria to help distinguish between adolescent turmoil and more malignant psychopathology. She discusses the level of functioning, constitutional predisposition, specific symptoms or behavior patterns, and environmental stresses. The author believes that early recognition and intervention may prevent deterioration through the bolstering of proper defenses.

Sol Nichtern analyzes the mind-and-body conflicts of adolescence and describes configurations that emerge reflecting both the nature of the conflicts and their resolution. He develops a psychiatric history of Mahatma Gandhi to illustrate one form of resolution—the victory of cognitive defenses over body impulses. Nichtern believes that the manner of resolution of adolescent turmoil is transmitted, developmentally and generationally, from one stage to the next.

Sidney Weissman and Rebecca S. Cohen address the significance of parenthood as a critical and ongoing experience of adulthood and describe the parenting alliance as a relationship vital to evolving parenthood roles and tasks. The authors focus on aspects of psychology of the self to clarify the developmental aspects of the parenting alliance and parenthood.

Nicholas Meyer poignantly explores his interest in art and his own personality development. Through the exploration of several characters in literature (Peter Pan, Henry Higgins, Sherlock Holmes), Meyer studies elements of his own emotional growth. The author concludes that where there is life, there is hope.

Meyer S. Gunther views serious, chronic, organic illness during adolescence as an integrated human experience. Such an experience is an expression of a basic human potential—the capacity of human beings to confront, transcend, and then grow when faced by a life-threatening, life-altering illness despite the monumental traumas and dilemmas in such adversity.

Irving N. Berlin presents a perspective on the incidence and dynamics of suicide among American Indian adolescents. He discusses data from national studies on suicide, sociocultural factors related to Native American adolescent suicide, and developmental issues in suicide and suicide attempts. He reviews problems in Native infant, preschool, school-aged children, and adolescents as well as intervention efforts. Berlin emphasizes, in approaching Indian adolescents, that tribal authorities must sanction and become involved in suicide intervention so that tribal traditions and concerns are communicated to the young persons.

John G. Looney, William Ellis, Elissa Benedek, and John Schowalter present a model core curriculum for training general psychiatric residents in adolescent psychiatry. The authors address the design of an optimal curriculum and its integration into the general training experience, and they outline what and how the resident should be taught.

John G. Looney reports the findings and recommendations of the Committee on Research of the American Society for Adolescent Psychiatry. The study documents the need for increased research efforts with adolescents, notes the temporary reliance on clinical psychiatrists to effect needed research efforts, and outlines important areas that need investigation. The report recommends that a national survey be undertaken to delineate those areas being studied in order to promote collaboration among researchers in adolescent psychiatry.

1 PUTTING IT ALL TOGETHER: A MULTIDIMENSIONAL ASSESSMENT OF PSYCHOTIC POTENTIAL IN ADOLESCENCE[1]

CLARICE J. KESTENBAUM

Some years ago, having just completed my psychiatric training, I was asked by a senior colleague to evaluate a seventeen-year-old girl. My colleague informed me that the patient was a professor's daughter, bright, gifted, and experiencing an identity crisis—"typical adolescent turmoil," he assured me. She had begun her first semester at an Ivy League school in a neighboring city. One night, three weeks after leaving home, she was brought to the student health emergency room in an agitated state and was hospitalized overnight. She had attended a party where she had been offered her first marijuana cigarette and apparently had experienced feelings of confusion and panic. Her parents, deciding that she was still immature, had her transferred back home where she enrolled in the local college.

I saw the young patient and, after taking a brief psychiatric history, began psychotherapy on a twice-weekly basis. I did not obtain a detailed family history other than to ask a few cursory questions regarding parental physical and mental health. The study of genetics had not been strongly emphasized during my training. I did not see the parents for the purpose of obtaining childhood developmental data because the patient did not want her parents to be involved in her treatment in any way other than to pay the bills, and I respected her wish for autonomy. I did not even obtain psychological tests because her grades had always been excellent. She had been, in fact, an A student.

Treatment proceeded smoothly for several weeks—too smoothly; in

0-226-24058-4/85/0012-0002$01.00

fact, the patient became extremely dependent on me, called me every day, and appeared in my office hours before her appointed session time. She discussed her wish to be a philosopher, her wish to meditate many hours a day, her growing isolation from peers, and her belief that she was somehow destined for greatness in a secret, mysterious way. She finally announced during her tenth session that she knew I was attempting to control her mind, "which is okay," she assured me, "since I like hearing your voice speaking to me from the radio or television."

At that point I called in her parents, who, despite my recommendation, refused to have their daughter hospitalized and removed her from my care. Three consultations later the patient finally forced her family to hospitalize her by stating that voices told her to kill herself. She was diagnosed as having paranoid schizophrenia. I learned from her physician that there was a strong family history of schizophrenia, that the patient herself had had numerous symptoms in early childhood, and that denial of any illness was customary in her family.

Adolescent Turmoil and Pathology

I present this case as an extreme example of misdiagnosis in order to illustrate the point that a distinction must be made between adolescent turmoil and more malignant pathology (Masterson 1968). Distinguishing features can help sort out those seriously disturbed adolescents into discrete groupings, permitting more accurate assessment, diagnosis, and treatment.

Holzman and Grinker (1977) have reviewed the literature on adolescent psychopathology (Block 1971; Offer and Offer 1973; Vaillant 1971). They conclude that "adolescence is *not* an intrinsically pathogenic period. Although some turmoil is discernible, there is no indication of major disruptions in young persons *whose earlier behavior was not deviant*" (p. 283; italics mine). They note further that, if a child has been competent previously, he or she will master the tasks of adolescence well despite transient periods of regression. Those adolescents, however, who demonstrate serious psychopathology have an underlying vulnerability usually manifested in some way earlier in life. The social and academic requirements of adolescence strain such individuals to the breaking point and frequently precipitate a psychosis.

The importance of taking an accurate developmental history in assessing an acutely ill adolescent cannot be overstated. The patient may have myriad symptoms, for example, anorexia, suicidal threats, violent rages. Awareness of the underlying personality and premorbid history is essential in establishing a diagnosis and treatment plan despite the fact that it is extremely difficult to give a definite label to a severe adolescent disorder. Many adolescents with moderate to severe illness are exhibiting early manifestations of schizophrenia or bipolar manic-depressive disorder. How, then, can one know if one is dealing with a passing adolescent "crisis" or the beginning of a serious illness?

There are some organic conditions that simulate a schizophrenic disorder, such as temporal lobe epilepsy, brain tumors (particularly of the frontal lobe), drug abuse, and rare inborn errors of metabolism. By and large, however, the adolescent who is prepsychotic (it is not infrequent to mistakenly label some of these individuals "borderline") is showing signs of either incipient schizophrenic or manic-depressive breakdown.

In attempting to sort out those factors that may predict which adolescent may become psychotic within either of these two domains, it is important to consider (1) level of functioning (neurotic, psychotic, borderline), (2) constitutional predisposition, (3) specific symptoms or behavior patterns, and (4) environmental stresses.

Level of Functioning

THE NEUROTIC LEVEL

In general terms, the neurotic level of personality organization, according to Kernberg (1967), is one in which the sense of identity is intact and firm and the capacity to test reality is preserved. Conflicts may result in mild symptoms, such as examination anxiety and periods of lowered energy and mood. Adolescence, the transition from childhood to adulthood, is well known to be a time of increased physical and psychological demands. It presents certain developmental tasks, as Erikson (1959) and Blos (1962) have noted, including solidification of identity in terms of gender and sex role, work and career choice, formulation of ethical values, loosening of parental ties and establishing new relationships, and developing the ability to think and act independently and to make realistic decisions.

As I noted earlier, recent research has demonstrated that many adolescents may experience the adolescent passage as one of intense struggle and conflict but only some adolescents allow such conflicts to interfere with their overall functioning. Most people involved with the neurotic adolescent would not consider his behavior pathological; he is well defended against anxiety and depression by employing "higher-level" types of defense, according to Vaillant (1971). Vaillant conceptualized defense mechanisms in the form of a hierarchy and considered that the highest-level, mature defenses, are employed by healthy individuals from adolescence throughout life. These defenses—which include sublimation (the channeling of unacceptable impulses into socially acceptable outlets), altruism, and humor—are based on mature cognitive functions and identification with appropriate role models. The next level, neurotic defenses, Vaillant contended, contains somewhat less mature defense mechanisms, characteristic of people from the age of three years throughout life. These include intellectualization (rational explanations of behavior divorced from expectable feelings), displacement (transfer of a feeling originally directed toward one person, object, or situation to another, which becomes invested with the emotional significance originally associated with the first), and reaction formation (transformation of objectionable impulses into their opposites). A neurotic adolescent faced with the task of leaving home, for example, may displace feelings originally directed toward idealized parents onto a new hero (or ego ideal) such as a football coach or science teacher. He may criticize his parents, calling them old-fashioned and lacking in understanding of the younger generation, although at the same time he retains his love for them and selects as new models for identification individuals whose value systems are not far from those of his family. The same adolescent spends more time with peers and may become involved in an intimate relationship—a "first love" with a member of the opposite sex—often as a safe way of separating himself from overinvolvement with his parents.

THE PSYCHOTIC LEVEL

It is obvious that the young woman I described earlier was functioning on a psychotic level. Her ability to test reality had disintegrated, she was delusional and experiencing auditory hallucinations, and she demonstrated illogical thought processes. According to Vaillant's formulation, she displayed psychotic defense mechanisms, including psychotic denial (unconscious repression of intolerable thoughts, wishes, and facts), distortion, and delusion—the narcissistic defenses. These are discernible in preschool children and continue in healthy adults in the form of fantasies and dreams. The psychotic adolescent has not been able to integrate the various aspects of a core identity. Identity formation may take on a delusional quality such as the belief that one has the powers of Jesus or the devil. Such adolescents may have much difficulty separating from their original parental love-objects and may employ a particularly malignant defense mechanism—reversal of affect, or turning love into hate (Freud 1958).

The sudden direction of intense hatred toward parents who have been loved earlier in life is in itself a sign of severe psychopathology. Cult leaders not infrequently serve as substitute parents for disturbed adolescents. The love-object choice of a psychotic individual may also be a popular figure such as a movie star or rock singer with whom there has been absolutely no personal contact. A delusional system based on fantasy about the idealized hero may develop.

THE BORDERLINE LEVEL

Kernberg's (1967) description of the borderline adolescent represents the intermediate variant between neurotic and psychotic organization. The critical points in his diagnostic spectrum are reality testing (adequate capacity to test reality in both interpersonal and nonpersonal realms) and ego integration (sharply contradictory and unassimilated attitudes about important aspects of the self and pathological internalized object relations).

Gunderson (1977) uses the following criteria: (1) clinging, manipulative, demanding relationships; (2) lowered achievement in school or work; (3) intolerance of being alone; (4) shifting attachments; (5) brief psychotic episodes; (6) rageful affect; and (7) manipulative suicide gestures. He also notes more antisocial patterns, drug abuse, and deviant sexual patterns among his young patients.

Some clinicians believe that the label "borderline adolescent" implies a constellation of behaviors that are stable over time and that the borderline adolescent will eventually become a borderline adult. I disagree with that position and believe that the diagnosis "borderline" embraces a heterogeneous group of overlapping syndromes that lead to a variety of psychiatric conditions later in life. The majority of borderline adolescents, I believe, are "on the way to becoming" psychotic—either schizophrenic, for example, or manic-depressive—and such seriously disturbed adolescents may be exhibiting the prodromata of a future major psychiatric disorder (Kestenbaum 1983).

Constitutional Predisposition

Increasing numbers of research projects during the past two decades have focused attention on those individuals who have a high probability of developing a major psychiatric disorder in adult life. These studies are subsumed under the rubric "risk research" and have been directed for the most part toward determining which people are most vulnerable to eventual schizophrenic illness. The children of schizophrenics, for example, are at greater risk for developing schizophrenia than are children in the general population (10–15 percent for the child of one schizophrenic parent compared with approximately 1 percent for the child of two normal parents [Rosenthal 1970]). "Vulnerability" implies that each individual is endowed with a degree of susceptibility to illness that will become manifest under certain circumstances. For an adolescent vulnerable to schizophrenia, for instance, periods of acute stress may result in a failure of coping mechanisms so that maladaptation results.

Schizophrenics are well known to constitute a heterogeneous group (e.g., paranoid, hebephrenic, catatonic, simple). There are marked differences among them in terms of genetics, biochemistry, symptom clusters, and outcomes. A schizophrenic individual may demonstrate some schizophrenic attributes without ever becoming psychotic (e.g., the nonpsychotic schizophrenic or schizotypal personality and the schizoid individual). If an adolescent becomes psychotic, it is important to know what the premorbid personality was like and whether the particular individual who is showing signs of an acute schizophrenic reaction had previously shown symptoms included in the schizophrenic spectrum (Stone 1980). The "schizotypal" individual (Spitzer and Endicott 1979) demonstrates serious disturbance in identity and communication, suspiciousness, magical thinking (e.g., clairvoyance, extreme superstition), undue social anxiety, hypersensitivity to real or imagined criticism, and social isolation. Waring and Ricks (1965) noted that the differences between the early histories of chronic schizophrenic patients and normal controls were a family history of schizophrenia and a schizoid premorbid personality. They noted an absence of close peer relationships. In another controlled study, Watt (1972) found that one-third of a group of fifty-four hospitalized schizophrenic adults had been identified by teachers as being deviant in childhood before they showed psychotic disorganization. Patterns of maladjustment for boys and girls differed. Boys who later became schizophrenic demonstrated primary evidence of unsocialized aggression and secondary evidence of internal conflict, overinhibition, and depression. Girls who later became schizophrenic demonstrated primary evidence of oversensitiveness, conformity, and introversion. Recent longitudinal studies of high-risk children (Erlenmeyer-Kimling, Cornblatt, and Fleiss 1979) have corroborated these findings and have demonstrated that some of the children of schizophrenics (but by no means all) demonstrate attention problems, low IQ scores, mild neurological defects, and social problems long before psychotic symptoms appear. It seems clear that a subgroup of children of schizophrenics is vulnerable to the disorder and could probably be helped by educational and psychosocial means many years before the stress of adolescence precipitates a psychotic episode.

Recent advances in the study of individuals with affective disorders (e.g., manic-depressive disorders) demonstrate that serious forms of the disorders are commonly encountered in childhood and adolescence (Cytryn and McKnew 1972). There is a high rate of lifetime prevalence among first- and second-degree relatives of patients with primary mood disorders compared with the general population: 6–24 percent versus 1–2 percent (Rosenthal 1970). Carlson and Strober (1978) contend that many young patients are often mislabeled schizophrenic when they are actually experiencing first manic-psychotic breakdowns. In examining the premorbid temperaments of these adolescents, Akisal (1981) noted that they displayed episodic and promiscuous behavior, alcohol and drug abuse, and uneven work and school records. These adolescents are often impulsive, unstable, and irritable and show intense unwarranted anger. They have problems being alone and frequently describe chronic feelings of emptiness and boredom. Such premorbid characteristics may indicate vulnerability to manic-depressive psychosis in late adolescence.

Specific Symptoms or Behavior Patterns

Symptoms are often the first indication for an outside observer that "something is wrong." Taken out of context, they do not provide enough information to ascertain the degree of psychopathology. School avoidance, for example, may be a sign of increasing academic difficulty, delinquency, or schizoid withdrawal. Compulsive handwashing may be a defense against masturbatory impulses in a neurotic, borderline, or psychotic individual.

A multidimensional approach, in which the premorbid personality and developmental history are taken into account, provides far more accurate diagnosis. Some symptoms are more common with certain types of disorders. For example, extreme shyness has been identified as a symptom commonly found in the early histories of some schizophrenic women. Likewise, unsocialized aggression has been correlated with schizophrenia in boys. A recent study by Inamdar, Lewis, Siomopoulos, Shanok, and Lamela (1982) found that 6 percent of a sample of hospitalized psychotic adolescents had been violent, 43 percent had been suicidal, and 28 percent had been both violent and suicidal. Violence was almost twice as common for boys as for girls. The authors concluded that "the disintegrative psychotic process, with its impact on cognition, affect, and behavior, most likely increases the risk of both outwardly directed violent behavior and self-distructive behavior." The authors believe that the combination of suicide attempts and aggressive assaults is a common behavioral manifestation of psychosis in adolescents.

Substance abuse may produce long-lasting psychotic states in vulnerable adolescents (Stone 1973). Such individuals are often exquisitely sensitive to narcotics and will relinquish them with greater reluctance than most nonvulnerable adolescents. Symptoms indicative of manic-depressive pathology may include irascibility, insubordination, temper outbursts, extreme arrogance, querulousness, and grandiosity. Anorexia nervosa may indicate the presence of masked depression.

It is obvious that the symptom complex represents but the tip of the iceberg, that the total personality and developmental history provide a firmer base on which a diagnosis can be made with any degree of accuracy.

Environmental Stress

Most researchers agree that environmental influences and stressors contribute to breakdown in genetically vulnerable individuals (Dohrenwend 1979). Stress may be acute, as with the death of a parent, or chronic, as with continuous child neglect and repeated acts of abuse.

In his study of children of psychotic parents, Anthony (1969) noted the effects of an ill parent on the child. He observed that sicker schizophrenic parents (diagnosed hebephrenic or catatonic) produced healthier children than was expected, whereas relatively healthier parents (diagnosed schizoid or borderline) produced more deviant children than was expected. He took into consideration the age of the child at the time of the parent's illness and the family support system in terms of other available members with whom the child could identify or become involved. He found that the most disturbed children were those symbiotically involved with the ill parent and that children under two, still in the phase of separation-individuation, were especially sensitive to the disturbing influence of the chronically ill mother. Whether the child internalizes or externalizes conflict, how compliant or negativistic he is, how prone to a *folie à deux,* and how identified with the ill parent determines his ultimate development. Anthony observed that the more disturbed children had a loss of ego skills by school age and exhibited such symptoms as nightmares, phobias, obsessions, and antisocial behavior. In a similar vein, Kauffman, Grunebaum, Cohler, and Gamer (1979) found "that the mother's current level of functioning is even more important than her diagnosis in understanding the impact of her disturbance on the child's later development. Women who are isolated from social contacts and who cannot function effectively in their adult social roles have children with lower competence." Thus environmental influences, particularly the paucity of supports, produced less competent children.

From the foregoing discussion it is clear that competence can be compromised by external environmental influences as well as by constitutional defects. It is not surprising, then, that the onset of puberty—with the resultant increase in sexual and aggressive drive activity, body changes, and academic and social demands—taxes the vulnerable adolescent beyond his ability to cope. Holzman and Grinker (1977) note that "the strain experienced by the typically maturing schizophrenic underscores issues of competence in already vulnerable people" (p. 284). Some young people may lose touch with reality as the disorganization becomes progressive (chronic schizophrenia). Others may seem superficially competent until completion of high school but may break down under the stress of leaving their familiar home to enter a new and unfamiliar environment (acute schizophrenia). The degree of stress cannot be measured as an independent variable without consideration of the individual's ability to defend against intolerable anxiety or depression. Some adolescents can cope with severe stress such as major illness or the loss of a parent, but others cannot handle a change of school or the move of a best friend.

Conclusions

The multidimensional approach to diagnosis embraces the four factors I have outlined: the level of functioning, constitutional predisposition, specific symptoms, and environmental stress. Conceptualizing a prepsychotic adolescent in such terms may, as Laufer (1977) says, "enable us to see more critically how the various contributions and views about development can be used in understanding . . . adolscent pathology" (p. 255). Such early recognition may actually help prevent further deterioration to a psychotic state. The young patient I presented above had a family history of schizophrenia and reportedly demonstrated numerous symptoms in childhood. She became disorganized three weeks after leaving home and experienced panic and confusion under the influence of marijuana. (Both the separation and the drug served as stressors for the vulnerable girl.) The patient had been a brilliant student but had had few friends and became even more isolated in college. She began to develop bizarre, omnipotent fantasies and eventually lost touch with reality in a delusional world of her own making.

Would early recognition of her premorbid condition have prevented her subsequent schizophrenic breakdown? One cannot know with certainty. The constitutional vulnerability would most likely have remained unchanged, but defenses against isolation, depression, and anxiety might have been bolstered by appropriate therapeutic intervention.

The child at risk for major psychiatric illness in adult life is at his most vulnerable point in mid adolescence. It is important for the clinician to make a careful assessment of the multiple variables that contribute to psychotic breakdown for the adolescent at risk to obtain the appropriate therapy. Laufer believes, as I do, that intervention in adolescence is not only desirable but "that it may be crucial in a person's future life" (p. 255). Certainly in cases of adolescents vulnerable to psychosis, it is essential to prevent breakdown whenever possible.

NOTE

1. Paper presented at the ESCASAP "Vicissitudes of Adolescence: Physical and Mental," Key Biscayne, Fla., September 23–25, 1983.

REFERENCES

Akisal, H. S. 1981. Subaffective disorders: dysthymic, cyclothymic and bipolar II disorders in the "borderline" realm. *Psychiatric Clinics of North America* 4:25–46.

Anthony, E. J. 1969. A clinical evaluation of children with psychotic parents. *American Journal of Psychiatry* 126:177–184.

Block, J. 1971. *Lives through Time*. Berkeley, Calif.: Bancroft.

Blos, P. 1962. *On Adolescence: A Psychoanalytic Interpretation*. New York: Free Press.

Carlson, G. A., and Strober, M. 1978. Manic-depressive illness in early adolescence. *Journal of the American Academy of Child Psychiatry* 17:138–153.

Cytryn, L., and McKnew, D. H., Jr. 1972. Proposed classification of childhood depression. *American Journal of Psychiatry* 129:149–155.

Dohrenwend, B. P. 1979. Stressful life events and psychopathology: some issues of theory and method. In J. E. Barrett, R. M. Rose, and G. L. Klerman, eds. *Stress and Mental Disorder*. New York: Raven.

Erikson, E. H. 1959. Identity and the life cycle. *Psychological Issues* 1:1–171.

Erlenmeyer-Kimling, L.; Cornblatt, B.; and Fleiss, J. 1979. High-risk research in schizophrenia. *Psychiatric Annals* 9:79–102.

Freud, A. 1958. Adolescence. *Psychoanalytic Study of the Child* 13:255–278.

Gunderson, J. E. 1977. Characteristics of borderlines. In P. Hartocollis, ed. *Borderline Personality Disorders: The Concept, the Syndrome, the Patient*. New York: International Universities Press.

Holzman, P. S., and Grinker, R. R. 1977. Schizophrenia in adolescence. *Adolescent Psychiatry* 5:276–290.

Inamdar, S. C.; Lewis, D. O.; Siomopoulos, G.; Shanok, S. S.; and Lamela, M. 1982. Violent and suicidal behavior in psychotic adolescents. *American Journal of Psychiatry* 139:932–935.

Kauffman, C.; Grunebaum, H.; Cohler, B.; and Gamer, E. 1979. Superkids: competent children of psychotic mothers. *American Journal of Psychiatry* 136:1398–1402.

Kernberg, O. 1967. Borderline personality organization. *Journal of the American Psychoanalytic Association* 15:641–685.

Kestenbaum, C. J. 1983. The concept of the borderline child as a child at risk for major psychiatric disorder in adult life. In K. S. Robson, ed. *The Borderline Child: Approaches to Etiology, Diagnosis, and Treatment*. New York: McGraw-Hill.

Laufer, M. 1977. A view of adolescent pathology. *Adolescent Psychiatry* 5:243–256.

Masterson, J. F., Jr. 1968. The psychiatric significance of adolescent turmoil. *American Journal of Psychiatry* 124:1549–1554.

Offer, D., and Offer, J. 1973. Normal adolescence in perspective. In J. C. Schoolar, ed. *Current Issues in Adolescent Psychiatry*. New York: Brunner/Mazel.

Rosenthal, D. 1970. *Genetic Theory and Abnormal Behavior*. New York: McGraw-Hill.

Spitzer, R. L., and Endicott, J. 1979. Justification for separating schizotypal and borderline personality disorders. *Schizophrenia Bulletin* 5:95–100.

Stone, M. H. 1973. Drug-related schizophrenic reactions. *International Journal of Psychiatry* 11:391–441.

Stone, M. H. 1980. *The Borderline Syndromes: Constitution, Personality, and Adaptation*. New York: McGraw-Hill.

Vaillant, G. E. 1971. Theoretical hierarchy of adaptive ego mechanisms. *Archives of General Psychiatry* 24:107–118.

Waring, M., and Ricks, D. 1965. Family patterns of children who became adult schizophrenics. *Journal of Nervous and Mental Disease* 140:351–364.

Watt, N. F. 1972. Longitudinal changes in the social behavior of children hospitalized for schizophrenia as adults. *Journal of Nervous and Mental Disease* 155:42–54.

2 GANDHI: HIS ADOLESCENT CONFLICT OF MIND AND BODY

SOL NICHTERN

Pubescence introduces a developmental crisis involving impulses, functions, and responses of mind and body in the progression toward maturity. This crisis generates inner conflicts of monumental proportions to the emerging adolescent, while family, culture, and religion impose their values on these developmentally determined conflicts. Often, resolutions of these conflicts blend these values with the features of the mind-and-body conflict of adolescence so that the values remain significant during adult life and there is a generational transmission of values. In some instances, however, either the body or the mind emerges victorious over the other, with one being sacrificed for the significance of the other. Configurations emerge with special features reflecting both the nature of the conflicts and their resolution.

Gandhi (1948) recorded such a struggle in his autobiography, *The Story of My Experiments with Truth*. He revealed in a highly personal way his intense internal conflicts, with the ultimate victory of his mind over his body and the influence of this outcome on his historical role within a nonviolent movement. Most of Gandhi's approaches to political struggle demonstrated his constant willingness to sacrifice his body for the beliefs of his mind. He adopted celibacy (*brahmacharya*) as the symbolic action of his growing morality and with the conviction "that truth is the substance of all morality." Gandhi made his truths (*satyagraha*) the goal of all his actions. His attitude toward political struggle demonstrated his constant willingness to sacrifice his body for his beliefs. He used the sacrificial threat of self-destruction by starvation effectively, repeatedly, and knowingly against friend and foe while advocating nonviolence (*ahimsa*).

0-226-24058-4/85/0012-0008$01.00

However, he used it in a timely manner within the structure of his family, culture, and religion, with the result that his actions and their meaning were understood by most and evoked support for and recruitment to his ideas and respect for his—and his ideas'—survival.

Gandhi offered a description of his evolution as a person devoted to nonviolence. In chapter 8 of his autobiography, entitled "Stealing and Atonement," he openly stated his prejudice. He had handed his father a written confession of his stealing "a bit of gold out of my meat-eating brother's armlet." He was fifteen years of age at the time of the incident, and yet it was more than he could bear. So he wrote a confession and gave it to his ailing father, who was confined to what was to be his deathbed. His father read the note, cried, and then tore it up; he never said a word. Gandhi cried with his father and then wrote this touching description of his truth: "This was, for me, an object lesson in *ahimsa*. Then I could read in it nothing more than a father's love, but today I know that it was pure *ahimsa*. When such *ahimsa* becomes all-embracing, it transforms everything it touches. There is no limit to its power" (p. 41).

In the prime of his adult political life, when he wrote his autobiography, Gandhi equated an event of his adolescence involving parental love and acceptance with nonviolence. Under such circumstances, only an examination of Gandhi's adolescence can reveal the nature of his *ahimsa*.

It is indeed significant to this theme of adolescent conflict that, in his autobiography, Gandhi limited his comments about his birth, parentage, and childhood to approximately six pages and then plunged into an elaborate search for early truths in the description of his adolescence, beginning with his child marriage. The few memories of childhood included one related to his teacher: "For I had learnt to carry out the orders of elders, not to scan their actions." Another related to the play, *Shravana Pitribhaki Nataka,* stressing Shravana's devotion to his parents and his constant search for the truth.

Gandhi and his bride, Kasturba, were thirteen years old at the time of their marriage. He lamented his father's injuries in an accident on his way to their marriage, expressed his devotion to his parents and his equal devotion to "the passion that flesh is heir to," and desired "that all happiness and pleasure should be sacrificed in devoted service to my parents." Thus, Gandhi quickly introduced his pubescent conflict between body and mind which was to plague him and haunt his existence until he found its resolution in a willingness to sacrifice body for ideals by his vow of celibacy.

This conflict was one of the principal themes of his autobiography. The descriptions of his adolescent and young adult life became the events of this recurrent theme. Later, his social and political actions reflected as much the resolution of his personal conflicts as they did decisions of the moment.

There are repeated vignettes of this struggle between mind and body. In his chapter "Playing the Husband," Gandhi commented on Kasturba's illiterate state: "I was very anxious to teach her, but lustful love left me no time. . . . I must therefore confess that most of my effort to instruct Kasturba in our youth was unsuccessful. . . . And when I awoke from the sleep of lust, I had already launched forth into public life" (p. 24).

In his chapter "At the High School," Gandhi said: "The reason of my dislike for gymnastics was my keen desire to serve as nurse to my father" (p. 27). And in his chapter "My Father's Death and My Double Shame," Gandhi told "of my carnal desire even at the critical hour of my father's death, when he demanded wakeful service. It is a blot I have never been able to efface or forget and I have always thought that, although my devotion to my parents knew no bounds and I would have given up anything for it, yet it was weighed and found unpardonable wanting because my mind was at the same moment in the grip of lust" (p. 45). Here is a suggestion of the conflict of mind and body interlocked with life and death. In Gandhi's thoughts, his mind-body conflict was becoming linked with the continuation of his life.

This was Gandhi's truth of the moment, but it also represents one of the truths of adolescent turmoil. The adolescent is preoccupied with the conflict of existence, with sexuality and death, and with ideals. Not until these conflicts are put to rest can the adolescent continue on toward emotional maturity. Not until Gandhi was able to put his inner turmoil to rest was he able to approach fully his leadership role, and he did this in the same manner that he resolved his personal conflicts: his body became subordinated to his ideals. Ultimately, Gandhi recruited his body as a symbol of political action by fasting. He clothed it as a symbol of his beliefs and his rejection of the physical and material world. He wedded it to the spinning wheel as a symbolic instrument of human existence, after renouncing his body as a sexual instrument. Often, he ignored his body at times of illness. His body was made the extension of his mind so that he could deny its significance to his physical being.

Gandhi's second shame was offered poignantly in the following description: "The poor mite that was born to my wife scarcely breathed for more than three or four days. Nothing else could be expected. Let all those who are married be warned by my example" (p. 46). Here was another painful statement of his conflict between body and mind in terms of sexuality and birth terminating in death. Gandhi's truth was his awareness of their linkage in his adolescent attempt at adult sexuality. His final resolution of the conflicts within this linkage was his abandonment of adult sexuality by his vow of celibacy and his acceptance of the parent-child model of relationship for all of his family, social, political, and religious interactions. This choice lent itself well to the two-tiered society of India, permitting Gandhi to emerge as a patriarchal religious leader within the village structure of ancient India and as a sophisticated leader of ideals and truths within the emerging political structure of modern India. Gandhi's description of his interactions with people constantly mirrored his passive acceptance of them and his simultaneous assertive pursuance of his own inner ideals and truths.

In his chapter "A Tragedy," Gandhi offered a vivid description of significant peer interactions challenging parental authority. The challenge was around the eating of meat and sexual activity. Both represented areas where strong religious, cultural, and family restrictions had been imposed on Gandhi. The conflicts generated by these restrictions were offered in exquisite detail as a tragedy. Gandhi's truth emerged as a continuing turmoil that plagued him until by his vow of celibacy he accepted as his own the parent-child values by which he became powerful parent or helpless child, as needed. It was in this chapter that Gandhi confessed once again to his lust and made reference to an adolescent incident with a prostitute and "four more similar incidents." Much later in his autobiography, Gandhi described one of these similar incidents of an "outing" to yet another house of prostitution in Zanzibar with a ship's captain. His childlike innocence in the adventure accompanied by his shame and strength to resist the temptation of the moment stood as vivid examples of the combination of helplessness and power that marked so much of his life.

The resolution of Gandhi's conflict of mind and body was vividly documented in several chapters of his autobiography devoted to his description of the circumstances leading to his vow of celibacy when he examined the nature of his relationship with his wife. Gandhi linked faithfulness to making his wife the instrument of his lust. Then he described his striving after self-control and the endless difficulties in the task, with the final resolution related to the cumulative effect of these unsuccessful strivings. Gandhi described his final resolution: "It became my conviction that procreation and the consequent care of children were inconsistent with public service" (p. 254). ". . . the idea flashed upon me that if I wanted to devote myself to the service of the community in this manner, I must relinquish the desire for children and wealth and live the life of a *vanaprastha*—one retired from household cares" (p. 254). Next, Gandhi recognized the importance of vows as a pathway to his commitment to life and ideals and freedom from his fear of death:

> I vow to flee from the serpent which I know will bite me. I do not simply make an effort to flee from him. I know that mere effort will mean certain death. Mere effort means ignorance of the certain fact that the serpent is bound to kill me. The fact, therefore, that I could rest content with an effort only means that I have not yet clearly realized the necessity of death and its action. But supposing that my views are changed in the future, how can I bind myself by a vow? Such a doubt often deters us but that doubt also betrays a lack of clear perception that a particular thing must be renounced. [P. 255]

Gandhi took his vow in 1906 and described his *brahmacharya* as providing him with the foundation for his truth. He offered the purity of his understanding within his search for truth as stemming from his vow of celibacy. He described his relief from the internal conflict and his achievement of peace, clarity of thought, and the dominance of mind over body: "Everyday of the vow has taken me nearer the knowledge that in *brahmacharya* lies the protection of the body, the mind and the soul. For *brahmacharya* was now no process of hard penance, it was a matter of consolation and joy. Everyday revealed a fresh beauty in it" (p. 257).

It is also possible to trace Gandhi's recruitment of fasting as an instrument of his struggles—personal and political—to this moment of his taking the vow of celibacy. He offered the idea of control of the palate and food intake as part of the observance of the vow: "Control of the palate is the first essential in the observance of the vow. I find that complete control of the palate made the observance very easy, and so I now pursue my dietetic experiments not merely from the vegetarian's but from the *brahmachari's* point of view" (p. 258). "As an external aid to *brahmacharya,* fasting is as necessary as selection and restriction in diet" (p. 258). Gandhi moved on to correlate religion with controls: "Nevertheless the existence of God within makes even control of the mind possible. Let no one think that it is impossible because it is difficult. It is the highest goal, and it is no wonder that the highest effort should be necessary to attain it" (p. 259).

Gandhi's acceptance of *brahmacharya* as the resolution of his personal conflicts permitted him to acquire a political posture derived from his victory of mind over body, from sacrificing his body for the principles of his mind, from recruiting fasting as an act of purification and resolution, and from experiencing his ideas with the religious conviction of purity and truth. It appears that Gandhi's resolution of his personal conflicts reflects a pattern within all of us during our adolescence, so that his social and political activity achieved wide popular appeal. This combination may have permitted him to emerge as a leader of thought and action in a nation attempting to achieve its own maturity and independence. Certainly, Mahatma Gandhi demonstrated a special skill for blending belief, timing, action, and ideas capable of recruiting others.

The force of his nonviolent movement led the way to an almost bloodless revolution against the mighty power of the British Empire. The magnitude of this movement can be appreciated only when it is seen in its historical context. The movement occurred during and between the two world wars and during one of the most violent revolutions of all times, the Russian Revolution. It took place during the Holocaust and the creation and explosion of the atomic bomb. These events resulted in the destruction of millions of human lives. In the midst of such destructive violence, Mahatma Gandhi developed his personal strivings for truth and nonviolence and integrated them with a religious and political process which brought into existence modern India. It was Gandhi's acceptance of his *ahimsa* and *satyagraha* that made him a powerful political leader. He embraced others with a fatherly love, while he viewed himself as being embraced by others in the same way. When challenged, Gandhi took actions which sought the approval of others. He constantly searched for the truth within all of his relationships and political struggles, for all represented his continuous search for resolution of his conflicts and his dedication to and need for nonviolence.

Conclusions

The intense conflicts of mind and body that were Gandhi's are common to most adolescents. Not all make the choices Gandhi did. But all adolescents are forced to respond to these conflicts with patterns of thought and behavior reflecting their universal nature. Many of these adolescent conflicts incorporate the transmission of developmental and generational values from one stage to the next. Thus, as with Gandhi, the resolution of the adolescent turmoil of mind and body may do much to determine the future of the individual as well as his or her functioning in adult life.

REFERENCE

Gandhi, M. K. 1948. *Gandhi's Autobiography: The Story of My Experiments with Truth*. Washington, D.C.: Public Affairs Press.

3 THE PARENTING ALLIANCE AND ADOLESCENCE

SIDNEY WEISSMAN AND REBECCA S. COHEN

The parenting alliance is a paradigmatic relationship vital to the evolving parenthood experience and other adult tasks. It encompasses interactions between spouses that pertain to child rearing, with the provision that these behaviors are appropriate to the developmental needs of children. It is a contributing process for the continuous mastery of developmental issues for the adults and children involved in it. The relationship which operates between the parental partners is the center about which family process evolves. The parenting alliance has been acknowledged both in psychoanalytic individual developmental theory and in family theories. The concept was derived operationally from clinical work with adolescents, their parents, and adult patients who are parents.

Before addressing the parenting alliance, we must acknowledge the significance of parenthood as a critical and ongoing experience of adulthood. In becoming a parent, the adult faces numerous contingencies of decision making; moreover, these decisions are made usually by an adult with another adult. Much has been written about the revival of earlier experiences with love, dependence, and helplessness which surface in the course of adult parenthood (Anthony and Benedek 1970; Benedek 1959). These revived or residual experiences may be experienced stressfully and differentially and mastered according to the particular phase of the life course in which the adult parent finds himself or herself. (We shall use the generic male pronoun form hereafter.) Parenthood is, therefore, a complex process which ushers in a course for development throughout adulthood (Michels 1981). The uniqueness of the parenthood experience lies in the

0-226-24058-4/85/0012-0003$01.00

complexity of the possible regressions in drives, affects, and self-esteem and adult effectiveness. We hope to demonstrate that the parenting alliance, as a self-selfobject relationship,[1] functions as a milieu for the resolution of the aforementioned reactivated developmental issues. This alliance plays a critical role in the continuous unfolding of the parenthood experience. It performs a sustaining function for the individual partners as each responds continuously to the developmental progression of the child.

Societal expectations may vary as each culture constructs different values and timetables by which growth and development are monitored. However, parental responsibility for the biologically and psychologically dependent child is universal. Whereas parenthood as a process may originate in procreative, libidinal forces (Benedek 1959), once a child is anticipated, a new experience develops between the parents and takes on a life of its own. In all human societies, parenting alliances develop, although the roles of each partner may vary. Nevertheless, a parenting alliance emerges when the decision is made to procreate or from the awareness of becoming a parent. This alliance proceeds out of the anticipation of mutual bonds to the child. Each partner anticipates a shared experience which will facilitate the performance of the tasks of parenthood. The fluidity of the child's needs creates continuous challenges, inconsistencies, and contradictions; hence the constant fear of regressive pulls. It is evident, therefore, that parenthood tests the capacity to endure frustration and delay. The parenting alliance is the significant aspect, or constituent, of the parenthood experience on which an adult can rely for affirmation and predictability when stressed by the seemingly endless frustrations and tensions that occur in the many contingencies of parenthood. Much of the parenthood experience that has been discussed in the literature identifies several of its aspects, including the dyadic relationship between parent and child and even the triadic aspects of parent-couple and child. However, what has not been addressed is the meaning of the experience of the parenting alliance not merely for the child's triadic relationship capacities but for the continuous maintenance of this triadic relationship for the adult parent.

Theoretical and Conceptual Considerations

The parenting alliance is that component of a marital relationship that is distinct from the libidinal object needs of the spouses for each other.

However, it clearly involves the issue of self-esteem and its vicissitudes, which can endanger the adult's feeling of competence, effectiveness, and well-being. The alliance consists of the capacity of a spouse to acknowledge, respect, and value the parenting roles and tasks of the partner. This capacity must be at once firm and resilient to permit the alliance to endure when one or both partners experience stress in the parenting sphere or in other pertinent aspects of life. The parenting alliance, as a construct, can be applied to family process when it is stable, or in flux, to determine or predict how parents and children will master or fail in response to family changes.

Unquestionably, the existence and aspects of the import of the interactions between the parents have been acknowledged in the writings of psychoanalytic and systems family process theorists (Bowen 1976; Lidz 1963, 1976; Meissner 1978; Minuchin 1974; Stierlin 1977). The process as a construct has been acknowledged but addressed largely as a derivative of libidinal drives and their resulting ties within family process. Therefore, as a process it is not conceptualized consistently; nor is it assessed independently from the entire emotional matrix of the family as a compendium of the interacting personalities of both spouses. When attempts were made to observe "parental coalitions" (Lidz 1976) as a distinct segment of family process, they could not be sustained because the underpinnings of most family theories are rooted in, or informed by, the concepts of psychoanalytic drive theory. It was apparent to us that, in order for this process, the parenting alliance, to be understood and utilized clinically, a differentiation has to be made between the marital relationship and the parenting relationship. The former is an experience of sexual and libidinal ties along with self-selfobject functions; the latter is a selfobject relationship between the parents that evolves as they engage in child rearing and encompasses the experiential and transactional aspects of self-esteem regulation. Psychodynamic family theorists have addressed the relationship between the parents within the frameworks of (1) the complementarity of their mutual needs and/or (2) their intrapsychic levels of differentiation of self from others (internal objects). When examined, their constructs do not help in understanding many situations that we observe in our offices or in our lives. These are the many instances we know wherein the marriages are stable, and yet children emerge with severe pathology. Conversely, we have observed marriages that are fragile and unsatisfactory, and yet the children emerged with capacities for competence and creativity. Family clinicians (Lidz 1976) have observed, along with us, that, when marriages dissolve, some parents are able to maintain a stable connection to sustain a mutual process of empathic parenting. In our construct, therefore, we have attempted to identify a part of the system that can and does continue to operate when the larger system and some of its components shift or change shape. We recognize that parents, either married or divorced, must have the capacity (or structure) for commitment to engage in the demands of the parenting process. This commitment, however, does not reside in the domain of the libidinal drives. We will present, in this chapter, an aspect of self-psychology theory which does illuminate the parenting relationship between two adults.

The early shared experience of child rearing for both parents lays down a nidus from which the alliance evolves and becomes a discrete process within the family structure. This early experience includes both parents with their initial responses to the ongoing, changing demands of the child that cannot be delayed. Our concept requires recognition that motherhood and fatherhood develop simultaneously and that the parent-child dyadic transactions of each proceed within the context of the alliance. Therefore, fathers participate psychologically and behaviorally from the beginning. Rather than contributing to triangulation by intruding on the mother-child symbiosis (Meissner 1978), they perform an important affirming and sustaining function for the mother whose empathic capacities are likely to be strained by the time-consuming, intimate contact of immediate nurturing.

Parenthood requires the commitment of adults to parent in the face of the child's unempathic relatedness. Under the best of circumstances, and at all developmental levels, children have difficulty in maintaining a stable relationship with more than one adult at a time. And yet they require the nurturing, empathic responses of both parents for the establishment of object ties, gender identity, self-cohesion, and drive integration. Empathy in parent-child interrelatedness flows in one direction. The child is essentially a nonempathic partner whose empathic capacities will become established in the future on the completion of a long and complex developmental process (Weissman and Barglow 1980). The parents' potential for self-esteem dysfunction and for other regressions in response to the impact created by the child's needs is ever present (Cohen and Balikov 1974). The mutual support (external and internal) of the parenting alliance sustains the parenting process by promoting the regulation of the heightened tensions inherent in the process of child rearing.

The parenting alliance can be observed and understood best, therefore, within the conceptual framework of recent advances in psychoanalytic theory. As indicated, self-psychology (Kohut 1971, 1977) has introduced the concept of self-selfobject relationships. The self-selfobject construct (self-sustaining functions) is useful in understanding the parenting alliance. Wolf (1980) describes a developmental line of self-selfobject relationships. These do not disappear with growth, but they become less intense and are subject to substitution as maturation occurs. Wolf describes, further, a continuous feedback process between the self and its selfobjects. This process results in continuous modifications of both. The selfobject requirements become less archaic over time, and, as Terman (1980) has indicated, they become nonobligatory. The uniqueness of the adult parenthood experience lies in its being located within a matrix of self and selfobject transactions between both parental partners and child. As a consequence, changes and expansions in the self are continuous for both parent and child, each in the phase-appropriate context.

For the adult parent, the seemingly dyadic parenting alliance involves transactions regarding a third individual. Thus, on an intrapsychic level, it is always a triadic process with its baseline resting on the parental transactions about a child whose needs are being attended to. Moreover, the child serves a selfobject purpose appropriate to adulthood affirmations of adult experiences of pleasure and competence which sustain self-esteem. In the initial oedipal triadic relationship, the child is the small undeveloped member of a triad wherein his fantasies do not match his capacities. In the parenting relationship, the parent's experience in the triad is quite different. In addition to dealing with the various emotional and cognitive capacities which are brought to bear on each parent's care of the child, the parent must support and interact with the other parent in this unique constantly evolving caretaking role. The child's growth and development arouse specific fantasies as the parent relives old fantasies, or resolves old problems, or experiences a new sense of self in responding to the constantly evolving relationship with the child. The relationship with the coparent, when husband and wife address issues of parenting, is not one of satisfying dependency needs or, as we have indicated, obtaining sexual gratification. In the parenthood experience, adults contend with the product of their sexuality and their ongoing needs for mutuality. Consequently, this is a new set of experiences which in turn can lead to further psychological development of the adult in a new universe of operations. Without the existence of the parenting alliance, the uniqueness of this experience may be lost for the adult's further psychological development.

(We believe that this is an area for further investigation.)

Cohler (1981), in describing the concept from self-psychology of maintaining self-cohesion, indicates that in this process "each person becomes a historian of the self, creating an internally consistent interpretation of the life cycle, so that past, present, and future appear to become congruent." We propose that, in the parenting couple, as the triadic parenthood experience is played out, the shared parenting alliance becomes part of each spouse's personal stance toward the future. As the life course proceeds within each partner, the parenting alliance becomes a part of that partner's personal history. This connectedness to the coparent within the parenting experience, if affirmatively maintained, can continue in the face of marital disruption. A parenting alliance, therefore, is not coterminous with a marital alliance.

The alliance begins prior to the arrival of the child. The psychological support and idealization by the father of the mother during pregnancy and the child's infancy are critical factors in this phase. In essence, each parent provides the other with support in the new experience of early parenthood. Currently, we see many mothers who return early to work. Here, the father's continued idealization of his wife as mother is as critical as the sharing of responsibilities. The alliance may operate to sustain parents during the toddler's rapprochement phase (Mahler and Furer 1968) or the transitional selfobject phase to either parent—but particularly to the mother. We know well the adult-appropriate soothing functions provided by the father for the distraught mother of the eighteen-month-old who is at once discovering the delights of the world and collapsing with rage and exhaustion because her competence is far below her reach. Clearly, each parent's role has specific values for a particular child. Each, however, needs the support of the other when the child's appropriate developmental forays erode a parent's empathic capacities. The emotional connectedness of the parents may be essential for creating an environment for the mastery of oedipal issues. The oedipal experience of exclusion is mitigated by the child's reliance upon the continuity of the parenting alliance. This alliance may be a significant facilitating force in promoting ego-ideal formation during the latency years.

The parenting alliance is of special significance for the adolescent. As he negotiates the psychological tasks and physiological shifts of adolescence, the presence of the parenting alliance provides a framework of consistency and support on which to rely. We suspect that some of the pathology attributed to adolescents, such as splitting the parents, may stem from the absence of a parenting alliance. As the adolescent integrates body changes, explores the world, and attempts to map out a route of his own, the existence of a parenting alliance makes it possible to acknowledge a variety of perceptions of the world. These can be reconciled into meaningful coexistence, just as varied perceptions can coexist between parents. In this milieu, the adolescent can proceed to adulthood. We suspect that, in families that have an effective parenting alliance, the adolescent process evolves smoothly. In such families, the adolescent is free to experiment with the range of newly acquired capacities undergirded by the coparent-child triad. Oedipal resolutions in adolescence hinge on the continuity of this parental couple–adolescent triad.

Let us consider some specific assets provided by the alliance for parents. Psychological or physical problems in a parent may limit effectiveness in caring for children. Such a parent is prone to suffer a loss of self-esteem. The parenting alliance may be the critical factor for sustaining the maximum parenting functions possible for the parent with such limitations. For all parents, the alliance assures each a relationship with an adult who serves as an ongoing selfobject in which to test responses, perceptions, hopes, fantasies, and ideals regarding the child.

The decisions made in raising children mobilize the totality of one's fantasies and self-perceptions. Whereas the reality of one's life is experienced in work and marriage, it is in the raising of children that one may entertain one's fantasies. In one's relationship with one's spouse, when the focus is on child rearing, one approaches these fantasies implicitly or explicitly. The parenting alliance is the means by which two adults can communicate meaningfully and share these fantasies and differing perceptions of the world. During periods in which parents are particularly vulnerable to the stimuli of regressive fantasies, the parenting alliance may be the critical factor for maintaining cohesion. To restate: the parenting alliance provides a substrate for the psychological growth and development of the parents.

We do not mean that parenting does not occur in the absence of a parenting alliance that is brought about by death, divorce, or illness. We recognize, moreover, that some adults become single parents by choice. In the absence of the parenting alliance, however, the adult must deal with the demands and stimulations of child rearing in isolation. We suspect that closer examination of single parenting will reveal that such individuals parent most effectively when they can establish parenting-type alliances with a family member or friend to sustain them in their roles as parents and adults.

Clinical Presentations

In the previous discussion, we described the theoretical foundation and heuristic value of the concept of the parenting alliance. We will proceed with clinical material to demonstrate the operational value of the concept. In the first vignette, we describe the development of the parenting alliance in a divorced couple.

CASE EXAMPLE 1

The identified patient was a thirteen-year-old boy who was living with his divorced mother. In the six months prior to the evaluation, the quality of his schoolwork had deteriorated seriously and he was not going to be promoted into high school. In the month before the evaluation, his mother became frightened that he would lose control, strike out, and hurt her. She took the initiative in requesting the evaluation. In her first interview, she was concerned about her son's school failure and expanded on her fear that he could lose control and hurt her. In the week prior to the consultation, the son had stopped going to school, and she was afraid to be home alone with him.

The identified patient was a muscular boy who appeared to be his stated age. He made it clear that he saw no reason for seeing a psychiatrist, that his mother had made him come, and that there was nothing wrong with him. He told the therapist to talk to his father who "agreed with him that he did not have any problems." When reference was made to problems at school, he responded angrily that there were none. Reference to his failing grades was greeted by silence. Inquiry into his feelings about his parents' divorce made him become slightly agitated, but he insisted that the divorce had no effect on him. He became increasingly angry during the interview and insisted that his father would help him so that he would not have to put up with a psychiatrist. After the initial interview with the child and his mother, a subsequent interview was arranged with the father, an attorney. There was no reluctance on the father's part to meet with the therapist. During the interview, with some hesitation, he spoke about the divorce, but the major focus was on his son's behavior. He reported that he had acted in much the same fashion when he was a teenager. Although he tended to dismiss the boy's problems as inconsequential and the usual issues faced by adolescents, he was concerned about his son and interested in the psychiatrist's view of the problem.

Following further evaluation, the psychiatrist advised the parents in a joint session that their son needed hospitalization because of serious psychiatric problems and the real danger that he could attack and harm the mother. The mother was relieved by this recommendation, but the father was baffled. He could not understand that his son's problems required hospitalization but indicated that he would support the recommendation. In planning the son's treatment, the therapist arranged to meet biweekly in joint session with the parents to focus on the unique needs of the son.

The boy was quite angry at being placed in the hospital. During the first few days of hospitalization, he insisted that he was leaving and called his father to take him out. The father was confused. He did not believe, yet, that his son should be in the hospital, but was not totally convinced that his ex-wife was wrong in being frightened of him; moreover, he, too, was concerned about the son's school performance. With much difficulty, he told his son that he would have to stay in the hospital, at least for a few weeks. The boy stormed out of the joint session with his parents and therapist that had been planned to discuss the course of his treatment. He refused, soon, to see the therapist individually, although he became comfortable in the hospital school. The parents continued to meet with the therapist. The son continued to attempt to convince his father that there was nothing wrong with him. He presented to the father the hospital treatment as a plot in which the therapist had allied himself with the mother to get him out of her house. At each visit, he insisted that his father do something to get him out of the hospital. The father was inclined, initially, to support this request, but before taking any action brought his concerns to the therapist and his ex-wife. Each time, in turn, the father came to understand better that his ex-wife's concerns about their son were related not to the old wounds from the failed marriage but more relevantly to the boy's developmental needs. As this occurred, the boy gradually gave up the attempts to provoke his father and became increasingly involved in the hospital treatment program. The therapeutic work with the parents focused solely on the developmental tasks faced by the son and the issues they presented to him in their coping together with his needs. And yet, as the work continued, their capacities to share with each other their experiences with their son increased.

About the eighth month of hospitalization, the psychiatrist and hospital team determined that a residential placement outside the mother's home was the most suitable treatment plan for the boy. The father reacted to this plan much as he had to the original plan to hospitalize the boy. Why was this necessary, hadn't the hospital been enough? This was dealt with, once again, in the joint session with his ex-wife. With some difficulty, we were able to arrange a placement at a youth center in another state. The agreement was made that, after the boy left the hospital, the parents were to continue to work with the therapist on a once-a-month basis.

The issues during the early months at the youth center were replications of the initial ones during the hospitalization. The patient again regarded the placement as a plot by the therapist and the mother to get rid of him. He attempted to enlist the father as an ally in his battle. Again, the consistent focus of the work with the parents was on the developmental issues faced by the boy and the reason for the placement. After a year, the boy settled down in the placement. He began to attend the off-campus public school near the youth center, where his schoolwork was clearly above average. When the father, who had remarried, planned a visit, he was able to talk to his ex-wife and the therapist about the advisability of visiting his son with his second wife. After discussing the issue with his ex-wife, he decided to visit his son alone first and talk to him about the remarriage. After three years in the center, the boy graduated from the local high school and enrolled in college. At that time, the joint sessions with the parents ended.

At the termination of the joint sessions, each parent had a clearer sense of the needs of the son. They were able to communicate with each other about these needs, in and outside of the joint meetings. Although the problems of an older daughter were not the focus of the work, they became better able to address these and develop strategies to assist her. The initially guarded communication was replaced by an openness and eagerness to hear what was happening with the son when he visited with the other parent. The parents also agreed on the choice of college and were pleased by their son's growth.

This case demonstrates that an individual can have serious interpersonal difficulties with a spouse but still maintain a relationship focused on the needs of the children. Here, a therapist was essential to nurture the latent alliance in these parents who were unable to function as effective parents prior to this intervention. The child's experience of the parenting alliance in a protected environment led to his subsequent growth and development.

The parenting alliance and the factors in the parents which allowed it to develop can be identified clearly. First, each of the parents had an investment in the son, with some recognition of his needs. The mother had a clearer perception of her son's needs than the father but did not know what to do. The father, although invested in the child, was not aware of the boy's special needs. Second, each parent valued the importance of the other parent in fostering the growth and development of the child. This view was shared by both parents, but the pain of the unsuccessful marriage and divorce prevented them from acting accordingly. The therapist, hospital, and youth center provided neutral ground for the parents to develop this area of the parenting alliance. Third, each parent began to respect and value the judgments of the other. The turmoil of the divorce had obscured their underlying capacities for mutual engagement. The mother communicated her investment in her ex-husband as the son's father by wanting to involve him in the son's therapy and life. The father, at first, did not hear or believe what she said. However, with the support of the therapist, he shifted from defensiveness to supporting the treatment process as well as his ex-wife's position. As the treatment proceeded, the father and mother became able to respect each other's judgments regarding the needs of the child without the therapist. Finally, an ongoing means of communication which maintains the alliance around the needs of the child must be established whether the parents are divorced or not. These parents, at the time the treatment ended, no longer needed the neutrality of the therapist and his office to communicate with each other and develop plans for their son. The parenting alliance subsequently provided a context, with the support of the hospital and residential treatment center, for a framework by which the parents could turn the anlage of a parenting alliance into a vibrant parenting alliance.

CASE EXAMPLE 2

The second case is that of a professional man in his mid-forties who was referred to the therapist when his bright eight-year-old son entered treatment with a child psychiatrist. The child's problems were poor peer relationships, multiple anxieties, and considerable irritability. Treatment for both parents was recommended by the child psychiatrist, but the mother refused. At the beginning of the father's therapy, he was concerned that he might interfere with his son's growth and development. His primarily personal reasons for obtaining psychotherapy were difficulties in being assertive at home and work. The patient presented a picture of his wife as a cold, angry, depressed woman in her forties. (This view of her corresponded to the diagnostic impression of the child psychiatrist.) In fact, the patient was concerned that, if he left his wife, she could become suicidal. In the therapy, he uncovered a similar relationship, as a child, with his mother—wherein he felt used as an "antidepressant." He felt that his anger toward his wife and estrangement from her contributed to his having extramarital affairs.

With his children, the patient was able to respond to their age-appropriate needs. In addition to the eight-year-old, the patient had two older sons, ages thirteen and fifteen. As treatment proceeded, with the passivity in focus, he was able to perceive subtleties in the children's needs and was able to facilitate growth along with provision for safety in setting limits and boundaries. As his ability to respond assertively to the children's needs expanded, he experienced increasing anger at his wife's detachment. He felt most assaulted by her depreciation of what she considered to be his increasing infantilization of the children. For example, she thought that his insistence on setting up reasonable hours for adolescents would keep them immature and that their initiative would be crushed. She implied, also, that he seemed to be clinging to the children, whose growth would be stunted, supposedly, just as his had been by his mother's handling of him during his childhood and adolescence. The wife regarded the patient's passivity to be the consequence of having been raised as a "sissy." He reacted to the wife's depreciation of his parenting as an assault on his masculinity and self-esteem.

On another occasion, substance abuse became an issue with the older boys, particularly the thirteen-year-old. The parents had good reason to suspect that the boy was involved, in some way, with a group of adolescent drug users. The patient suggested to his wife that they inform their son of their concern so that they could have an open discussion and let the boy know about their disapproval. The wife was as concerned as the father, but she believed that to forbid drug use in the home would drive the boy away or that he would become overly anxious and cautious. She regarded the patient's efforts as proof of his lack of sureness of himself as a man. The patient, nevertheless, did confront the boy, who revealed considerable depression and anxiety. At this time, the boy was referred for therapy. Once it had been done, the wife was relieved that her husband's assertiveness had been successful.

As the patient continued to deal with his children, he became aware of a desire to talk to his wife about his feelings as a parent. The wife responded by absenting herself from these attempted conversations. Although she could not involve herself with her husband in the subtle process of sharing experiences and expectations concerning their children, she was a concerned parent and supported treatment for the children. She had, however, no ability to invest in a parenting dyad within the context of a triadic relationship involving a child. The wife's detachment caused the patient to experience a lack of affirmation in his parenting role. The lack of feedback and continuity in the parenting sphere, wherein such interactions are necessary for the parenthood experience to be creative and expansive, left him depleted and doubtful about himself as a parent. Exclusive of the parenting relationship, the patient admired his wife's commitment to her public life, and they shared many values, ideals, and pleasures in recreational activities. His wife admired his many talents and encouraged their development.

The treatment proceeded with twice weekly psychotherapy for four years. After termination, the patient returned twice to his former therapist. Each visit focused on parenting issues. One is of particular interest. The patient's older sons were approaching late adolescence during the days of the anti–Vietnam War demonstrations. Both parents approved of their planned participation in a march on the Capitol. Once the sons announced that they planned to attend the march, the wife was not interested in discussing their concerns. In the days immediately prior to the march, she refused to discuss the boys' fears and to participate with them and her husband in planning how they could cope with the potential dangers. The patient became outraged by his wife's response. He asked to see his former therapist for two sessions in order to affirm the appropriateness of his responses to his sons in the face of an absent alliance with his wife. He was concerned that possibly he had been overprotective of his sons, yet he did not depreciate their needs for parental support. Exploration of the events and activities involving him, his wife, and their sons revealed a concern that the sons could be physically hurt. As a young man, he had also participated in demonstrations and had seen people hurt, and he recalled his fears and his shame about them.

Although the patient and his wife approved of their sons' activities, they could not mutually experience either pleasure or concern about the activities. In the absence of a parenting alliance with his wife, the father utilized the therapist for the necessary feedback in parenting tasks. This enabled him to assess, in a neutral setting, his concerns about his sons and to disentangle his identifications with them from his own youth. The therapist's confirming supportive stance enabled him to counsel and support the sons in a more effective parenting role. The therapist served, transiently, in a parenting-type alliance when the man's rage at his wife and his self-doubt threatened his sense of appropriateness with his children. Perhaps the positive therapeutic outcome led this man to seek a substitute when he was unable to get from his wife a mutual pride as well as concern as his sons took on mature tasks. In addition to the therapist, he utilized colleagues for the needed reflection around parenting tasks.

In this case, we see how a parenting alliance can be established with a therapist. This need not be regarded as extraneous to the process of intensive psychotherapy if adult developmental needs are conceptualized appropriately. The case illustrates that, as a parent becomes aware of the phase-appropriate needs of children and is able to disengage his needs from theirs, he continues to need a milieu for child rearing in which he can feel valued and affirmed in a feedback process. As this patient became more sensitive and empathic, he became invested increasingly in becoming an effective parent, just as he had struggled to become more effective in his career. In order to achieve this ideal, he sought actively for the kind of milieu which would help him sustain the gains he had made. In the example cited, the milieu was created most economically by a short return to his therapist. We suspect that many such short-term alliances are created when a parent meets with a child's therapist to provide developmental gains for the child.

CASE EXAMPLE 3

This case will demonstrate, also, the problems in a family where a parenting alliance did not exist. The identified patient was a sixteen-year-old boy who was referred by a school counselor for truancy from school, drug abuse, and minor delinquent activities. The boy came readily to the therapist's office. Early in the therapy, he described a disrupted family situation and estrangement from his father. He elaborated that his father was actually his stepfather, that his mother and father had divorced when he was an infant, and that he never knew his biologic father. He was adopted by his mother's second husband. He had a stepsister at home in addition to his parents. The patient insisted that there was nothing that he could do to please his father. He believed that his father cared about him only as long as he did not get into any trouble and was no bother. The boy described himself as unhappy and said that he used drugs. He insisted that there was nothing significant about it, that all his friends used drugs. He promised that, if his parents gave him another chance, he would not get into any further trouble.

On the basis of the boy's involvement with his parents and his desire for an improved relationship with them, and to learn more about the family, the therapist arranged an appointment with the boy and his parents. At this meeting, the boy voiced his complaints about his parents, and they, in turn, expressed their concern about his behavior. Father expressed anger at the boy for disrupting the family. As they spoke about their problems, they interrupted each other, and neither could listen to what the other person said. At the end of the hour, when the therapist proposed a second meeting to look further into some of the family problems, the father said that he saw no need to come back. All he wanted was that his son not cause any trouble; he was not going to become any more involved than necessary. After further discussion with his wife, who said that she felt that the meeting had been helpful and wished him to return, he repeated that he did not care and saw no reason to do so. The session ended with the patient startled by the outcome, the mother in tears, and the father restating he did not want to have any more to do with the boy.

Unlike the first case, the foundation for a parenting alliance and the capacity of the parents to work jointly with their child regarding his difficulty did not exist. The father did not share the mother's investment in the boy and did not see himself behaving as a father. Nor did he value the mother's concerns or her request that he become involved with the boy. Essentially, the father devalued his wife's parenting role as well as his own.

CASE EXAMPLE 4

The parenting alliance and its absence have special implications in the hospital treatment of an adolescent. In the first case, although the parents were divorced, they were able to develop and stabilize a parenting alliance. Because of the stability that the parenting alliance brought to their relationship, they were able to facilitate the development of an effective therapeutic plan for their son. In this case of a hospitalized adolescent girl, the parents did not have a parenting alliance and were unable to use the assistance of the child's psychiatrist or the social worker involved in the case to develop a parenting alliance.

Here, we can observe a marital relationship that was threatened with disruption by the push to develop a parenting alliance. The patient, a fourteen-year-old girl, was referred for hospitalization after being unable to attend school regularly and telling her parents that she was extremely frightened about leaving the house. In the initial meeting with the psychiatrist, the patient, who appeared to be much younger than her age, was extremely frightened and at times would rise out of her chair and stare out the window, shaking. She spoke very few words. She would mutter something about some sexual experience and the need to be punished. Although she appeared acutely psychotic at the time of admission, in the absence of any prior psychiatric history and in view of the potential report of some sexual encounter, a decision was made not to immediately use a neuroleptic agent. In the first two weeks of her hospitalization, she continued to remain quite frightened and was convinced that something terrible would happen to her or someone at home, although she could not elaborate precisely what the terrible event could be. She said that she had had a sexual relationship with a member of her family but could not clearly elaborate what precisely occurred. Initially, it was not clear whether some traumatic sexual experience had occurred or whether the report was a delusion. Later exploration with the family and the daughter led to the view that there had not been any sexual interaction with a family member, but that this was part of an acute delusional system involving her family and her importance to the family. The delusion gradually changed to the fear if she did not leave the hospital one of her parents would die. This view was held by the daughter throughout the remainder of her hospitalization, and she insisted daily that she needed to leave the hospital.

The patient was involved in individual therapy, and the patient's parents were seen both by the hospital social worker and by the patient's primary psychiatrist. Initially the father, as in the first case presented, opposed this child's therapy. Even after a neuroleptic drug was prescribed, he tended to minimize aspects of her difficulties. As the patient began to improve and the delusional thinking, although present, was not observed manifestly, the patient began to participate in the hospital's activities and began to attend the hospital school. At this point the father insisted that there was no real need for his daughter to remain in the hospital. The girl's mother supported the father's view, insisting that she would be able to provide all of the support and structure that the girl needed. The parents openly supported the child's desire to return home in spite of their having been informed of the girl's reasons for wanting to leave. In individual sessions the girl could address some of her fears of returning home and her fears of the future, but these could not be addressed in the presence of her parents. Since the patient was functioning at a higher level than on admission and not formally psychotic, she was discharged to the care of her parents.

The meetings with the parents revealed little involvement between the father and mother. The father worked for a large corporation and traveled a great deal. The girl was a companion to her mother in father's absence from home, and in more recent years family activities were planned without him. Mother was quite pleased to describe the activities she and daughter did together and would do when she returned home.

This case demonstrated that the parents did not have a parenting alliance. Neither of them could acknowledge the severity of the child's difficulty and communicate his or her concern to the other parent. Instead, they supported each other's denial and were not able to address the essential parenting tasks. In spite of the child's clear and persistent impairment at time of discharge, the parents focused only on her improvement and ignored the hospital staff recommendation for a lengthier hospitalization.

We can understand their actions as revealing a pseudoparenting alliance. Both parents were agreed on a specific action regarding their daughter. However, the action was inappropriate to the daughter's needs. The parents' agreement did not serve the interest of the child, but rather, stabilized the parents' unsteady marital relationship. In acknowledging the daugher's illness and addressing daughter's needs, they would have had to jointly function in the parenting relationship. If the daughter had remained in the hospital and did not provide companionship for mother, they would further have had to contend with serious issues that would inevitably have strained the marriage. The pseudoparenting alliance served to maintain a status quo in the marriage without addressing the needs of the child.

The child in this family served as a selfobject for the mother. The child, not the father, served to provide an essentially supportive environment for the mother so that she could maintain cohesive and stabilized functioning. In effect, the girl's preoccupation that someone at home would die if she remained in the hospital was based on her unconscious awareness of how she was utilized by the mother. To the outside world, the daughter's statement would appear to be a delusion, but in her absence, the mother was psychologically dead. When living at home, the daughter served as a selfobject for the mother. The selfobject role limited mother's potential for psychological fragmentation. The apparent delusion was the daughter's only way of presenting the reality in which she lived. Without the parents' readiness to assess their own needs or to acknowledge their need to use the child, the child cannot be engaged in or sustain a psychotherapeutic process.

In assessing a parental couple for the presence of a parenting alliance, therefore, it is critical to determine whether they are in agreement on the parenting task and whether their responses are appropriate to the child's needs. If the agreement is for an inappropriate parenting response, this response may serve to foster a denial of the child's disorder, and the reasons for this denial must then be explored. In this case, the parenting response served to develop a pseudoparenting alliance to enable the parents to avoid stress in the marital relationship. This led to an impasse with the daughter. She left the hospital, prematurely rupturing her therapy but leaving her parents' marital relationship undisturbed.

CASE EXAMPLE 5

A final clinical vignette will demonstrate the import of the parenting alliance for the family and the therapist in determining the course of clinical interventions, particularly with adolescents. A young adolescent girl was referred with urgency because of suspected turbulence in the home. The desperate concerns of the mother were the girl's "active" promiscuity and "widespread" drug abuse. Both parents had psychological sophistication commensurate with their high educational and social status. They had great expectations because of satisfaction with the outcome of an earlier therapeutic experience involving another child, a boy three years older than the referred patient. There was, also, a six-year-old son.

From everyone's account (except the girl's) of her behavior and her tenacious involvement with a "bad crowd," the therapist expected to find a seriously disordered girl. Initially, the mother and daughter were seen together, then separately, with the girl being seen first. She was an attractive, sullen girl who knew about her parents' concern and depreciated her mother for being overly anxious. Though guarded, she gave many indications of an intact personality structure. She knew she had to see the therapist because her parents did not know what else to do with her. During individual psychotherapy, the girl revealed her depression, obstinacy, and provocativeness and the rather narrow scope of the acting out. The mother, an attractive, dependent, and rigid woman, was devastated by fears that the girl's life was ruined. She revealed her many anxieties because of emotional problems in both her parents' families.

She reported that the son's adolescence did not trouble the parents and that he had a good relationship with them. She conjectured that perhaps the daughter was missing the old times with father, who was described as being currently very preoccupied with serious matters in his business. (This the daughter had mentioned, too.) From the mother's perspective, the parents had a compatible marriage and had maintained a good parenting alliance in the past. The daughter's adolescence created a threat to the mother's equilibrium for which psychotherapy was eventually recommended.

To clarify the family situation, the therapist saw the father alone for an evaluation. He appeared to be a caring, thoughtful, somewhat rigid man, successful in his business but recently engaged in a critical expansion to which he was devoting much time. He recognized his wife's exaggerated response to the girl's activities and was supportively aware of the historical reasons. He regarded highly her parenting efforts and was pleased that the therapist had wanted to see him. He was pleased to feel needed and became accessible to a better understanding of the daughter's developmentally appropriate longing for him and her need for a more stable alliance between the parents. For obvious reasons and others that cannot be presented here, the therapist believed that the girl required individual psychotherapy. To facilitate the girl's treatment and create a more benign family process, the therapist worked with the parents in three sessions for the specific task of promoting a better alliance. The therapist continued to work with the girl, who soon became aware of how her anxieties, disappointments, and conflicts contributed to her acting out. She maintained responsibility for her twice-weekly sessions and seemed able to deal with the parents without further intervention by the therapist.

In this case, both parents were invested in the child and with each other as parents. The parenting alliance was strained by the father's preoccupations, leaving the mother vulnerable to regression. Although there was disagreement about discipline, their mutual respect for their needs and judgment remained intact. Each wanted communication with the other, and both were amenable to dealing with the developmental needs of their daughter. The mother decided to reduce the intensity of her concern with the daughter by engaging in more community work, and this was supported by the father. The girl felt affirmed by their reengaged parenting and became pleased by her mother's successful activities. The therapy became remarkably smooth, with only occasional flare-ups emanating from the mother's intrapsychic stress. Had psychotherapy for the mother been immediately recommended or had family therapy been instituted, we are doubtful that the family could have settled into dealing with the appropriate issues and achieving some relief.

The mother's anxieties, self-esteem problems, and close tie to the daughter could have interfered with the therapy and the family equilibrium without the reestablishment of the alliance. Clearly, the parenting alliance could not serve as the sole therapeutic agent for the mother's threatened intrapsychic disruption. It can be credited, however, with cooling down the family, shifting the imbalance, and providing sufficient self-esteem support for the mother to seek her own therapy—which she had considered for many years. By pointing out their responsibilities to the parents, the therapist laid the groundwork for permitting the girl to take responsibility for her behavior.

We suspect that a gap is created often by recommending therapy for the family, or the parent(s), and/or the adolescent without proper focus on the vicissitudes of the parenting alliance. With a good enough parenting alliance, parents are freer to attend to intrapsychic issues for which they need time for mastery. With the alliance in place, an adolescent has an advantage which enables him to address his developmental or intrapsychic problem in psychotherapy, as is demonstrated in this case.

Conclusions

We regard the parenting alliance as a process that is critical for the study of adult development. Until recently, it has not been possible to conceptualize it so as to understand its explanatory power. Largely, it has appeared in the literature to amplify clinical understanding of child development or of seriously disordered young adults. Indeed, the relationship between the parents has been noted frequently when it is in disarray or absent. It is often the case that we note the existence of a structure or function only when it is absent. So it has been in our clinical work from which we derived the concept of the parenting alliance.

To review: Therapists can assist parents in establishing a parenting alliance if: (1) each parent is invested in the child; (2) each parent values the other parent's involvement with the child; (3) each parent respects the judgments of the other parent; and (4) each parent desires to communicate with the other.

The parenting alliance is an adult life-course process that both amplifies and is amplified by the self-psychology concept of self-selfobject relationships. Moreover, it can identify factors that promote creative growth in adulthood. We recognize the danger of overloading the concept but propose it, nevertheless, as a significant, interpersonal, and intrapsychic process in assessing adult development and family cohesion and in planning therapeutic intervention.

NOTES

This paper is based on "The Parenting Alliance," a chapter by Rebecca Cohen and Sidney Weissman, in *Parenthood: A Psychodynamic Perspective,* ed. R. Cohen, B. Cohler, and S. Weissman (New York: Guilford, 1984).

1. The concept of the self-selfobject relationships was initially developed by Kohut (1971, 1977) to describe a specific transference relationship that he observed in the psychoanalysis of certain patients. As his observations continued, the psychology of the self was developed. The self-selfobject construct was extended to normal development. We now regard the intrapsychic operation in which one individual (object) sustains his or her self-esteem regulation and psychological intactness by use of another individual (object) in a specific situation or relationship as a self-selfobject relationship. The individual may or may not be aware of the importance of the other in maintaining his psychological equilibrium.

REFERENCES

Anthony, E. J., and Benedek, T. 1970. *Parenthood: Its Psychology and Psychopathology*. Boston: Little, Brown.

Benedek, T. 1959. Parenthood as a development phase. *Journal of the American Psychoanalytic Association* 7:389–417.

Bowen, M. 1976. Theory in the practice of psychotherapy. In P. Guerin, Jr., ed. *Family Therapy: Theory and Practice*. New York: Gardner.

Cohen, R., and Balikov, H. 1974. On the impact of adolescence upon parents. *Adolescent Psychiatry* 3:217–236.

Cohler, J. 1981. Adult developmental psychology and reconstruction in psychoanalysis. In S. E. Greenspan and G. H. Pollock, eds. *The Course of Life: Adulthood and the Aging Process*. Washington, D.C.: National Institute of Mental Health.

Goldberg, A., 1980. *Advances in Self-Psychology*. New York: International Universities Press.

Kohut, H. 1971. *The Analysis of the Self*. New York: International Universities Press.

Kohut, H. 1977. *The Restoration of the Self*. New York: International Universities Press.

Lidz, T. 1963. *The Family and Human Adaptation*. New York: International Universities Press.

Lidz, T. 1976. *The Person*. Rev. ed. New York: Basic.

Mahler, M. S., and Furer, M. 1968. *On Human Symbiosis and Vicissitudes of Individuation*. New York: International Universities Press.

Meissner, W. W. 1978. The conceptualization of marriage and family dynamics from a psychoanalytic perspective. In T. J. Paolino, Jr., and B. S. McCrady, eds. *Marriage and Marital Therapy*. New York: Brunner/Mazel.

Michels, R. 1981. Adulthood. In S. I. Greenspan and G. H. Pollock, eds. *The Course of Life: Adulthood and the Aging Process*. Washington, D.C.: National Institute of Mental Health.

Minuchin, S. 1974. *Families and Family Therapy*. Cambridge, Mass.: Harvard University Press.

Stierlin, H. 1977. *Psychoanalysis and Family Therapy*. Cambridge, Mass.: Harvard University Press.

Terman, D. M. 1980. Object love and the psychology of the self. In A. Goldberg, ed. *Advances in Self-Psychology*. New York: International Universities Press.

Tolpin, M. 1971. On the beginnings of a cohesive self: an application of the concept of transmuting internalization to the study of the transitional object and signal anxiety. *Psychoanalytic Study of the Child* 26:316–352.

Weissman, S., and Barglow, P. 1980. Recent contributions to the theory of female adolescent psychological development. *Adolescent Psychiatry* 8:214–230.

Wolf, E. 1980. On the developmental line of selfobject relations. In A. Goldberg, ed. *Advances in Self-Psychology*. New York: International Universities Press.

4 LOST BOYS WANDERING AROUND THE PETER PANTHEON

NICHOLAS MEYER

While it is generally acknowledged that the primary purpose of art is to make us feel rather than think, it is also true that certain artistic enterprises stay in our minds long after their sentient impact has made itself felt. Satisfied on a noncerebral level, when our emotions have subsided and our heartbeats returned to their normal cadence, we sometimes replay the experience in our memories and there may discover some lurking meaning which may serve to explain or to enhance our feelings of enjoyment.

Thus, while the tragedy of *King Lear* moves us to instinctive empathetic tears, it is forever after the fact of the play that men and women have attempted to dissect its components in order to learn precisely what it is in *Lear* that moves us so profoundly. In Aristotelian terms, one might simply say that *Lear* is a perfect imitation of life, and it is in the perfection of imitating life—as Aristotle was apparently the first to observe—that we derive the most acute pleasure. It is sometimes fun, and occasionally instructive, however, not to leave it at that. This is because, in asking ourselves to think about what we have felt in connection with an artistic encounter, we may learn something about ourselves as well as the work which has provoked the train of associations.

One time, several years ago, I borrowed from my brother-in-law a copy of the Mary Martin cast album of *Peter Pan*. My brother-in-law put the record into my hands, saying, "Have you ever thought about *Peter Pan*—I mean *really* thought about it?" I said I hadn't, but, prompted by the twinkle in his eye, took the record home, played it, was charmed again

0-226-24058-4/85/0012-0039$01.00

by it—moved to tears, in fact—and then sat back and took my brother-in-law's advice.

Peter Pan is the story of a boy who refuses to grow up; *the Boy who wouldn't grow up* is the play's subtitle. The part of Peter Pan is always played by a girl. This fact, remembered almost at once, is an arresting one. (Nor was this the only play written by Peter Pan's creator, the playwright J. M. Barrie, in which a male youth is thus impersonated: in 1936, a year before his death, Barrie wrote his last play, *The Boy David,* for Elizabeth Bergner.)

Peter Pan arrives at the London home of Mr. and Mrs. Darling and spirits away their three children—though the principal emphasis is on the oldest, the girl Wendy—to a magical kingdom where Peter lives called Never-Never Land.

They get there after Peter teaches the three children how to fly. Once in Never-Never Land they have wonderful adventures. They meet the tomboy Indian princess, Tiger Lily, and Peter's friends, the parentless Lost Boys, and escape the villainous Captain Hook, Peter's archenemy, before returning to London and reality, which includes growing up. Peter promises to return for Wendy, who begs him not to forget her, but Time stands still in Never-Never Land, and by the time he comes back, Wendy is a grown woman with children of her own. As a sort of consolation prize, Peter borrows her oldest daughter, Jane, for an excursion with him to his magical home.

The principal relationship in the play concerns Peter and Wendy. Where Wendy's affections are concerned, Peter has two principal rivals, one in the real world of London and the other in Never-Never Land. Peter defies Wendy's father, Mr. Darling, by spiriting off his daughter in a sort of fantastical elopement (chaperoned by her two obliging brothers), but in Never-Never Land, he must save Wendy from the greedy possessiveness of the terrible Captain Hook, who, like Peter, wants "the Wendy," as he calls her, bestowing a generic significance on her given name. Both Peter and Captain Hook want the Wendy for the same purpose: "to be our mother."

Just as it is challenging to note that Peter Pan is always played by an actress, it is equally suggestive to recall that the benign Mr. Darling (his name is an apt description) and the terrible Captain Hook are always portrayed by the same actor. It is not too difficult to see the implication here, namely, that Mr. Darling and Captain Hook are one and the same person, or, more accurately, that they are the two separate halves of one person, the sweet Mr. Darling, who is kind to those who treat him with respect, and the monstrous pirate Captain, who, though comically drawn, is nevertheless capable of instilling a very lively fear on the part of boys and girls in the audience. His name, Captain Hook, incidentally, derives from a murderous appendage which replaces one of his hands. It is not hard to imagine to what dark purpose this terrible device will be put if the Captain ever gets hold of Peter Pan. (In fact, considering that Peter Pan is being played by a woman, it is possible, in a sense, to argue that Hook has already succeeded.)

The only thing Captain Hook truly fears is a crocodile which has swallowed a perpetually ticking clock. It takes no great leap of the imagination to understand that Hook's real fear is the same as every father's; devouring time, for which playwright Barrie could hardly have devised a more potent image. In time all fathers will be supplanted by their sons. Peter Pan, then, would seem chronologically destined to win the Wendy.

But in Peter Pan's refusal to grow up, the audience is treated to the odd and moving story of one for whom puberty, adulthood, and sexual responsibility (obliquely described in the play with every image of adulthood except references to sexual capacity—smelly pipes, constricting neckties, etc.) are apparently too much to handle. The fact that Peter Pan was always intended to be played by an actress (the play won't work any other way) shows to what an extent Peter has been prepared by his creator to abrogate his sexual privileges. The boon companionship of the Lost Boys and the initiation of Wendy into Never-Never Land—followed some years later by the initiation of Jane, who, presumably, will be followed at some point by another and then another in an endless string of girls on the threshold of womanhood whom Peter will "borrow" for a while—form the pattern of Peter Pan's endless life.

In a way this is kind of sad. Never-Never Land at first seems such a wonderful and magical place, as viewed from the perspective of Wendy, Michael, and John. But from Peter Pan's view, it seems finally to be a kind of curse, although he may defiantly insist that things are just fine and that he wouldn't have them any other way. As long as he is truly immortal and as long as one accepts the premise that all preadolescent girls are interchangeable, perhaps this is true; yet somehow there is a lurking sense of unease attached to these conditions for Peter's claim of perpetual happiness.

What is certainly true, however, is that the play/musical *Peter Pan* is an artistic masterpiece, a modern fairy tale which has entered our world with all the built-in conviction of a myth.

What is certainly true is the miracle of art which has taken place and in which the painful personal life of Peter Pan's creator, James M. Barrie, has been transformed through his inspired genius into a deathless work of enchantment which has beguiled generations who have never needed to probe too deeply or to be told just what it was that was moving them so pleasantly. Seen as the nostalgia for lost innocence and make-believe, experienced like an Impressionist painting—agreeably out of focus—it is not necessary to formally outline the oedipal struggle of a boy unsuccessfully battling his father for the affections of his mother and, fatally wounded by the attempt in some way we do not know, choosing—as Barrie chose—to retire from the fray. One of the Lost Boys himself, he adopted his own family of Darlings, or rather (as in the play), permitted the Darlings to adopt him, with, as it happened, unimaginably tragic consequences.

It is the stunning miracle of art that, like alchemy, it is capable of turning such base and irrelevant materials into the stuff of enduring and universally appealing magic.

Without being quite sure why, I thought of *Peter Pan* again, when, a week ago, I watched the excellent revival of *My Fair Lady* with Rex Harrison re-creating his original portrayal of the irascible Professor Henry Higgins and Cheryl Kennedy bringing to marvelous life the cockney flower girl Eliza Doolittle, whom Higgins remakes into a "consort for a Prince," in his words. I was very moved by the play and found myself weeping for much of the performance.

Later, turning over the experience in my mind and trying to understand what it was that had touched me so deeply, I found myself puzzling over several things and eventually found my way back to *Peter Pan*—although not without some interesting detours.

My Fair Lady is, of course, based on the play *Pygmalion,* by Bernard Shaw (which derives, in turn, from the Greek myth of the sculptor who falls in love with his own statue, Galatea). The sculpting process in *Pygmalion* involves the remolding of the drab flower girl into a lady by chipping away at her cockney accents until she talks beautiful English. (She is also washed.)

Now Shaw is a completely paradoxical literary figure, whose plays exist and are performed for reasons entirely unrelated to his writing of them. A dedicated Fabian Socialist, Shaw wrote his plays (and the lengthy, witty prefaces that accompany them) to teach and not to entertain. It is a curious fact of theatrical life that audiences, for the most part, are never taught by anything of Shaw's, whereas they are almost invariably entertained. The social issues so dear to Shaw are obscured by his characters, so colorful and so real that they take precedence in our attentions over the peppery Irishman's dry and trenchant social lessons. Thus, while Sylvia Fine chose several musicals to discuss on public television recently and proposed to treat those plays which addressed social topics (*Lady in the Dark*—psychoanalysis; *Finian's Rainbow*—racial prejudice; *South Pacific*—ditto), it seems not to have occurred to her that *My Fair Lady,* which some have dubbed the perfect musical, was equally worthy of her consideration, being almost exclusively about social issues, namely, the class system—how the fact of one's speech affects one's placement in that class system, and how women are treated by society.

On second thought, it is perhaps no fault of Miss Fine that *My Fair Lady* did not occur to her as an example of the socially relevant musical. I doubt very much if most audiences come out of the theater mulling over the issues that Shaw wished to raise (although, after twenty-five years of "consciousness-raising" by the women's movement, some of Higgins's male chauvinism is more deeply felt today than when the show first opened).

Poor Shaw, an entertainer in spite of himself! A playwright whose social concerns were overwhelmed by his own theatrical genius. So much luckier than his great hero, Ibsen, whose creaky social dramas may occupy a space in theatrical history because of their ground-breaking sociological significance, but whose work seems doomed to popular extinction because the personages of Ibsen's dramas have not the one essential ingredient which Shaw was able to confer on his characters: life.

My Fair Lady is almost exclusively derived from Shaw's *Pygmalion,* with one curious and happy exception: the ending. In *Pygmalion,* Eliza Doolittle appears to walk out forever on the charming but tyrannical Professor Higgins, and audiences from the first night of the play have disputed the author's ending. Shaw, writing in a postscript to the play, insisted that Eliza and Higgins could never ever get together. Writing about Miss Doolittle as if she were a real person, Shaw postulated her eventual marriage to the ineffectual Freddie, a projection which was happily seized upon by Alan Jay Lerner and used to advantage in the musical. In his essay on the subject, Shaw adduced a great many reasons and precepts to argue his case for the separate fate of Miss Doolittle, but the very fact that he was obliged to argue it invites closer examination. Audiences may be stupid, but they are never wrong. When Prokofiev first mounted his ballet version of *Romeo and Juliet,* the lovers at the end of the story danced happily ever after. This proved to be a great miscalculation; audiences protested, and the composer was compelled to change his ballet back in conformation to the original play. This example is useful because it also illustrates that audiences are not mindlessly addicted to happy endings; therefore the consistent and persistent notion on the part of thousands of people that Higgins and Eliza are made for each other—and the authors of *My Fair Lady* understood this perfectly and did what Shaw refused to do—ought to suggest that we look again at the playwright's obdurate insistence that Higgins and Eliza as a couple are doomed to be apart.

Even if they get together, it is admittedly questionable on just what basis Higgins and Eliza will cohabit. Certainly it will not be a sexual relationship. Higgins is clearly an asexual sort of man—"a confirmed old bachelor and likely to remain so" is his assessment—set in his way and mistrustful of women except in quasi-maternal roles: fetching his slippers, cooking his meals—keeping house, in other words. (The same function Peter Pan has in mind for the Wendy.) When Higgins asks Eliza to come live with him and she wants to know what for, he answers engagingly, "For the fun of it." Fun, I think, is not intended as any sort of sexual euphemism. Higgins literally means fun, in much the same way Peter Pan wants to take Wendy (and/or her successors) to his "apartment," or home, Never-Never Land, to be likewise instructed, initiated, and created—so that they may eventually mother him. Like Peter's arrangements with Wendy, Higgins's offer to Eliza is elaborately casual. They can both leave, he says, whenever either of them feels like it. Peter Pan displays some of Higgins's casualness when he unwittingly allows ten years to elapse before remembering to return for Wendy as he pledged; his bittersweet resignation at finding her transformed in his absence into a grown-up might easily be compared to Higgins's reluctant melancholy when Eliza refuses to play the game under his roof by his rules anymore. By the time he locates her, Eliza, like Wendy, has done some growing up; but like the youth-teaching Peter Pan, Higgins's specialty is the unformed, the rough clay. Lest it be forgotten what Peter Pan teaches Wendy, it may be recalled again that he teaches her to fly. Flying has long been equated with sex in symbolic terms. The song "Fly Me to the Moon," as well as an advertising campaign for a well-known airline in which attractive stewardesses smilingly invite prospective customers to "fly them" to Miami and other locations, are two examples of this accepted linkage. In the recent film version of *Superman,* the Man of Steel woos Lois Lane by taking her flying. Before leaving the ground, he looks meaningfully at her and makes a faintly derisive reference to the flying which takes place in *Peter Pan* as being for children; his voice is full of anticipatory relish, as though what is about to follow will in some way be the Real Thing. (It is, however, oddly, almost touchingly like the same scene in *Peter Pan*. Like Wendy, Lois Lane appears dressed for bed when she is taken flying, but for all its implied sexuality, the scene is as demure as anything in Barrie's play.)

Higgins is not much different. If he can teach Eliza to talk properly, he emphasizes, there is nothing she cannot do, nowhere she cannot go. Like Peter Pan, Professor Higgins is a flying instructor.

It is now not too difficult to make a case for Henry Higgins as a kind of overage Peter Pan; a man, yes, but one who has seemingly never made a sexual connection with another human being, and in this sense a virgin or young boy like Peter. He is impish, delightful, clever, and boastful—like boys—as well as being willful, spoiled, and stubborn. It would be incorrect, I think, to infer the presence of much in the way of homosexuality in the relations between Higgins and the Lost Boy chaperone of *Pygmalion,* Colonel Pickering. Pickering is a boon companion to Higgins; he exists to feed the Professor's not inconsiderable vanity with a constant flow of admiration and approval. Higgins lives in what might be described as a presexual world. He never relates to Pickering except as a chum, and, by his own admission, he can barely relate to Eliza as a person, much less a woman! (At one point he actually likens her to a parcel, suggesting that she be wrapped in brown paper while awaiting her new clothes.) When Eliza, pushed to her limits, abandons Higgins, he runs to his mother, as though he were a small boy, deprived of a playmate; he wants her to fix it for him, to make Eliza come back for more sleep-over dates. As for Eliza, he wants her to be one of the boys. ("Why can't a woman be a chum?" he sings plaintively in the musical.) It is interesting to note that in all their exchanges, Higgins's mother treats him as though he were a child, and not a particularly good child at that. When Higgins shows up at her box at Ascot and she points out that he is not dressed for the occasion, the dignified professor of phonetics replies defensively that he changed his shirt. This is funny, but surely much of its impact is attributable to the inherent infantilism of the remark, coming from a supposedly grown man.

In fact, Higgins has many of the traits of a little boy, including the desire to astonish grown-ups with his cleverness. When he stands outside Covent Garden Opera House and gleefully flabbergasts passersby by telling from their speech where they were born, they react, as Pickering does, with delighted surprise and amusement, much as grown-ups do when approached by a child carrying a deck of cards—"Pick a card, any card ———." They are dutifully and perhaps genuinely impressed by the feat of magic when the correct card is identified by the youngster, but then they go about their business, to their homes, wives, husbands, families. Higgins, one senses, is left stranded on the street corner, waiting for the next person to amaze. Colonel Pickering has the agreeable virtue of having no home to get back to; he will always be around to be astonished and to applaud.

It is surely no accident that when Eliza, in *My Fair Lady,* satisfies an audience craving by returning to Higgins and his world, he greets her—smiling with ecstatic wonder and relief—with the words, "Eliza—where the devil are my slippers?" This is certainly I-Love-You in Henry Higgins talk, and it was shrewd of Alan Jay Lerner, in his adaptation of the play, to recognize that this was probably as close as Higgins—or any other boy—could come to acknowledging romantic passion. (While its male chauvinism is strikingly apparent, so, too, I think is its infantilism, which may suggest an entirely separate series of associations. One might bear in mind, however, the fact that young boys are prone to pulling the braids of the girls they like as a manifestation of their interest and affection.) Eliza, it is clear, is expected by Higgins to pick up after him, like a small boy's mother. That she may be quite prepared to do this is matter of another essay; here we will confine ourselves to noting that she too runs to Higgins's mother in a time of crisis and distress.

In reading about George Bernard Shaw, it is interesting to discover that his relations with women did not appear to be of a sexual nature. By his own account, he did not lose his virginity until he was twenty-nine. He was married but disabled immediately prior to the wedding by a bout with tuberculosis and immediately afterward on his honeymoon was incapacitated by a fall which required that an arm be immobilized in a sling. Charlotte, his wife, is seldom mentioned, and the couple produced no children. Much more commented on is the playwright's voluminous correspondence with such actresses as Ellen Terry and Mrs. Patrick Campbell, for whom the part of Eliza Doolittle was written.

It is downright fascinating to discover that, as a child, Shaw lived with his father and mother, who was a singer, in a house that also contained her singing teacher and mentor, one Professor Vandaleur Lee.

So great was Lee's influence with Shaw's mother that eventually she abandoned her husband (who drank) and her son and took her two daughters with her to live with Professor Lee in London. Young Shaw was separated from his mother for five years before rejoining her unconventional menage. Although the model for Higgins was ostensibly a phonetics teacher, one Henry Sweet, it seems evident—at least on an unconscious level—that the real model was the man who won Shaw's mother from her husband and, in a sense, from Shaw himself. His mother's middle name, incidentally, was Elizabeth.

Now we can make a guess as to why Shaw was so insistent on the fact of Higgins and Eliza's irreconcilability. It had nothing to do with social issues so dear to Shaw's Fabian mind so much as it was the correction of a highly personal and objectionable state of affairs in the playwright's heart and in his past. Unable to tolerate the fact of his mother's being the mistress of Professor Lee, Shaw is perversely blind to the inevitability of the relationship, so readily apparent to all the audiences that watched his play and kept trying to tell him that he got the ending wrong. Shaw's refusal to acknowledge this fact, indeed, the desperation with which he denied it, suggests the torment the memories of his own childhood must have caused him, in which he lost possession of his mother to one who could not—in his child's perception—rightfully claim her. His love of music, by the way, was equaled only by his ambivalence toward teaching as a profession. "Those who can't do teach" is a barbed Shavianism. One could spend hours pondering the word *do* in that sentence.

But it takes no hours to ponder the fact that, once again, artistic alchemy has taken place. Bernard Shaw has unraveled the tangled skein of his own life and rewoven the threads therefrom to make a magical flying carpet atop which Henry Higgins and Eliza Doolittle are destined to float in the popular imagination forever.

Of course, the Greek myth of Pygmalion and Galatea was not the only source of Shaw's inspiration. Creativity, as we know, is an enormously mysterious and complex process, in which a great many ideas, impressions, and bits of knowledge are intermingled by the artist to form a new distillation of art. At least one other major contributor to Shaw's play was the great detective hero of Sir Arthur Conan Doyle, Sherlock Holmes.

Indeed, the resemblances between Holmes and Higgins—beginning with their last names—are so many and so striking and so obvious as to be, well, almost embarrassing.

Like Higgins, Holmes is a detective. But whereas Higgins's sole specialty is deducing a person's origins from his speech, Holmes's expertise enables him to astonish clients by telling everything about them—occupation, past, as well as their problem. Like Higgins, Holmes might be described as a charming if irascible bachelor, mistrustful of women, whose rooms, like the professor's, are presided over by a motherly sort of housekeeper—Mrs. Pierce of 27a Wimpole Street; Mrs. Hudson of 221b Baker Street. (Wouldn't those two ladies find it interesting to compare notes!)

Like Higgins, Holmes has a boon companion, Dr. Watson, who admiringly chronicles his friend's achievements while not distracting Holmes with any particular needs of his own. If Colonel Pickering has just returned from India, Dr. Watson has just returned from Afghanistan. There seems little question that Shaw, writing *Pygmalion* in 1912, was well aware of the most popular fictional character ever created, whose exploits were then at their height. And like Higgins and Pickering, I don't think homosexuality is to be properly inferred. Just because heterosexuality is absent does not imply its counterpart. Holmes evinces no physical interest in Watson, or indeed in anyone, save for the physical clues they present which may be relevant to the case under investigation. Indeed, Watson goes off and gets married. (Holmes refers to this as Watson's only act of betrayal, but clearly, in my understanding, the word "betrayal" is a half-serious taunt referring to the abandonment of companionship, not a sexual defection.) In any case, dependable Watson returns to his old Baker Street digs at every opportunity, for more adventures with Holmes. "For the fun of it," as Higgins might say. Holmes, "who never spoke of the softer passions save with a gibe and sneer" (reminiscent of the contempt with which preadolescent boys scoff at any expression of affection for girls, making life miserable for older brothers and sisters), might be characterized as yet another incarnation of Peter Pan, having adventures in his own magical kingdom of London, where things are not always as they appear. Beneath and around the placid facades of the secure bastion of Victoriana are to be found scurrilous doings, murders, abductions, robberies—adventures, in short, not unlike the pirates and their evil machinations in Never-Never Land. The converting of a benign landscape into a war-torn terrain is a common practice among boys playing cowboys and Indians and a dozen other similar games of fantasy. It is surely not without meaning that most readers are introduced to Sherlock Holmes at this impressionable prepubescent stage of life. Holmes's creator understood this perfectly when he wrote

> I have wrought my simple plan
> If I give one hour of joy
> To the boy who's half a man
> Or the man who's half a boy.

With these sentiments thus expressed, it should come as no surprise to learn that Arthur Conan Doyle enjoyed a warm friendship with his contemporary, the playwright J. M. Barrie. It seems almost too good to be true when one learns that the creator of *Peter Pan* and the creator of *Sherlock Holmes* actually collaborated on an opera, but they did. (It flopped, but Barrie got a droll two-page Holmes parody out of the experience.)

Women in the Holmes saga are treated with cautious reverence approaching the cult of the Virgin. Irene Adler, the love of Holmes's life, is known by him as *The* Woman, rather like the Wendy. Holmes seems no more capable of nor disposed toward an adult union with her than Alfie P. Doolittle's sly insinuations have any bearing on Henry Higgins's true appetites where Doolittle's daughter is concerned. ("Men of the world, is it?" Higgins patronizingly echoes Doolittle's choice of words, but there is no evidence that he is a man of the world in that sense, unless one acknowledges that he talks a good game. When Pickering asks Higgins if he is a man of good character where women are concerned, Higgins banteringly rejoins by asking the colonel if he has ever met a man of good character where women are concerned. While this reply is witty enough, it smacks of locker-room braggadocio. Certainly there is nothing in the rest of Higgins's history to support the implied claim of vast experience, or, at the least, knowledge.) Sex does not enter into the lives of Holmes or Shaw's imitation of him.

Don Quixote and Sancho Panza belong in this chaste Peter Pantheon, as well; like Holmes, Quixote is a deducer, not of things as they are, perhaps, but certainly as they ought to be. In identifying windmills as giants, he has taken the cowboys and Indians fantasy to a wild extreme, converting all of Spain into his own Never-Never Land. He sallies forth to do battles with ogres and monsters—for knightly honor and the fun of it—accompanied by the loyal and quizzically admiring Sancho, who, like Watson and Pickering after him, takes endless delight in allowing his friend to explain the world. Quixote—and his real self, Alonso Quiana—is also a bachelor, holding all women in the revered esteem that is the role of true preadolescent knights, a code which defines Holmes's behavior toward women, his muttered misgivings notwithstanding.

The British author Trevor Hall, in a brilliant piece of his own deducing, postulated the murder of Holmes's mother by his father as a means of accounting for much of Sherlock's character, his distrust of women (his mother, Hall suggests, had a lover), and his choice of profession, etc. I found this idea sufficiently convincing to incorporate into my Sherlock Holmes novel *The Seven-Per-Cent Solution*.

Which brings me to myself, to my own interest in Peter Pan, Henry Higgins, Sherlock Holmes, and to what we can learn about ourselves through art. As I write these lines, I am two days away from my thirty-fifth birthday. I am a bachelor, but despite numerous love affairs, I have never married. Many women in my life have since gone on to marry. At least two that I know of have had children. They have, in a word, grown up, while I seem destined—so far—to remain stuck in Never-Never Land. As I mentioned earlier, Peter Pan's fate may not seem grim if he is truly immortal and will never grow old; it may not seem grim if all woman are interchangeable. . . .

But in reality, we do grow old, and all people are by no means interchangeable. My repetitive enactment of conquest and/or initiation, in which I carry off some young woman and seduce her, perhaps even live with her for a time, has never yet gone beyond the initial elopement to my own Never-Never Land. I am always in search of more Wendys, but as the years roll on and take their inevitable toll, my role as Peter Pan fits less and less comfortably and I find all the more poignant the story of Peter Pan, the play *Pygmalion,* and its musical offspring, and perhaps that is why my own imitations of Sherlock Holmes have been so kindly received: I write about Holmes with elements of the same unconscious kinship displayed by his great originator, Sir Arthur Conan Doyle. Space does not permit a full discussion of the singular relationship enjoyed by that curious odd couple—imagine trying to kill off a literary creation who won't stay dead—but the fact that Doyle did succeed in marrying and having children I take as some sort of cautiously hopeful omen. Perhaps the first step in this direction for me has been my tentative recognition of a syndrome in which I can watch my pattern of action objectified in various plays and books.

I do not mean to imply in this essay that I have covered or cataloged all the meanings in the plays and stories discussed. On the contrary, I am pleased to know that I have barely touched them. The wonderful thing about the greatest art is its onion-like capacity to unfold, revealing layer after layer of inner meaning, ad infinitum—and, like an onion, make you cry in the process.

And if some irate person angrily demands of me what Shaw's childhood has to do with *Pygmalion* or what J. M. Barrie's has to do with *Peter Pan,* I answer unhesitatingly: nothing.

But *Peter Pan* and *Pygmalion* have a great deal to do with the childhoods of Barrie and Shaw.

And, as I have lately come to learn, with my own.

REFERENCES

Barrie, J. M. 1950. *Peter Pan*. New York: Scribner, 1950.
Doyle, A. C. 1930. *The Complete Sherlock Holmes*. Garden City, N.Y.: Doubleday.
Lerner, A. J. 1956. *My Fair Lady*. New York: Coward-McCann.
Shaw, G. B. 1940. *Pygmalion*. New York: Dodd Mead.
Weissman, P. 1965. *Creativity in the Theater: A Psychoanalytic Study*. New York: Basic.

5 ACUTE-ONSET SERIOUS CHRONIC ORGANIC ILLNESS IN ADOLESCENCE: SOME CRITICAL ISSUES

MEYER S. GUNTHER

Serious chronic illness in adolescence confronts the clinician with a basic dilemma: Which ones, among the vast number of relevant variables, are crucial? A sensible solution to this dilemma begins with the recognition that serious chronic illness in adolescence must be viewed as a unique but integrated human experience. Such an experience is an expression of a basic human potential: the capacity of human beings to confront, transcend, and then grow when faced by a life-threatening, life-altering illness despite the monumental traumas and difficulties inherent in such adversity.

Psychoanalytic interest in serious chronic illness, especially with visible body damage and clear-cut alteration in life-role activities, has been sketchy. Existing reports are anecdotal, frequently drawn from lengthy individual analyses. Calef (1959) reported a panel describing the analysis of children and adolescents with major life-threatening illnesses and congenital lesions. Tourkow (1974) reviewed a workshop on psychic consequences of loss and replacement of body parts. In 1977 an anthology of studies from *The Psychoanalytic Study of the Child* on children with major disabling illnesses was issued, entitled *Physical Illness and Handicap in Childhood* (Eissler, Freud, Kris, and Solnit 1977). Occasionally there have been other publications on special aspects of severe traumatic illnesses or body defects (Bergmann and A. Freud 1965; Castelnuovo-Tedesco 1980, 1981; Earle 1979; Horwitz 1976; Lipton 1962; Lussier 1980; Moore 1975; Niederland 1965; Solnit and Priel 1975; Yorke 1980)

0-226-24058-4/85/0012-0009$01.00

as well as a host of organ transplant studies (Blacher 1978, 1982; Castelnuovo-Tedesco 1978; Muslin 1971).

The yield of these articles is significant but disparate. It encompasses such commonly understood issues as separation, regression, introversion, anxiety, dependency, overcompensation, grandiosity, infantile narcissism, and other fixations, but especially identity and body image problems—issues familiar to all clinicians. Much of this literature on chronic, severe, life-threatening, life-altering illness—congenital or acquired—focuses on the specific interference of illness in normal development. The emphasis is on induced alterations from normal which occur to various parts of the psychic apparatus and not on the massively traumatic disorganizing and disruptive effects of the disease experience as a special variable with uniquely primary effects on an established stable set of personality configurations.

The reasons for this are multiple and speculative. Few such people come to the attention of psychoanalysts. There is undoubtedly a reaction of universal abhorrence to individuals whose visible physical deficits or handicaps are so upsetting and so therapeutically frustrating that they pose special countertransference burdens for all who work with them. There is also the question of the cohort problem. Many investigations treat all severe acute-onset chronic illness as if it were part of a single dynamic cohort. They assume all psychological meanings are the same regardless of the specific pattern of onset and prognosis, the severity of the treatment, or the sequelae. Equally troublesome has been a tendency to use the normal psychology of the able-bodied as an absolute standard against which psychological issues of people who are handicapped or who suffer from disabling chronic illnesses are measured and evaluated. This dubious assumption of a "universal normality" may have become commonly accepted because of the developmental plasticity of children, as if it were true of adolescents and adults as well. In addition, the limitations of ego psychology as a fully adequate explanatory framework have probably served to frustrate investigators attempting to understand the special meanings experienced by people who suffer either congenital lesions or major, traumatic, or chronic lesions. With the elaboration of the concept of massive psychic trauma in regard to the Holocaust studies (Krystal 1968; Niederland 1981), the concept of current life situation trauma as an independent variable of monstrous proportion and monstrously destructive effect on the core of human personality has gained respectability in psychoanalytic thinking. The work of Kohut (1971, 1972, 1977), his followers

(Goldberg 1978, 1980), and other self psychologists (Gedo 1979, 1981; Klein 1976; Stolorow and Lachman 1980) have come to offer an additional framework for thinking about these atypical human experiences.

Serious Chronic Organic Disease—Some Generalizations

A serious chronic disease may be defined as a life-threatening, life-altering, interminable, continuing process which affects selective but vital aspects of the victim's body, mind, and/or behavior. Like psychoneurotic symptoms, it is experienced as unexpected, unwelcome, and alien. In the ultimate sense, however, it is not curable. Neither altered anatomy nor physiology can be restored to pre-illness normalcy. (Certain parallels to aging are self-evident.) A crucial characteristic of a serious chronic disease is that in some ways it irrevocably alters one's capacities and competencies for basic life roles—the roles defining activities of daily living, as well as social, sexual, familial, and vocational activities. Consequently, if significant self-expression and self-fulfillment are to be achieved, it is imperative that one revise aspects of one's self-system, especially the pattern of life aims and the body image (or body components of one's self [Gunther 1971]).

An appropriate long-term therapeutic approach is one modeled on rehabilitative principles and not simply on expectations of cure. Rehabilitation focuses on maximizing remaining resources by altering their integration and deployment, conceivably uncovering or adding new ones, as well as slowing down the progression of the chronic disease as much as possible. Such an approach involves the principle of optimal matching of the individual to new aims, to new life activities, and, above all, to new methods or processes of living if a life of some quality is to be achieved.

A serious chronic illness involves an experience of repetitive developmental and problem-solving struggles as each new phase in the life cycle is encountered. Several psychological qualities are typical:

1. A self-oriented shift in the deployment of one's life energies occurs; one becomes more "narcissistic." Self-protective, self-assertive, and self-gratifying activities have priority.

2. There is some difference, if not distortion, in overall developmental pattern compared with that of the presumed norm. It arises from diminished opportunity for life experience, for stimulus input, for problem-solving activities, as well as from different defensive needs. It evolves through the interplay between disease-related adaptational struggles and

normally programmed developmental tasks. Above all, it is related to the meanings which the individual attaches to these disease-connected experiences and the reciprocal effect of these meanings in influencing one's ordinary life struggles. These meanings focus not merely on the disease and its alterations in one's body and one's life but also on concerns over the treatment and fear of the ultimate effect on one's longevity. These differences particularly affect issues of self-esteem regulation.

3. Finally, there is another quality which characterizes a serious chronic illness. In the context of decent human relationships, someone very close to the patient—a parent, spouse, lover, sibling, or a child—worries a great deal about the victim of a serious chronic illness. Ultimately he or she must learn to deal with the chronic worrisome anxiety which the illness engenders. This is accomplished most often by the worrier's changing his or her relationship with the disease victim.

How would a serious chronic illness be rated? On a scale of one to four, the four-plus illnesses are closed head injuries, spinal cord lesions, malignancies, some cardiac illnesses, limb amputation, burns, and degenerative neurological disorders of congenital origin. Somewhat less severe would be seizure disorders, juvenile diabetes, and chronic asthma. Two diseases which are chronic and incurable but which rate only a one-plus on my scale are hay fever and nearsightedness.

Common Reactions to Serious Illness—Acute or Chronic

If one observes victims of serious, acute illness or the acute-onset phase of a chronic illness at almost any age and under almost any circumstances, one will see some, but not necessarily all, of the following psychological phenomena:

1. *Affects.*—Frequent are such things as anxiety of multiple origins, anger, guilt, surprise, and resentment. Helplessness, hopelessness, and other depressive feelings of varying intensity are quite common.

2. *Fear.*—Depending on the age, fears of separation from loved ones and familiar routines, fears of the unknown, fears of pain, fears of treatment, and fears of future uncertainty are typical.

3. *Regression.*—Some degree of regression in object relations, self-system, defenses, and cognitive function is universal when one encounters a serious illness. This is partly situationally induced but primarily of intrapsychic, that is, adaptive, origin.

4. *Introversion.*—Withdrawal and turning inward to a more narcissis-

tic, self-protective, self-concerned orientation with the temporary loss of investment in one's usual relationships and activities are very common.

5. *Attitudes toward medical caretakers.*—Attitudes tend to vary depending on age and personality, but typical are mixtures of dependent trust, magical hope, and self-object idealization, on one hand, alternating with angry disappointment and irritable resentment about everything connected with the illness. Thus, caretakers are recipients of complex projections as well as needs.

6. *The problem of aggression.*—A heightening of aggressive feelings is frequent. This is related to physical restriction, to regression, and to an effort at restitution through intensified discharge. Such discharge is in the service of attempts to influence one's world to overcome feelings of helplessness. Direct expression may be modified by reaction formation and passive-aggressive attitudes.

7. *Defensive functioning.*—Regression, the formation of dependent self-object transferences, passive withdrawal, compulsive rituals, reaction formations, the use of magical thinking, and some degree of denial or projection and turning against the self are common defensive maneuvers when one faces a serious illness.

Some Specific Adolescent Adaptations

Adolescent adaptations to confrontation with a severe chronic illness are notoriously varied. First, I shall describe ominously bad adaptations. It can be argued that division of these into four semiseparated syndromes is artificial—that all these are varieties of the same adaptive processes with different quantitative intensities or phases occurring at different times in one long, complex process.

1. *Disorganization and peculiar regression.*—It is characterized by some depressive affect, pseudostupidity, and childishness, together with shallow noncompliance that seems to originate from something other than aggressive defiance. These youngsters recognize the existence of the illness and the need to participate in medical rehabilitative learning but seem unable to learn. Everyone who works with them is convinced that they are trying, but they appear self-defeating. Apparently they undergo an atypical regression as a means of defending themselves from their terrible fears of abandonment in consequence of the threat of an uncontrolled outpouring of aggression. Their only solution appears to be a "false self" defense (Winnicott 1960a, 1960b)—an ambivalent effort to remain "the

good kid" while unknowingly undermining this adaptation even as they attempt to carry it out. In terms of treatment, they retain some capacity for introspection and appropriate responses if the medical caretakers offer significant holding environment responses to their aggressive anxieties.

2. *Serious depression with the potential for suicide.*—These adolescents are sullen and withdrawn, hopelessly pessimistic about themselves and their future. They, too, recognize the existence and seriousness of the illness, but they consistently reject offers of help and medical procedures as either useless or too difficult. Their most persistent attitudes are negativism and apathy, although they may flare into rage attacks if confronted. They may have been previously designated for the role of the bad kid or the wastebasket for the deposit of the family's psychopathology, if not its cause. The thoughtful observer gains the impression that they view the occurrence of physical illness as if it were predetermined and, therefore, something to be accepted submissively as a means of living out their true fate. They convey a subtle sense of using the illness for revenge against the parents who failed them. Their illness becomes the vehicle for focal discharge of all manner of aggression toward their parents and the adult world, that is, retribution via self-sacrifice. There is a hint of a disguised plea for help, but it is very difficult to engage. They require major psychiatric intervention involving either psychiatric hospitalization or intensive treatment in a totally structured medical milieu—a solution almost impossible to achieve.

3. *Impossibly provocative.*—Adolescents with this syndrome are much more openly aggressive than the preceding group, as if they had been engaged in a chronic power struggle with the world all their lives. Their attitude toward the illness is that of manifest disbelief in the fact either that they are sick or that they need anything from anybody. There is a persistent magical belief that everything is okay combined with a defiant distrust of all authorities. The underlying conflict may have to do not only with the fear that they are going to lose contact with their new bodies and hence never grow up but also with deeply rooted conflicts over dependent needs. Partly as a desperate protest, sexualization of everything lurks just behind the surface. Thus, they find it intolerably dangerous to consider that they may need any caretaking assistance from the medical authorities, especially if treatment involves continuing physical dependence, intimate contact, or frequent medical examinations. For all these reasons, they reject the very help they need most. Although they are vigorously defended against their true anxieties, in their negativistic way they really are implicitly engaged with the medical milieu. They will re-

spond to a firm, authoritarian structure and a similar form of confronting adolescent psychotherapy. As with all of the adaptations, but especially in this particular group, parental counseling is very helpful.

4. *Omnipotent regression with maximal narcissistic pathology.*—Like the last group, these adolescents are characterized by openly defiant, provocative, negativistic hostility but with the addition of a monumental capacity for manipulative, impulsive self-gratification. The existence of the illness is recognized and rationalized as the excuse for this behavior. All responsibility is projected onto the staff and the parents through the use of complex splitting processes. In their eyes neither family nor staff can do anything properly, a projection which originates in their rage at the part of themselves that has become ill or damaged. This part of themselves is then projected not simply to defeat the caretakers but to feel better by making the caretakers suffer what they are suffering. An even more pathological fantasy is that by making the caretakers (or parents) sick, they will make themselves well. Thus, although they are not openly suicidal, self-destruction via self-neglect is a serious danger. These youngsters have regressed to a level of structural disorganization defended by reawakened primitive grandiosity or paranoid/magical thinking. From the point of view of help, like the last group they require maximum firmly structured environments as a context for vigorous psychotherapy in which superego functions of the therapist substitute for what is so inoperative in themselves. Psychiatric hospitalization is sometimes necessary in the light of limited ability to structure the medical milieu.

To offset the ominous picture presented up to this point, there are normal but irritating adolescent adaptations to illness. In contrast to the preceding adaptations, these adaptations all involve more consistent efforts to confront the reality of the illness and its tasks and to begin to struggle to master them. In addition, these adaptations often become the model for patterns of future lifelong struggle. In contrast to the preceding group, these youngsters have not got lost either in an overwhelming outpouring of painful affects and frightening disorganization or in pathological efforts to defend themselves against such dangers.

1. *The "superstar" syndrome.*—This is the patient who excels at responsibility, self-protective activities, and new learning. The trouble is that he or she has to do it his own way, that is, better but differently from the medical authorities' wish. These youngsters constantly need to establish the uniqueness of their capacity to cope with "anything that comes along." Obviously there is some degree of counterphobic-like denial implied in this adaptation, but, overall, it is a constructive one.

2. *The passionate attachment syndrome.*—This is the adolescent who defies parents, doctors, and major medical personnel but picks some other caretakers, typically a lower-echelon allied health person or perhaps a fellow patient, and makes that person the sole source of all authority for recommendations about treatment and various decisions regarding life plans. Intensely attached to that person, the adolescent will work only for that person. Everyone else is considered dumb, worthless, or evil. Dynamically, it probably represents a transitional step in the renunciation and working through of the intensely ambivalent relationship to the parents with some of that having spilled over to the adjacent medical caretakers. Like the first adaptation, some individuation by negation seems to be involved.

3. *The syndrome of selective withdrawal.*—These are the youngsters who spend a great deal of time temporarily withdrawn into a world of the secret self of childhood. This serves as a respite for reorganizing and rebuilding, not just for evasion. When the youngsters come out of it in their own good time, they participate reasonably in learning and treatment activities and become reliable self-managers.

4. *The syndrome of selective avoidance and selective overcompensation.*—This involves an idiosyncratic phobic-like avoidance of certain life-role activities where the illness or its visible consequences are more likely to be noticed unfavorably by others. This would be especially true of sufferers from orthopedic, neurological, or skin lesions. This behavior is coupled with an intense effort to develop a special skill or creative capability in a particular area, often to excess, as compensation for the losses in other areas. Unfortunately, these overcompensatory, often grandiose, efforts are sometimes rooted in nonexistent or at best mediocre abilities. Nevertheless, by utilizing selective denial and selective overcompensation, these adolescents manage to come to terms with some of the more basic losses and to continue the struggle with life. But the price they pay in so doing is renunciation of certain interpersonal activities and, at times, painful distortion in others.

Normal Adolescence in Relationship to Serious Chronic Illness

Although the following list is incomplete and subjectively defined, these five issues may be viewed as constituting commonly acceptable adolescent developmental problems:

1. The experience of the new body with its genital libido, leading to fundamental changes in the body-self as a basis for tender and sensual pleasures—changes that, in turn, dramatically alter the adolescent's way of relating to his body.

2. The parents as primary love objects must be given up. In turn, parental introjects as sources of control and regulation must be revised. More reliable and neutralized sources of inner guidance and judgment must be evolved. Ultimately the superego must be fundamentally reworked as a basis for new relationships with the parents as well as with the responsibilities of adulthood.

3. A wide variety of new life aims and new life investments must be confronted. Decisions regarding a host of activities, interests, and goals must be struggled with and integrated to form a new self.

4. New capacities for inner autonomy, regulation, and management must be developed. These must be interwoven with qualities of authenticity, firmness, and resiliency leading to further cohesion of the new self—a self which will now facilitate a variety of new experiences that can be welcomed, managed, and eventually enjoyed.

5. Aspects of old childhood structures and identifications must be harmonized with the new self as a "second individuation" experience in order to evolve appropriate adult integration.

What happens in the course of efforts to achieve these aims when such tasks are complicated by the unexpected occurrence of a life-threatening, life-altering, chronic organic illness? First, the normal hypercathexis of the new genitalized body is complicated by the development of shifting, fuzzy relationships among the old body self, the now-changing body, and the defective parts or functions of the damaged body. Without question, this is upsetting, guilt evoking, and disorganizing, and, in consequence, a variety of dangers develop with respect to the stability of higher cognitive processes. Regressive or desperate defenses are formed against this experience of genital flooding, and so it becomes easy to avoid all experimental self-oriented activity with the new body and its potential for sensory gratification. Normal trial-and-error investigations which might be utilized to provide a pathway for the stepwise integration of the new body-self may be postponed endlessly. Second, there occurs a more than usually ambivalent struggle to renounce old identifications and regulatory processes. The normal renunciation of old learning capacities is much more problematic because the need for new learning is now so vital for survival. The normally occurring intensification of instinctual tensions is further heightened because discharge opportunities are limited. In addition, the temporary cognitive deregulation attendant on normal regression with reversion to primary process and magical thinking is further intensified by the illness and body focus. All of these factors produce an intensification of the normal reinstinctualization of many personality processes, especially cognitive ones. Third, there is often an ambivalent clinging to the parental substitutes—the medical caretakers—as a defense against the frightening narcissistic implications of these special experiences, particularly as a defense against the injury, pain, and trauma of these illness tasks, let alone against the normal developmental burdens. Yet, at the same time, there is a rejection of the caretakers not only because of the intensification of displaced incestuously based guilt but also as a result of the enormity of the disappointment and rage at all parental-like figures—feelings ascribable to outrage at the occurrence of the illness and necessity for treatment and not simply to ordinary adolescent developmental conflicts. Finally, all the usual adolescent maneuvers designed to evade facing unpleasant tasks are intensified: denial, avoidance, isolation, displacement, projection, and acting out.

To complicate these special tasks of confronting a serious chronic illness, if the adolescent has to accomplish this in the context of an acute-onset lengthy hospitalization, the following milieu circumstances serve to worsen things considerably. The necessary work of self-transformation, new learning, and growth must now be initiated: (1) in an atmosphere of social relationships that invites regressive renunciation of inner controls and mature aspirations while substituting overtly authoritarian externalized superego figures not only as the source of control but also as the source of future salvation; (2) in an atmosphere of maximum stimulation to conflicts over dependency, intimacy, and sexuality, especially the anxiety of sexual damage, that is, residual castration anxiety; (3) in an atmosphere in which each new lifesaving or life-altering procedure or rehabilitation technique is experienced as a new trauma which tends to reawaken all old traumas in connection with the illness and, therefore, to threaten further regression and disorganization. At the same time, reliably available cognitive capacities for new learning are expected by the caretakers; (4) in a situation of very limited discharge opportunities, particularly for aggressive tensions—let alone sexual tensions; (5) in a social and interpersonal atmosphere that frequently favors projection, splitting, disavowal, and magical thinking as attitudes toward parts of one's body and the new body-self; and (6) in an atmosphere where the familiar and at least partially protective images and reality presence of the parents are either unavailable or have failed, a situation experienced as gross, intensified abandonment.

It is apparent that many of the tasks of normal adolescent development have parallels in the tasks of struggle with an acute-onset severe chronic illness. In many ways the tasks are negatively synergistic, especially when hospitalization is involved. The adolescent sufferer from an acute illness which is on its way to becoming a chronic life-altering disease may be asking himself the following hypothetical questions. About the illness itself: "Why am I sick? What or who failed to protect me? What have I done to deserve this?" About the new body and its altered functions: "How will I learn to value it? How will I learn to understand and integrate its differences from what I was led to expect and from what all my peers are experiencing? How will I learn to regulate myself, to manage all the strange sensations, new activities, and new tasks that this altered body of mine now requires?" About the medical caretakers: "How will I learn to develop a set of workable relationships with the medical authorities, people who are different from my parents—more authoritarian, more demanding—who so often deal with me as if I am a child or as if I am deliberately out to frustrate them and to render them incapable of helping me? Yet, some of them do seem to like me, and I guess I do really need them." Regarding the new self: "How will I develop a new self-concept—one without any model in my own previous developmental experience and one without any comparative basis in my peers' experiences? How will the terrible new burden of my illness affect my still uncertain life aims—ones that may now have to be different from what I had been led to expect and hope for? Will I ever become a whole person, comfortable with myself?"

From the preceding descriptions, three tentative inferences may be specified regarding the unique negative synergy of adolescent development issues with the tasks imposed by a serious chronic organic illness: (1) Sooner or later, the adolescent must begin to engage the world of rehabilitation learning tasks as well as his own developmental issues; no matter what anxieties, ambivalence, or avoidance techniques are utilized initially, eventually the realities of both tasks must be confronted. (2) Anxieties about aggression in its protean manifestations seem to be a recurrent and universal issue for these adolescents. (3) Relationships with the caretakers appear to have a crucial, reciprocal role in determining the adolescent's capacity to engage the tasks constructively.

The Psychology of the Caretakers

The adolescent's struggles do not take place in an interpersonal vacuum. They occur in the context of intense relationships with parents and medical caretakers, among others. What are these crucial individuals experiencing in response to the adolescent's illness and his struggles?

Parents attempt to be selflessly available and endlessly responsive by disavowing or otherwise controlling their own anguished feelings. On the surface they remain involved with the adolescent, focusing their efforts on maintaining the child's hope and offering support. At a deeper level they are beset with myriad contradictory, ambivalent, and often counterproductive feelings and attitudes, usually not conscious. They are stirred by all of the usual anxieties of parents of adolescents plus some crucial additional ones. They may be battling with terrible feelings of loss—the loss of the wonderful adult that the child was expected to become someday and now may never be. They may be experiencing a variety of emotions—anger, rage, disappointment, loss, resentment, and fear of the future. Above all, they must struggle with their own misplaced sense of responsibility and guilt for the youngster's illness. There is the deeper dilemma: How can they become new objects in a new relationship for a changed, profoundly self-absorbed adolescent whom they hardly know? Should they go back to the safety of being the more authoritarian parents of the preadolescent youngster who in retrospect now seems to have been so much easier to relate to? To complicate things, they oscillate between clinging to the medical authorities for instruction, guidance, and reassurance and yet desperately resisting the very counsel which they apparently seek.

What are the medical caretakers experiencing? If the adolescent is in a major hospital for any period of time, he is being cared for by residents, interns, nurses, and allied health personnel who are probably within ten years of his age. Thus, the caretakers may still be struggling with their own postadolescent consolidations. As a consequence, the caretakers frequently have immediate and intense identification/counteridentification problems (or transference/countertransference problems) with the adolescent. Typically, there is considerable resistance to offering relationships of friendly closeness, selfless response, and realistic expectations and an exaggerated tendency to merge with the sick adolescent instead. At the other extreme are angry rejection and moral manipulation. The more mature and empathic caretakers sense that, despite desperation and ambivalence, the adolescent is turning to them as a source of new object experience, new instruction, new protection, new solutions.

In the situation of therapeutic responsibility for major serious illness that is life threatening and life altering, the caretakers have other burdens as well. They have their own complex professional expectations, an intense need to cure, to experience concrete performance success with their patients, combined with fear of exposure and failure. Narcissistic humiliation under these circumstances is an obvious danger. Because of this, they are often driven to place unrealistic, self-serving, and grossly insensitive expectations on their young patients. Complicating this, authoritarian medical institutions tend to make the patient's most immediately responsible caretakers especially fearful of and sensitive to the issues of impulse control, emotional lability, and negativistic acting-out behavior on the part of the patients. This leads psychologically unsophisticated caretakers, especially those at the bottom of the therapeutic pyramid, to become rigid, authoritarian, punitive, moral disciplinarians at times. All this creates a counterproductive, countertherapeutic milieu for the adolescents.

The preceding description of the reactions of patients, parents, and caretakers to the shared catastrophe necessitates consideration of the ways in which all three groups share certain similar painful affects and distorted reactions. (1) All three groups tend to deal with each other around unrealistic, wish-influenced expectations involving such things as idealized motives, the presumed dominance of objective logic and sweet reason in the cognitive sphere, and possession of magical power to transform. (2) At the same time, all three groups fear they will be unable to influence the others in regard to these expectations. In particular, the secret fear of their own helplessness looms in the background, compounded by anxieties regarding the consequences of failure of these self-expectations. (3) All three groups suffer some tendency to displace, externalize, or project responsibility for their own failures to achieve expected levels of influence in regard to the goal of alleviating some of the personality consequences of the illness, if not its anatomic/physiologic consequences. (4) Privately, and perhaps with some feeling of shame, all three groups suffer from some degree of intrusion of unexpected, unwelcome, painful feelings and upsetting thoughts which they cannot consciously control, much like individuals suffering from a posttraumatic (anxiety) syndrome.

Conclusions

What major issues will influence outcome significantly? Which and how much of those issues can we influence? In the following list, the first six are subject to little influence.

1. How soundly have the tasks and burdens of childhood development been traversed? How soundly and flexibly have basic identifications, capacities, and values been laid down? In metaphoric terms, how well formed are the parts; how good is the glue; how reliable is the assembly blueprint?

2. How sound has the relationship with the mother been, in terms of the crucial issues of protection from trauma and reliability of response? This is critical because of the modeling effect which this relationship has on future relationships with medical caretakers.

3. What basic malfunctions or alterations in body functions has the disease produced? How do these changes work "psychologically" in terms of losses or alterations in expected life-role capacities and life aims and in one's physical appearance and mobility? What is the meaning to the victim of such things as patterns of onset, progression, treatment, and ultimate influence on longevity?

4. To what degree are the profound, disease-related body changes predictable, knowable, and concretely experienceable? In contrast, how much anxiety-ridden unpredictability, uncertainty, and inherent unknowability will there be for the victim regarding the effects of the disease on his body and life?

5. How do the special burdens of the chronic illness mesh with the victim's preexisting personality strengths and vulnerabilities as well as with current developmental tasks and struggles? Are there resources available for potential mastery of the burdens and changes? Are the losses in anatomy and physiology so extensive and irremediable that even compromise mastery is impossible?

6. How extensive will be the ultimately residual, irreduceable dependency—physical, psychological, and social—as a result of the illness? Dependency on the caretakers may be the major long-term limiting influence—an issue which exerts its influence after all of the other adaptive problems have been confronted.

7. The initial acute treatment or onset phase of the chronic illness: has this been supplemented by a rehabilitation-oriented approach conceptualized around the goal of maximizing the patient's potentials for

facing his myriad life tasks and assisting his everyday efforts to master those tasks? Or is the therapeutic approach a lesion-focused, cure-oriented one, limited to assisting the patient in terms of medical competencies only, rather than overall needs? And is the medical care/rehabilitation facility going to be available, if needed, for the rest of his life?

8. The medical caretakers: do they understand and accept their role as "new objects" in providing a responsive consistent milieu which can substitute for missing personality functions while at the same time offering developmental opportunities for the patient? In particular, do they understand and accept Winnicott's (1960a, 1960b) concept of the holding environment, that is, the responsibility of the caretaking objects in the milieu to provide an illusion of safety and protection to contain the profound aggression and its derivatives, so that both the patient and the caretakers are safeguarded from the destructive outpouring of such aggression? If this baseline function is not fulfilled, the twin tasks facing the adolescent suddenly confronted with a serious chronic illness—normal adolescent transformations plus the new learning or rehabilitation—will be profoundly impaired if not doomed to failure. If the firm foundation for these tasks is missing or compromised, then efforts to accomplish them will flounder on an endless series of power struggles, mutual manipulations, and irreversible regression. If the caretakers (and their administrators) do not understand or accept this function, will they at least tolerate our attempting to educate them to its nature and virtue?

9. The family—how reliable is it? After coming to some settlement of its own complex, overdetermined struggles, does it return to a relationship of reliable albeit selective involvement with the sick youngster as long as is necessary? Or does it gradually disinvolve itself, using one or another rationalization?

10. Psychotherapy—a subject which merits a paper of its own. Many youngsters need treatment to stay alive through the combined traumas of adolescence and a major chronic organic illness, let alone master them. Yet the capacity to use such help (Newman 1981) has numerous difficulties and barriers. Many competently trained adolescent therapists are often handicapped by their lack of pertinent illness-related conceptual tools for dealing with massive psychic trauma. Seriously ill youngsters are often monumentally resistive to accepting any psychotherapeutic help even if it is part of the medical milieu, let alone if it is from the outside. To afford the best therapeutic opportunity to such youngsters, a comprehensive combination of medical, psychotherapeutic, and milieu-structuring

expertise is necessary. In addition, special organizational arrangements may be necessary with regard to issues such as who is going to be responsible for which medical, psychological, learning, and living needs of the patient.

Is it any wonder that there is an enormous variability in adolescent adjustment reactions to the onset of a serious chronic illness that is life threatening and life altering? Is it any wonder that the adolescent in the situation of the acute hospital, the rehabilitation hospitals, or posthospital home recovery is characterized by enormous moment-to-moment mood and cognitive swings; by shifts from relatedness to withdrawal; from elements of progressive maturity and thoughtful reorganization to elements of ominously grandiose, prepsychotic regression and disorganization? And, finally, is it any wonder, therefore, that acute-onset, serious, chronic illness in adolescence constitutes maximal burdens for all concerned—the patients, their families, and their medical caretakers?

REFERENCES

Bergmann, T., and Freud, A. 1965. *Children in the Hospital*. New York: International Universities Press.

Blacher, R. 1983. Death, resurrection and rebirth: observations on cardiac surgery. *Psychoanalytic Quarterly* 52:56–72.

Calef, V. 1959. Report of a panel: psychological consequences of physical illness in childhood. *Journal of the American Psychoanalytic Association* 7:155–162.

Castelnuovo-Tedesco, P. 1980. Ego vicissitudes in response to replacement or loss of body parts. *Psychoanalytic Quarterly* 47:381–397.

Castelnuovo-Tedesco, P. 1981. Psychological consequences of physical defects: psychoanalytic perspectives. *International Review of Psychoanalysis* 8:145–154.

Earle, E. M. 1979. The psychological effect of mutilating surgery in children and adolescents. *Psychoanalytic Study of the Child* 34:527–546.

Eissler, R.; Freud, A.; Kris, M.; and Solnit, A. J., eds. 1977. *Physical Illness and Handicap in Childhood: An Anthology of the Psychoanalytic Study of the Child*. New Haven, Conn.: Yale University Press.

Gedo, J. E. 1979. *Beyond Interpretation*. New York: International Universities Press.

Gedo, J. E. 1981. *Advances in Clinical Psychoanalysis*. New York: International Universities Press.

Gedo, J. E., and Goldberg, A. 1973. *Models of the Mind: A Psychoanalytic Theory*. Chicago: University of Chicago Press.

Goldberg, A., ed. 1978. *The Psychology of the Self: A Casebook*. New York: International Universities Press.

Goldberg, A. 1980. *Advances in Self-Psychology*. New York: International Universities Press.

Gunther, M. S. 1971. Psychiatric consultation in a rehabilitation hospital: a regression hypothesis. *Comprehensive Psychiatry* 12:572–585.

Horwitz, M. 1976. *Stress Response Syndromes*. New York: Jason Aronson.

Klein, G. S. 1976. *Psychoanalytic Theory: An Exploration of Essentials*. New York: International Universities Press.

Kohut, H. 1971. *The Analysis of the Self*. New York: International Universities Press.

Kohut, H. 1972. Thoughts on narcissism and narcissistic rage. In P. H. Orustein, ed. *The Search for the Self*. New York: International Universities Press, 1978, Vol. 2.

Kohut, H. 1977. *The Restoration of the Self*. New York: International Universities Press.

Krystal, H. 1968. *Massive Psychic Trauma*. New York: International Universities Press.

Lipton, S. D. 1962. On the psychology of childhood tonsillectomy. *Psychoanalytic Study of the Child* 17:363–417.

Lussier, A. 1980. The physical handicap and the body ego. *International Journal of Psycho-Analysis* 61:179–186.

Moore, W. T. 1975. The impact of surgery on boys. *Psychoanalytic Study of the Child* 30:529–548.

Muslin, H. 1971. On acquiring a kidney. *American Journal of Psychiatry* 127:1185–1188.

Newman, K. 1981. The capacity to use the object. Presented to the Fiftieth Anniversary Celebration, Chicago Psychoanalytic Society and the Institute for Psychoanalysis, November 7, Chicago.

Niederland, W. G. 1965. Narcissistic ego impairments in patients with early physical malformations. *Psychoanalytic Study of the Child* 20:518–534.

Niederland, W. G. 1981. The survivor syndrome: further characteristics and dimensions. *Journal of the American Psychoanalytic Association* 29:415–426.

Solnit, A. J., and Priel, B. 1975. Psychological reactions to facial and hand burns in young men. *Psychoanalytic Study of the Child* 30:549–566.

Stolorow, R., and Lachman, R. M. 1980. *Psychoanalysis of Developmental Arrests*. New York: International Universities Press.

Tourkow, L. P. 1974. Report of a panel: psychic consequences of loss and replacement of body parts. *Journal of the American Psychoanalytic Association* 22:170–181.

Winnicott, D. W. 1960a. Ego distortion in terms of true and false self. In *The Maturational Processes and the Facilitating Environment*. New York: International Universities Press, 1965.

Winnicott, D. W. 1960b. Psychiatric disorders in terms of infantile developmental processes. In *The Maturational Process and the Facilitating Environment*. New York: International Universities Press, 1965.

Yorke, C. 1980. Some comments on the psychoanalytic treatment of patients with physical disabilities. *International Journal of Psycho-Analysis* 61:187–193.

6 PREVENTION OF ADOLESCENT SUICIDE AMONG SOME NATIVE AMERICAN TRIBES

IRVING N. BERLIN

For many years the frequency of suicide among Native Americans has been viewed from two conflicting perspectives. One is that there has been an alarming increase in suicide among Indian adolescents; the other, that overall Anglo and Indian suicide rates have essentially been equal. What has become clear from detailed studies of attempted and completed suicide among different tribes is that the suicide rate varies from tribe to tribe; in some it is very high, while in others it is below the average for the United States as a whole. Therefore, one cannot describe a typical suicidal Native American adolescent, since there is no such pattern (Dizmang, Watson, May, and Bopp 1974).

It is safe to say, however, that for many tribes and pueblos suicide has greatly increased (Hopi Health Department 1981; Levy 1965; Ogden, Spector, and Hill 1970; Peters 1981; Shore 1975; Shore, Kinzie, Pattison, and Hampson 1973). Alcoholism, drug abuse, solvent abuse, single-parent families, child abuse and neglect, spouse abuse, violent death in auto accidents, and death through violence among peers quarreling while under the influence of alcohol have also increased greatly among young people in these communities (Beiser 1981; Green, Sack, and Pambrun 1981; Johnson and Johnson 1965; Krause and Buffler 1979). There is agreement that suicide is completed primarily among males and suicide attempts occur mostly among females (May and Dizmang 1974; Peters 1981).

It is also clear from a number of studies done in communities with a high suicide and attempted-suicide rate that there are some common fac-

0-226-24058-4/85/0012-0001$01.00

tors. Where good case studies have been done with incompleted suicides or with families of suicides, these factors have been validated. Dizmang et al. (1974) found that six factors were most important: (1) Seventy percent of the suicides had more than one significant caretaker before age fifteen as compared with only 15 percent of controls. (2) Forty percent of the primary caretakers of the suicide group had had five or more arrests, compared with 7.5 percent of controls. (3) Fifty percent of the suicide group had experienced two or more losses by divorce or desertion, compared with 10 percent of controls. (4) Eighty percent of suicides had had one or more arrests in the twelve months before the suicide, compared with 25.5 percent of controls. (5) By age fifteen, 70 percent of suicides had been arrested, compared with 20 percent of controls. (6) Sixty percent of suicides attended boarding school before the ninth grade, compared with 27.5 percent of controls.

Data from National Studies on Suicide

The clinical research findings by Teicher (1979) at Los Angeles General Hospital on adolescent suicide and suicide attempts amplify some of the issues described in Indian adolescent suicide. He has described two kinds of factors which seem to be etiologic in suicide. The first are developmental and chronic factors that may predispose the adolescent to either a precipitating event or cumulative pressures which result in an attempted or successful suicide. He also delineated acute stress factors which lead to impulsive suicide attempts.

Like many researchers in suicide, Teicher emphasized that, for the general adolescent population, it is the second highest cause of death and that the approximately 4,000 actual suicides recorded each year are a gross underrepresentation since many auto accident deaths (from the history of the adolescents gathered from parents) are probably suicide attempts. This appears to be true also of Native American suicides, which are often coupled with auto accidents following a drinking binge. There are approximately a half-million suicide attempts among all U.S. adolescents, up over 200 percent in the last decade.

Teicher described a three-stage process leading to a suicide attempt: a long-standing history of problems from childhood to adolescence, a period of escalation of problems related to adolescence, and a final stage of weeks or days prior to an attempt with a rapid breakdown of the adolescent's contacts and associations with friends, peers, and family. Teicher listed ten factors which can be integrated with the factors May and Dizmang (1974) isolated for the Indian adolescent who attempts or commits suicide: (1) Twenty percent have a parent who attempted suicide. (2) Forty percent have a parent, relative, or close friend who attempted suicide. (3) Seventy-two percent have one or both natural parents absent from home, divorced, separated, or deceased. (4) Eighty-four percent who have a stepparent have felt severe conflict with the stepparent and alienation from the family. (5) Fifty-eight percent have a parent who has been married more than once. (6) Sixty-two percent have both parents working; and in one-parent families, that parent worked. (7) The adolescent has undergone serious environmental changes—among others, parental remarriage, hospitalization of family members, death in family, change of school, being sent to foster care, and juvenile detention. (8) In 16 percent of suicide attempts, parental alcoholism has caused serious interpersonal problems. (9) Large numbers live without care from parents, in foster families, or with relations. (10) Families have marked residential mobility that makes enduring ties to peers, teachers, and other family members impossible.

Acute stresses leading to acute attempts in an otherwise well-functioning adolescent are:

(1) Death in immediate or extended family.
(2) Divorce of parents or sudden illness of a parent with major loss of support.
(3) A major family move with separation from peer group at a critical developmental period. A number of important considerations:
   (*a*) In early adolescence, peer-group associations are very important; they help with the development of feelings of closeness and intimacy, and they help the adolescent deal with sexual feelings by sharing fantasies and concerns.
   (*b*) Moves which break up such peer relationships disrupt a critical phase of development. It is almost impossible for most young adolescents to reestablish peer relationships in another setting.
   (*c*) Feelings of loneliness, isolation, ineffectiveness, and loss, with poor self-esteem, are major problems.
   (*d*) Parents who are unable to understand and empathize with or support the adolescent's sense of loss or isolation and the

loss of self-esteem greatly exacerbate the acute feelings of hopelessness or helplessness that often precede a suicide attempt.

(4) Loss of a romantic attachment, either by a physical separation (a move) or disruption for other interpersonal reasons.
  (*a*) The intense attachment is often a substitute for previously close relationships with parents which have been disrupted by the adolescent independence strivings.
  (*b*) The romance provides an intense, close, supportive all-consuming relationship. When the relationship fails, the adolescent has no one to turn to and feels abandoned and isolated.

(5) The onset of an acute or chronic disease in adolescence, such as diabetes, anorexia nervosa, ulcerative colitis, cardiac disease, leukemia, and so on, often makes adolescents:
  (*a*) feel hopeless about their future because they feel no one would want to associate with a defective person;
  (*b*) feel a change in body image so that other adolescents of opposite sex will not find them attractive;
  (*c*) alter their self-expectations in adult life, influencing their decisions about a job or profession, marriage, and so on;
  (*d*) increase their dependence on their family and halt the drive for independence.

(6) Adolescents with chronic diseases from childhood perceive themselves as damaged, with decreased self-esteem and a deformed body image that will, they feel, repel adolescents of the opposite sex as well as peers of the same sex. These perceptions often increase dependence on parents who are trying to effect separation and independence for the adolescent; he responds by feeling a lack of support from anyone.

(7) The adolescent's equilibrium may be upset by a move from a small school to a large high school or from a small high school where he has done well and been popular (a big frog in a small pond) to a college with a large group of very bright students. If the adolescent begins to feel lost, with no sustaining relationships, and if he does not know how to study and fails his first midterm examinations, he may well respond with a suicide attempt. Particularly for Indian adolescents, going off to a large boarding school may lead to feeling lost and unsure of one's self.

> This often reduces self-esteem and brings on scholastic failure, with the sense of letting the family down and being worthless.

Teicher (1979) described the adolescent dilemma for parents: the change of the adolescent from a nice, social, fun, agreeable preadolescent to a demanding, opinionated, and volatile person whom the parent does not know how to handle. The adolescent feels he or she is not understood and is being inappropriately punished. The result is often rebellion or withdrawal.

Among many Indian cultures, the increase in divorce, family mobility, breakdown of extended family, increase in alcoholism among adults, and breakdown in the involvement with tribal religious and clan traditions often leave the adolescent without anyone to turn to for help when chronic problems or stressful situations arise. The feeling of helplessness and hopelessness is characteristic of the adolescent thinking about suicide. Any new family stress, extra demand, or feeling of increased helplessness because an authority figure, such as a teacher, family member, or friend, does not understand or gets angry with the adolescent may precipitate a suicide effort.

Sociocultural Factors Related to Native American Adolescent Suicide

The research on suicide on a national scale provides additional insights applicable to Native American adolescent suicide. May and Dizmang (1974) emphasized the sociocultural factors that may be causative: social disorganization, breakdown of traditional social systems, great stress on individuals, and increased low self-esteem (Townsley and Goldstein 1977). The pressures to belong to one's native culture and adjust and, at the same time, to "make it" in Anglo culture pose contradictory values. Family and extended-family breakdowns have occurred among many tribes and pueblos, resulting in chaotic families, with divorce, desertion, and alcoholism frequent in adults (Leighton 1971; McDermott 1967). The psychosocial needs of neither the adults nor their small children are met. It has been shown that the more traditional the tribe, the fewer the suicides, and vice versa (May and Dizmang 1974; Ogden et al. 1970; Stratton, Zeiner, and Paredes 1978; Teicher 1979; Townsley and Goldstein 1977).

Levy (1965), Levy and Kunitz (1971), and May and Dizmang (1974) defined traditional tribes as those who maintain their religious rituals, societies, priesthoods, and methods of government without substantial change over many generations. In many Southwest pueblos, the secret societies, religious rites, puberty ceremonies, and religious and healing heirarchies have remained essentially unchanged since these tribes have resided in pueblos. For some tribes, despite being moved from reservation to reservation, these traditions, at least among the elderly, are largely unchanged. In contrast, there are tribes which no longer have a religious heirarchy, societies, or religious leaders. Their governance in the past was based on war, with hunting and war chiefs as clan rulers. Both governance and religious leadership have deteriorated since relocation on their present reservations, and substitutes for these have been borrowed from the Anglo society. The clan and extended families are no longer organized or functional. Alcoholism appears to have become a major problem for some of these tribes, and inhalant and alcohol use are major adolescent problems (Johnson and Johnson 1965; Levy and Kunitz 1971; May and Dizmang 1974).

Loss of employment has also been found to be an important factor, and the role of chronic depression in suicide is stressed by several authors (Department of Health and Human Services 1981; Johnson and Johnson 1965; Krause and Buffler 1979; Levy and Kunitz 1971; Ogden et al. 1970).

Developmental Issues in Suicides and Suicide Attempts

My own observations of infant- and child-rearing practices among Native American communities in Alaska, the Pacific Northwest, and now the Southwest span a period of twenty years. There is a great variation in the methods of child rearing among various tribes. The traditional tribes have many common practices related to child rearing, especially as it functions as a tradition bearer. This function defines many of the adult-child relationships. There are similar adult-pubescent-young-adolescent relationships related to puberty rites.

Thus, in some tribes it is evident that the infant is cherished and tenderly attended to by adults and older children of the nuclear and extended family. The separation-individuation process, becoming independent and self-sufficient, occurs with traditional supportive involvement of elders in the family or clan (Berlin 1978).

In tribes where suicide and suicide attempts are high, the infant and small child experience family chaos. There is often no primary caretaker the infant can become attached to and learn to trust; thus, the infant's needs are not predictably met. This situation is often brought about by alcoholism in one or both parents.

In many instances, female adolescents become the family caretakers, and often they leave home in anger at the family's demands that they care for the other children and the adults dependent on alcohol or drugs. These female adolescents are angry and emotionally very needy of someone's love and caring, and they often become pregnant. They then frequently discover that their infant's needs and demands are too great without help from the extended family. These adolescents, still children themselves, may become abusing parents, particularly if they find little satisfaction and little care being provided by the males with whom they live (Beiser 1981; Department of Health and Human Services 1981; Green et al. 1981; Hopi Health Department 1981).

Problems in Native American Infants and Preschool Children

Common signs of problems in infancy are constant irritability, crying, inability to be comforted, patterns of decreased sleeping, and refusal to eat. These symptoms make the mother or caretaker even more upset, since her angry or impatient attention does not quiet the infant or help it sleep or eat. Such mothers feel they are bad parents, and often they turn more and more to alcohol for escape and comfort.

Preschool children, when dealt with by alcoholic, depressed, unhappy, or angry parents, are not allowed to explore and learn about the world around them. Disturbed parents expect children who walk and talk to be little adults. When they do not respond promptly to requests or demands, the parents' anger quickly turns to physical abuse or neglect, such as leaving them alone or with other children while they depart to gain comfort elsewhere. These children then feel scared and hateful toward adults, whose lack of concern causes them to feel unloved and not worthwhile. Such children may fail to learn to become independent and feel the world is safe (Erikson 1964; Kempe and Silver 1959). They frequently do not learn to play with other children. There often is no extended family to teach them when they are open and hungry for adult teaching about the culture which makes up their heritage. Later, they may gain little comfort from the philosophy of their ancestors when elders finally do present it and may resist acquiring an understanding of their heritage because their distrusted parents and other indifferent adults represent their culture (Department of Health and Human Services 1981; Shore et al. 1973; Shore and Manson 1981).

Problems of Native American School-aged Children and Adolescents

The Native American school-aged child often finds that his parents and relatives are unconcerned or too busy to be interested in his learning in school, which often turns him off on learning. Evidence from many studies show that parents' interest and concern about schoolwork and learning constitute the single most important factor in a child's being an effective learner (Mindell and Maynard 1967). At school age, a child who is a product of a chaotic family with little nurturance or concern from parents often finds learning difficult and may turn to drugs, alcohol, and—recently—to inhalant abuse (Department of Health and Human Services 1981; Kaufman 1973; Krause and Buffler 1979; Oetting and Goldstein 1978; Peters 1981; Van Winkle 1981).

In some communities where schools are not concerned with teaching the values and ways of viewing the world which are part of an ancient heritage, the children learn little about their own people at a time when they are most ready (Bryde 1970; Department of Health and Human Services 1981).

During school, also, children who have biological defects that influence their learning are often not identified. Poor hearing or vision, poor coordination caused by neurologic problems, and frequent hyperactive behavior are not identified and treated. These children are then frustrated in their learning throughout school—in fact, often for life, with increasing anger at others, feelings of isolation, sadness, and depression. Further, boarding schools rarely educate or relate to students as human beings, thus contributing to the students' uninterest in or dislike of learning (Kleinfeld and Bloom 1977).

I have had opportunities to make both official and unofficial observations of a number of boarding schools in the Northwest and Southwest, and, with very few exceptions, the schools are overcrowded, neither student nor learning oriented, and dangerously understaffed. In several schools, the dormitory aides who spend the most time with the students were overwhelmed by a ratio of one aide to fifty to ninety students. Understaffing is further complicated by the fact that many of the students have been sent to boarding school because of serious acting out, delinquent behavior, or serious emotional problems, especially depression, which are troublesome to the tribe. Some students come from communities at some distance from their reservation and find no Indian teacher or aide who speaks their language. Some boarding schools have requested help. Several investigations of boarding schools have occurred because of constant running away, serious acting out, and delinquent actions, both in the school and (especially) in neighboring communities, and a rash of suicide attempts or suicides. The schools have no trained mental health personnel; thus, along with the severe shortage of teachers—and especially dormitory aides—the lack of mental health resources adds to the problems of students and adults (Berlin 1978; 1982; Bryde 1970; Kinzie, Shore, and Pattison 1972; Kleinfeld and Bloom 1977; Mindell and Maynard 1967).

Few schools on or off the reservation teach children how to learn to solve problems; thus, learning never becomes interesting or has a purpose. Problem-solving learning was clearly basic to dealing with the ancient and traditional ways of supplying food, water, and shelter to a tribe. In Anglo society, in general, there is little effort to focus the learning process on how one assesses and begins to solve academically oriented problems and issues in math, history, and so on. All of science and other subjects taught by project learning methods can be designed to help students learn how and where to gather data, to assess their relevance to their project, and then to use the data to answer questions in the inherent and defined tasks posed by teachers and students for their project. Problem-solving learning in school prepares the young person to use problem-solving methods in other areas of his or her living, especially as a young adult (Berlin 1981; Block 1971; Coche and Douglas 1977; Elkind 1975; Mindell and Maynard 1967; Shure, Spivack, and Jaeger 1971).

Adolescence

In adolescence, the primary task in development is to become independent of the family and be one's own person while not deserting the family. The adolescent must also learn to relate to persons of the opposite sex in tender, loving ways if both are to enjoy marriage and parenthood. To become a respected and valued adult, one must find work or study for a vocation or profession. When the economy makes such a task impossible, adolescents fail to grow into mature, responsible, and caring adults.

Adolescents in all cultures need adult models. In religious areas, such models exist for most Indian adolescents but may not have maximum effect, since the modeling does not carry over into daily work and living as it did many years ago (Blos 1967).

It is clear that those Indian children who are adopted by Anglo families find, when they become adolescents, that they have no roots in either the Anglo or their native culture. Their suicide rate is twice as high as that of Indian youth on the reservations (Berlin 1978; Blos 1967; Mindell and Gurwitt 1977).

Thus we can see that development for some Indian children is not healthy. There are delays and distortions in infancy, preschool, school age, and adolescence, usually because adults in each period of development are unable to adequately parent because of their own troubled, depressed, and isolated feelings, which often result in alcoholism. As parents, they are, therefore, unable to be dependable and loving or to give their child a secure, wanted feeling. Troubled parents cannot enjoy the toddler's exploration of the world or take pleasure in the school-age child's excitement about learning or the adolescent's efforts to become an independent individual and significant to his people (Attneave 1979; Beiser 1981; May and Dizmang 1974; Townsley and Goldstein 1977).

Intervention Efforts

Several different kinds of interventions into suicide have occurred. Certainly one of the most effective, described by Shore and co-workers (1972), was a suicide prevention center. This was a twenty-four-hour holding facility where youth who would otherwise go to jail for drinking or minor offenses and perhaps commit suicide and those who had threatened or attempted suicide were housed. The tribal police cooperated in case finding. Tribal counselors, usually elders, were assigned to stay in the same room with the suicidal adolescent and talk with him about his problems as representatives of the tribe concerned about him. They remained available to the youth after his twenty-four-hour stay in the center and made an appointment for a subsequent meeting. The suicide rate was greatly reduced (Shore, Bopp, Waller, and Dawes 1972). Some suicide prevention centers that had no holding facilities were not as effective. Education about suicide for adolescents in school has also been described as helpful (May and Dizmang 1974).

One of the most potentially effective prevention methods is being tried in a large all-Indian high school. There, pregnant adolescents are kept in school, enrolled in classes on practical child care and parenting, and exposed to stimulation experiences in a day-care center, along with seminar discussions about infant and child development (Caldwell 1972). They learn what the infant and child require, to develop effectively, from parents. In this setting, some of the fathers-to-be have begun to attend the practical sessions and seminars because they are interesting. So far it is clear that these soon-to-be parents will be more effective parents than their own parents. Part of the seminar experience is learning about both the parents' and child's role according to the customs and traditions of the tribe (Berlin 1980; Blos 1967; Elkind 1975; Kohler 1971).

Alcohol treatment and counseling centers and mental health centers may be helpful to adolescents who drink and feel depressed or hostile and angry, especially if these helping places are sanctioned by the tribal government and the healers and elders of the tribe and also employ native mental health workers who can spread the word about the concern of the centers with adolescents thinking about suicide (Berlin 1979; Kinzie et al. 1972; Shore et al. 1973).

A first offender's program for alcohol- and drug-abusing adolescents and their parents has been effective (Snyder 1981). The tribal court sentences the adolescent and both parents to ten group sessions in which several families are involved in examining common problems. With a native counselor's help, an effort is made to find out how family fights usually start and how they can be reduced. The adolescent and parents get to understand each other better and in these sessions learn by practice how to solve problems better. It is probable that reduction in family problems and reduced drug and alcohol use also mean reduction in suicides or attempts.

In another community, all pregnant women are asked by health authorities and native healers to attend child development courses where there are practical opportunities to interact with babies and young children and learn about their development.

An effective early intervention program has been started in another community for all new mothers and their infants. They meet two to three times a week to share their problems with other mothers and to learn how to play with and stimulate their babies so that crying, sleeplessness, and fussiness are reduced. It has been found that such babies do well with frequent massage of limbs and body, being rocked in a rocking chair, and being bounced gently on an air mattress. These are babies who need a great deal of neuromuscular stimulation to overcome neurological handicaps. The mothers have been proud of how well their babies have done when measured against the nurses' or doctors' written predictions of development. Most infants in this program have done better than predicted (Kohler 1971).

In this program, mothers also exchange babies with other mothers for a half-hour once a week and find that it is hard to stimulate these strange babies by singing, visual stimulation with bright moving objects, or rocking. These delight their own infant but often do not make a strange baby happy. They are glad to return to their own infants. Most of the infant stimulation is consistent with baby handling traditional to many tribes (Berlin 1981).

Mothers and fathers are helped to learn that each person views the world differently, depending on whether eyes, ears, or skin and muscles are the best way he or she can understand the environment. It is clear that artists see and feel the world, musicians seem to hear the world, while athletes, sculptors, carpenters, and craftsmen understand the world best through their fingers, hands, and muscles. These basic tendencies can be demonstrated in very young babies. They can then also be taught to enjoy the other ways of understanding their world, using their primary method of taking in their environment as a starting place (Berlin 1981; Kohler 1971).

In another setting, adolescents at risk have been identified and worked with in groups. One group consisted of girls in a boarding high school who were bright, attractive, and chosen to be the cheerleaders, debate captains, and so on. The Native American tradition of not standing out or not indicating that one is better had resulted in harassment of these girls by other adolescents and caretaking adults. Several of these girls made suicide attempts. Tribal leaders were brought in to sanction the need to become good learners and leaders because their people needed it. Support groups of parents, leaders, and counselors have been very effective in helping these young women to do well and in discouraging those adolescents who would harass them (Berlin 1982; Department of Health and Human Services 1981).

In another project, adolescents were picked to take special training in child care and in counseling new mothers. Those picked for the project were all adolescents at high risk: females who had left home because of family troubles and had histories of problem drinking and females who had dropped out of school and were drinking and getting into trouble with the law. In their training as counselors, they were paid to work in a nearby tribal day-care center with the most difficult children, who were either overactive or very withdrawn. They learned about these children and their problems as they met and talked with their teachers and parents. These young women then began to want to understand the reasons for problems. Slowly, they also began to talk with their co-workers about some of their own family problems and gained insight into the needs of young children from their parents (Berlin 1980, 1982; Blos 1967).

In each prevention-intervention activity described above it was necessary to get tribal sanction and to be clear about issues of confidentiality and the sensitivities of families to others knowing about family problems, despite arrests and hospitalizations for alcohol abuse, drug problems, or suicide attempts. It was necessary to help the workers from the tribe to be very circumspect about confidentiality (Berlin 1979; Kinzie et al. 1972; Shore et al. 1973).

Among other prevention efforts are those which recognize depression in grade school as an indicator of later depression and possible suicide attempts. Groups of youngsters identified as sad and alone did well in group therapy. It has also been helpful to encourage Native American counselors to reach out to adolescents who recently have lost a family member or to form groups of adolescents who come from families where there have been parental deaths, divorce, or desertion so they can share common problems. Also, as adolescents begin to work together on practical learning of trades and art skills, their self-esteem increases, they appear less depressed, and they are able to work more easily with other young people in a variety of tribal projects (Department of Health and Human Services 1981).

Conclusions

The prevention of Native American suicide depends on recognizing high-risk infants, children, and adolescents and providing them with help and nurturance in a tribally accepted way. Identifying school-age children at risk and promoting attachment to counselors or teachers who can act as parent substitutes have appeared to be helpful.

In the process of identifying schoolchildren and adolescents at risk, community mental health, health, and education workers become attuned to and identify problems earlier.

Each tribe's governing body must sanction these projects and receive reports on their effectiveness. Such information enables the governing body to be aware of problems and the efforts being made to meet them. Tribal governments concerned with these issues can support those that offer their people the best results.

Work as a way of feeling values is a necessary part of prevention efforts.

There is no single most effective prevention program, but several programs presented here seem to have promise in suicide prevention.

A key factor in prevention and intervention is the recognition that tribal authorities must not only sanction each program but also enable respected elders to become involved in these programs. Thus, tribal traditions and concerns are communicated to children or youth, and they become better-integrated members of that tribe or pueblo.

REFERENCES

Attneave, C. L. 1979. The American child. In J. B. Noshpitz, ed. *Basic Handbook of Child Psychiatry*. New York: Basic.

Beiser, M. 1981. Mental health of American Indian and Alaska native children: some epidemiologic perspectives. *White Cloud Journal* 2(2): 37–47.

Berlin, I. N. 1978. Anglo adoption of Native-Americans: repercussions in adolescence. *Journal of the American Academy of Child Psychiatry* 17(2):387–388.

Berlin, I. N. 1979. Mental health consultation to child serving agencies as therapeutic intervention. In J. Noshpitz and S. Harrison, eds. *Basic Handbook of Child Psychiatry*. Vol. 3. New York: Basic.

Berlin, I. N. 1980. Opportunities in adolescence to rectify developmental failures. *Adolescent Psychiatry* 3:231–243.

Berlin, I. N. 1981. Problem solving and creativity: a family school collaboration. In I. N. Berlin, ed. *The International Year of the Child, 1979–80*. Albuquerque: University of New Mexico Press.

Berlin, I. N. 1982. Prevention of emotional problems among Native-American children: overview of developmental issues. *Journal of Preventive Psychiatry* 1(3):319–330.

Block, J. 1971. *Mastery Learning: Theory and Practice*. New York: Holt, Rinehart & Winston.

Blos, P. 1967. Second individuation process of adolescence. *Psychoanalytic Study of the Child* 22:162–186.

Bryde, J. D. 1970. *The Indian Student: A Study of Scholastic Failure and*

Personality Conflict. Vermillion: University of South Dakota Press.

Caldwell, B. M. 1972. What does research tell us about day care? *Children Today* 1:1–5.

Coche, E., and Douglas, A. 1977. Therapeutic effects of problem solving training and play reading groups. *Journal of Clinical Psychology* 33:820–827.

Department of Health and Human Services 1981. *Report of the Third National Indian Child Conference: The Indian Family—Foundations for Future*. Albuquerque, N.M.: Indian Health Service, Office of Mental Health Programs.

Dizmang, L. H.; Watson, J.; May, P. A.; and Bopp, J. 1974. Adolescent suicide at an Indian reservation. *American Journal of Orthopsychiatry* 44(1):43–49.

Elkind, D. 1975. Recent research in cognitive development in adolescence. In S. E. Drogastin and C. H. Elder, Jr., eds. *Adolescence in the Life Cycle*. New York: Halstead.

Erikson, E. H. 1964. *Childhood and Society*. Rev. ed. New York: Norton.

Green, B. E.; Sack, W. H.; and Pambrun, A. 1981. A review of child psychiatric epidemiology with special reference to American Indian and Alaska native children. *White Cloud Journal* 2(2):23–36.

Hopi Health Department. 1981. *Report of the First Hopi Mental Health Conference*. Oraibi, Ariz.: Hopi Health Department.

Johnson, D. L., and Johnson, C. A. 1965. Totally discouraged: a depressive syndrome of the Dakota Sioux. *Transcultural Research* 1:141–143.

Kaufman, A. 1973. Gasoline sniffing among children in a pueblo Indian village. *Pediatrics* 51:1060–1064.

Kempe, C. H., and Silver, H. K. 1959. The problem of parental criminal neglect and severe physical abuse of children. *American Journal Diseases of Children*. Abstract. 98:528.

Kinzie, J. D.; Shore, J. H.; and Pattison, E. M. 1972. Anatomy of psychiatric consultation to rural Indians. *Community Mental Health Journal* 8:196–207.

Kleinfeld, J., and Bloom, J. 1977. Boarding schools: effects on the mental health of Eskimo adolescents. *American Journal of Psychiatry* 134(4):441–447.

Kohler, M. 1971. The rights of children: an unexplored constituency. *Social Policy* 1:36–43.

Krause, R. F., and Buffler, P. A. 1979. Socioculture stress and the American native in Alaska: an analysis of changing patterns of psychiatric illness and alcohol abuse among Alaska natives. *Culture, Medicine and Psychiatry* 3:111–151.

Leighton, A. 1971. Cosmos and the Gallup city dump. In B. H. Kaplan, ed. *Psychiatric Disorder and the Urban Environment*. New York: Behavioral Publications.

Levy, J. E. 1965. Navajo suicide. *Human Organization* 24:309–318.

Levy, J. E., and Kunitz, S. J. 1971. Indian reservations: anomie, and social pathologies. *Southwestern Journal of Anthropology* 27:97–128.

McDermott, J. F. 1967. Social class and mental illness in children: the diagnosis of organicity and mental retardation. *Journal of the American Academy of Child Psychiatry* 6:309–320.

May, P. A., and Dizmang, L. H. 1974. Suicide and the American Indian. *Psychiatric Annals* 4(9):22–28.

Mindell, C., and Gurwitt, A. 1977. The placement of American Indian children: the need for change. In S. Unger, ed. *The Destruction of the American Indian Family*. New York: Association on American Indian Affairs.

Mindell, C., and Maynard, E. 1967. Ambivalence towards education among Indian high school students. *Pine Ridge Research Bulletin* 1:26–31.

Oetting, E. R., and Goldstein, G. S. 1978. *Drug Abuse among Indian Adolescents*. Report to National Institute of Drug Abuse. Grant R01054. Fort Collins: Colorado State University.

Ogden, M.; Spector, M. I.; and Hill, C. A. 1970. Suicides and homicides among Indians. *Public Health Reports* 35(1):75–80.

Peters, R. 1981. Suicidal behavior among Native Americans: an annotated bibliography. *White Cloud Journal* 2(3):9–20.

Piaget, J., and Inhelder, B. 1969. *The Psychology of the Child*. New York: Basic.

Plowden Report. 1966. *Central Advisory Council for Education (England)*. Vol. 1. London: Her Majesty's Stationery Office.

Shore, J. H. 1975. American Indian suicide—fact and fantasy. *Psychiatry* 38:86–91.

Shore, J. H.; Bopp, J. F.; Waller, T. R.; and Dawes, J. W. 1972. Suicide Prevention Center on an Indian reservation. *American Journal of Psychiatry* 128(9):76–81.

Shore, J. H.; Kinzie, J. D.; Pattison, E. M.; and Hampson, J. 1973. Psychiatric epidemiology of an Indian village. *Psychiatry* 36:70–81.

Shore, J. H., and Manson, S. M. 1981. Cross-cultural studies of depression among American Indians and Alaska natives. *White Cloud Journal* 2(2):5–12.

Shure, M.; Spivack, G.; and Jaeger, M. 1971. Problem-solving thinking and adjustment among disadvantaged preschool children. *Child Development* 42:1791–1803.

Snyder, R. 1981. The first offender program: children and our future. In I. N. Berlin, ed. *The International Year of the Child, 1979–80*. Albuquerque: University of New Mexico Press.

Stratton, R.; Zeiner, A.; and Paredes, A. 1978. Tribal affiliations and prevalence of alcohol problems. *Journal Studies on Alcohol* 39:1166–1177.

Teicher, J. D. 1979. Suicide and suicide attempts. In J. B. Noshpitz, ed. *Basic Handbook of Child Psychiatry*. Vol. 2. *Disturbances of Development*. New York: Basic.

Townsley, H. C., and Goldstein, G. S. 1977. One view of the etiology of depression in the American Indian. *Public Health Report* 92(5):458–461.

Van Winkle, N. S. 1981. *Native American Suicide in New Mexico: A Comparative Study (1957–79)*. M. A. thesis. University of New Mexico, Albuquerque, Department of Sociology, July.

Westermeyer, J.; Walker, D.; and Benton, E. 1981. A review of some methods for investigating substance abuse epidemiology among American Indians and Alaska natives. *White Cloud Journal* 2(2):13–21.

7 TRAINING IN ADOLESCENT PSYCHIATRY FOR GENERAL PSYCHIATRY RESIDENTS: ELEMENTS OF A MODEL CURRICULUM

JOHN G. LOONEY, WILLIAM ELLIS, ELISSA BENEDEK, AND JOHN SCHOWALTER

No medical residency program can incorporate the teaching of all necessary medical knowledge and skills; consequently, important core elements may be neglected in some training curricula in general psychiatry. The authors are concerned that one of these neglected core areas is preparation for the skillful management of adolescents, since, in a recent national survey, general psychiatrists who were from one to three years out of training stated that preparation for the treatment of adolescents was one of several areas neglected in many training programs (Looney 1980). Although an articulate position statement about the importance of training in adolescent psychiatry was published by the American Society for Adolescent Psychiatry in 1971, the authors feel that now, more than a decade later, an explicit reemphasis on its importance needs to be made, with specific suggestions about elements of such a core curriculum.

A brief review of some present practice patterns of psychiatrists documents the need for attention to adequate training in adolescent psychiatry. A survey of members of the American Psychiatric Association revealed that 65 percent of the respondents treat adolescents and that 35 percent spend more than ten hours per week with adolescent patients (Arnhoff and Kumbar 1973). Treating adolescents is therefore common. The respondents in this survey included those who had been trained in child psychiatry. Yet, if all trained psychiatrists treated adolescents, they

0-226-24058-4/85/0012-0061$01.00

would account for less than 20 percent of the positive responders. Another survey of psychiatrists identifying themselves as particularly involved in treating adolescents revealed that only 47 percent had been trained in child psychiatry (Weisberg 1978); thus, the care of adolescents is often provided by general psychiatrists.

Another argument for adequate training in child psychiatry is based on census and epidemiological data. In 1960 the twelve- through nineteen-year-old age group constituted 12.8 percent of the American population, but in 1970 the percentage had increased to 15.5 percent (U.S. Bureau of the Census 1973). Also interesting was the concomitant finding that those Americans who would become adolescents—that is, children less than twelve—constituted 22.3 percent of the population in 1970. Although compilation of the 1980 census data remains incomplete, it can be estimated that at present almost a fifth of our population is adolescent.

The most pertinent statistic in this regard would be the number of adolescents needing psychiatric care. Unfortunately, no definitive data on this issue are available. However, clinical impressions of the continuing high prevalence of suicide among adolescents, the increasing number of school dropouts, increasing antisocial behavior, and the like would suggest that large numbers of teenagers are in need of such care. Past data on this subject are of interest. One federal agency measure of psychiatric care utilization noted that in 1971 one-fourth of all psychiatric clinic patients were adolescent and that the number of adolescents hospitalized for psychiatric problems had increased 500 percent in the case of boys and 150 percent in the case of girls during the preceding fifteen years (American Society for Adolescent Psychiatry 1971). The military maintains accurate psychiatric epidemiological data, and in the U.S. Navy the incidence of psychopathology serious enough to require hospitalization in the seventeen- through nineteen-year-old age group was found to be 1,954 per 100,000 (Looney, unpublished observations, Naval Health Research Center, 1976). This incidence figure is an average for the four years 1968–1971, during which the military procured young men primarily by means of the draft lottery, a method that assured a random sampling of American youth of the period. If it is assumed that the incidence of psychopathology in American adolescents of all ages is the same as it is in this older group in the military (a conservative estimate, since military inductees are routinely screened for obvious psychiatric illness), it could be inferred that more than 600,000 adolescents yearly develop the need for psychiatric care. Other evidence of the large number of adolescents needing care comes from the Task Force on Adolescence of the President's Commission on Mental Health (Anthony, Miller, and Offer 1978). The Task Force estimates that as recently as 1976 almost 4 million adolescents needed some form of mental health treatment.

Since the treatment of teenagers must be an important part of the professional activities of psychiatrists, a careful consideration of the design of a curriculum for training the general psychiatrist in adolescent psychiatry is the purpose of this chapter.

A Suggested Curriculum

WHAT THE RESIDENT SHOULD BE TAUGHT

Suggestions regarding the design of a curriculum in adolescent psychiatry must address the two very basic questions of what an optimal curriculum would be and how it should be integrated into the general training experience. Although these two issues are related, they will be discussed separately for purposes of demonstrative clarity. The design of the curriculum will be outlined in somewhat greater detail. A description of what should be taught will be presented with regard to the acquisition of a body of knowledge as well as the development of clinical skills.

A. BODY OF KNOWLEDGE TO BE TAUGHT

Important areas of basic knowledge with which the resident needs to be familiar are (1) the normative adolescent developmental process, (2) the institutions or social organizations to which adolescents relate, (3) the adolescent's role within the family, (4) abnormal developmental syndromes, (5) modalities of treatment, (6) the skills possessed by other professionals who work with adolescents, and (7) ethical and legal issues of adolescent psychiatric treatment.

In most training programs the childhood developmental processes are taught, information which is necessary for understanding the subsequent developmental process of adolescence. However, this latter topic is often neglected in general psychiatry curricula, and it must be included if the resident is to become competent in dealing with teenagers. Care must be taken to differentiate between the normal developmental processes of adolescent boys and girls as well as between those of teenagers in early, mid, and late adolescence. In addition, the different dimensions of the adolescent developmental process must be presented with regard to their concurrent evolution. One conceptualization of these concurrent developmental processes would include (1) the physiological, (2) the psychological, (3) the cognitive, (4) the sexual, and (5) the social. It should be noted that instruction in the physiological processes of puberty and adolescence is often neglected, an unfortunate deficiency in view of the fact that physiological development is the basic process that presages the others.

The resident should be taught early on that, with regard to the evolution of the psychic apparatus, adolescence is a time of massive change. Normative differences between early and late adolescence are as great as those between toddlers and elementary school children. For example, the nature of normal worries changes markedly, since very young adolescents may be seriously concerned about the normal physical developments of puberty or the manifestations of sexual excitement, whereas late-stage adolescents are more likely to be concerned with serious boy-girl relationships, problems of emancipation from the family, or vocational and educational pursuits. The process of reorganization of the defenses used to deal with the resurgence of the drives needs to be traced through the continuum of adolescent development. An understanding of the changes in the ways that the adolescent deals with dependency is also important. The likelihood of decreasing behavioral impulsivity and a concomitant increase in the capacity for verbal expression should be noted. Changing moral solutions to various problems of living, changing body images, and changing sense of identity are other issues important to an understanding of this developmental process.

Changes in cognitive abilities during adolescence are also important. Particularly significant is the development of the capacity for abstract thinking, and appreciation of this development is important if one is to understand how adolescents meet the increasing challenges of the educational system.

The changing nature of sexual experience during adolescence is another important dimension of development. Changing fantasies, changes in masturbatory practices, and preparedness for or experience with sexual intercourse need to be seen in a normative perspective.

Social development during this period can be viewed in terms of changes in the adolescent's investments in parents, peers, and nonparental adults. It should be noted that there are normative differences among different socioeconomic, racial, and cultural groups with regard to these social changes.

The resident should also become familiar with the social institutions and informal social organizations that have an important effect on the course of adolescent development. Educational and vocational systems and the judicial system are especially important institutions in this regard. It should also be noted that there is a grouping tendency in adolescents that makes possible the development of organizations having either positive or negative purposes, these being represented by athletic teams and gangs of delinquents, respectively. One social institution that plays a crucial role in adolescent development is the family. The resident should become familiar with the effects on adolescents of growing up in different types of families—for example, intact versus fragmented and pathological versus optimal.

After developing an understanding of the normative adolescent developmental process, the social institutions affecting adolescents, and the effects of the family environment, the resident should be made aware of abnormal syndromes he is likely to encounter in adolescent patients. Criteria that discriminate the various disorders must be made clear. It is important to note the relative prevalence of different types of disorders and the expected course and outcome of these disorders with and without therapeutic intervention. The resident should become acquainted with the types of transient situational disturbances that can result from such stresses as moves, loss of important peer relationships, death, and parental discord or divorce. An understanding of the myriad symptomatology of the neuroses as they may emerge during adolescence is important.[1] Both unipolar and bipolar types of affective disorders may make their first appearance during adolescence, and symptomatic expressions of depression are somewhat different in young people. Certainly, risk factors conducive to or suggestive of suicide or accidental death should be well described. Personality disorders often emerge full-blown during adolescence. Particularly problematic in boys is severe antisocial behavior involving significantly dangerous actions; such severe disturbances should be distinguished from less problematic, group-oriented delinquency. In girls, promiscuity is often a prominent symptom. In both sexes drug and alcohol abuse often obscure the symptomatology of personality disorders. Borderline and psychotic disorders and homosexual tendencies often first appear during adolescence. Psychosomatic syndromes such as anorexia nervosa and obesity also commonly first manifest themselves during this period. Adolescent pregnancy, although not a diagnosed psychopathologic syndrome, is also often a serious problem. Psychological problems are often associated with chronic physical disabilities and with the mental retardation syndrome.

A knowledge of the theoretical underpinnings of the wide range of therapeutic modalities available for the treatment of disturbed adolescents is also important. Since teenagers often present in crisis situations, a thorough knowledge of crisis intervention theory is crucial. Theories of individual, group, and family psychotherapy should be outlined, as should the criteria for pharmacologic treatment of adolescent disorders. Special methods of treating educationally handicapped and mentally retarded adolescents need to be stressed.

Two other considerations are also important. One is that other professionals, such as educational specialists, psychologists, and social workers, possess their unique knowledge and skills. Meeting the needs of a troubled adolescent and his family is usually expedited by working with these professionals.

A second area requiring the resident's attention is the adolescent's unique legal status. The adolescent is clearly between childhood and adulthood with regard to his gradual accumulation of rights under the law, and his legal status also seems to be constantly redefined through court adjudication. The resident should be made aware of such issues as the prudent and ethical management of confidential information given by the patient and the rights of the adolescent to refuse treatment.

B. SKILLS TO BE TAUGHT

After being presented with this information, the resident should be allowed to develop clinical skills based on it; supervised practice with a sizable number of patients and their families is essential. Guidelines are useful in delineating expected areas of clinical skillfulness. One such guideline was developed by the Committee on Child Psychiatry of the American Board of Psychiatry and Neurology (McDermott, Maguire, and Berner 1976), and although this guideline was developed primarily to outline expected competence with children, it is also useful for discussing clinical expertise with adolescents. The following is an outline of the expected areas of competence that it considers: (1) competence in patient-care roles, including skill in (*a*) gathering information, (*b*) formulating a differential diagnosis, (*c*) therapeutic planning, (*d*) therapeutic management, and (*e*) recording information; (2) competence in nonclinical roles, including skill in (*a*) consultation, (*b*) administration, (*c*) evaluating research, and (*d*) teaching; and (3) professional habits and attitudes, including ethical behavior. Although the resident will have the opportunity in the course of his clinical training with adults to gain competence in gathering information, formulating a differential diagnosis, therapeutic planning, therapeutic management, and recording information, he must become familiar with the special aspects of these clinical functions that are most effective with adolescents. For instance, in gathering information he must be prepared to carry out an adequate assessment under chaotic circumstances, since adolescents are so commonly brought for evaluation when they are in crisis. It is also important to learn basic techniques of eliciting trust in these young patients, who often have significant problems in trusting adults. Also important is the ability to assess the meaning of behavioral expressions of distress, since adolescents, especially younger ones, rarely express their problems by verbal means. The resident must assess the family in a way that does not undermine the potential for development of trust with the adolescent; he must not be seen by the patient as being an agent of or in collusion with the parents. Cultural factors affecting the presenting symptoms must be assessed. In gathering information, the trainee must learn when to ask for consultative assistance, such as testing by a psychologist or an intensive family evaluation by a family-specialist colleague.

Skill in formulating a differential diagnosis is developed gradually, as the resident, under supervision, sees adolescents with a wide variety of disorders, and he or she must develop a sensitivity to the types of clinical symptoms that are seen in adolescents developing the major psychopathologic syndromes. In formulating a treatment plan, the trainee also must develop a sensitive awareness of which treatment modalities or combination of treatment modalities are most effective in treating different types of disorders. In addition, the resident must consider whether or not intervention is also needed at the level of the family and/or at the level of the social organization within which the patient functions.

In developing skill in therapeutic management of adults, the resident will develop modifications of treatment techniques that are also helpful in the therapeutic management of teenagers. The importance of skillful crisis management has been stressed. In individual psychotherapy, careful resolution of the sometimes tenuous therapeutic alliance is crucial. Adolescents' increased propensity for acting out must be handled. Modifications of the techniques of group and family therapy are necessary. The resident must be practiced in the use of pharmacologic agents. The trainee must develop sensitivity to indications for residential or hospital treatment, the most effective way of developing this sensitivity being to treat patients in these settings. The physical, educational, vocational, and social needs that are so important for development of the adolescent patient must also be met.

In recording information about adolescents, the resident must learn the importance of accurate descriptions of behavior, since alloplastic behavioral expressions will often be the strongest clues to the nature of underlying conflicts. Another important aspect of recording information about adolescents is the careful notation of the progression of development from the physiologic, psychologic, cognitive, sexual, educational/vocational, and social perspectives.

With regard to the development of competence in nonclinical roles, it is to be hoped that acquisition of administration, evaluation research, and teaching skills will be part of the general training experience; although it may well not be taught, skill in consultation with agencies dealing with adolescents is important since such consultation may be the most important means of gaining access to a population of normal adolescents. It is particularly important that the trainee be allowed to consult broadly within an agency so that he or she will have a feel for what it is like to do case consultation, consultation with a director, or consultation with a whole agency. Consultation can occur in a wide variety of community settings, including juvenile courts, penal institutions, probation departments, schools, foster-home agencies, welfare departments, mental health agencies, and various civic organizations.

Competence in ethical and legal issues related to adolescents is also important. The trainee must be skillful in dealing with the adolescent in terms of his increasing legal rights. The importance of developing a confidential relationship with the patient has been stressed, but the trainee must also learn when he must convey information to those outside of the therapeutic setting, such as when dangerous behavior is probable.

HOW THE RESIDENT SHOULD BE TAUGHT

The teaching of knowledge and skills must be carefully integrated into the broader training experience. Since this integration often requires a skillful use of administrative process, it would be helpful if a faculty member with some power within the educational hierarchy—someone with knowledge of and interest in adolescents—assumes primary responsibility for it. In large training programs having both adult and child divisions, a great deal of controversy can develop concerning which division should assume the major teaching duties, and skillful cross-divisional management is necessary to resolve the issue.

The integration of the teaching of knowledge and the teaching of skills can best be done during the existing four-year psychiatric residency program, an approach preferable to forcing the resident to undertake a brief, crash-course rotation. Teachers skillful in treating adolescents must be responsible for demonstrating and supervising those modifications of standard treatment modalities that are most effective with adolescents. Clearly, the trainee must have access to adequate numbers of adolescent patients and their families throughout the training experience. One exception to the practice of integrating the learning experience into the entire four-year period might be to provide a block rotation on an adolescent inpatient unit.

Conclusions

The authors have stressed that teaching general psychiatry residents the skillful management of adolescent patients should not be neglected and have presented ideas about the design for a comprehensive curriculum in adolescent psychiatry. Careful consideration must be given to the basic body of knowledge that the resident must acquire, and equally careful attention must be devoted to ensuring that the resident has the opportunity of complementing this knowledge with practical opportunities to develop clinical skill. The authors have also noted the complex administrative problems of integrating experience in adolescent psychiatry into the general curriculum and have stressed that psychiatrists knowledgeable about adolescents should first help training directors design effective curricula and then serve in the equally crucial role of teaching residents.

NOTE

1. There has been intense debate over whether the neuroses meet diagnostic criteria consistently enough to be included in DSM III. Irrespective of this conceptual conflict, the resident must learn both that unconscious conflicts do occur in adolescents and that they have a troublesome symptomatology.

REFERENCES

American Society for Adolescent Psychiatry. 1971. Position statement on training in adolescent psychiatry. *Adolescent Psychiatry* 1:418–421.

Anthony, E. J.; Miller, D. H.; and Offer, D. 1978. Report of the Task Force on Adolescence for the President's Commission on Mental Health. Unpublished report.

Arnhoff, F. N., and Kumbar, A. H. 1973. *The Nation's Psychiatrists: 1970 Survey*. Washington, D.C.: American Psychiatric Association.

Looney, J. G. 1980. Psychiatrists' transition from training to career: stress and mastery. *American Journal of Psychiatry* 137 (1):32–36.

McDermott, J. F.; McGuire, C.; and Berner, E. S. 1976. *Roles and Functions of Child Psychiatrists*. Evanston, Ill: American Board of Psychology and Neurology.

U.S. Bureau of the Census. 1973. *Characteristics of the Population*. Washington, D.C.: Government Printing Office.

8 RESEARCH PRIORITIES IN ADOLESCENT PSYCHIATRY: REPORT OF THE COMMITTEE ON RESEARCH OF THE AMERICAN SOCIETY FOR ADOLESCENT PSYCHIATRY

JOHN G. LOONEY

A concurrent report in this volume (Looney, Benedek, Ellis, and Showalter 1984) documents the need for an increased emphasis by psychiatric training programs on skillful clinical management of adolescent patients and outlines a suggested core curriculum that would assist the psychiatric resident in achieving clinical competence with adolescents. The following basic assumptions are implied in that report: (1) increased psychiatric manpower is needed to treat troubled adolescents in the present and in the future; (2) there are core elements of knowledge about the development of adolescents and core clinical procedures, both of which can be taught; and (3) residents should have available to them curricula that impart this clinical knowledge and develop their clinical skills.

The fact that these assumptions about clinical training can be stated documents that adolescent psychiatry has evolved into an important subdiscipline within general psychiatry. At this state of development of this subdiscipline, an important question must be answered. To what degree has the development of adolescent psychiatry been based on the evolutionary process of clinical trial and error and to what degree has it been based on methodically tested research hypotheses? The answer is not a simple one. The published contributions of some skillful clinicians are unquestionably extensive. There are also some sound research studies. However, the primary assumption offered in this report is that an as-

0-226-24058-4/85/0012-0062$01.00

sessment of the relative contributions of these two bases of knowledge demonstrates the overwhelming preponderance of clinical contributions in providing the foundation for the subdiscipline of adolescent psychiatry. The purpose of this report, therefore, is to carry out the following important tasks: (1) to document the need for increased research efforts with adolescents; (2) to suggest that, since there is no existing cadre of established researchers in psychiatry willing or able to shift their efforts into the field of adolescent psychiatry, this research effort must come from psychiatrists whose primary roles are clinical ones; and (3) to outline some important areas in adolescent psychiatry that need investigatory efforts.

Documenting the Need for Increased Research

Let us begin by reexamining the assumption that human adolescent development is still relatively unstudied from a data-based perspective. If one reviews the ten published volumes of the *Annals of the American Society for Adolescent Psychiatry* (1971–1982), one discovers that fewer than 5 percent of the contributions are research based. Yet, the *Annals* are by definition *Adolescent Psychiatry: Clinical and Developmental Studies*, so that a preponderance of research studies would not be expected. But if we look elsewhere, can research studies be found? To a limited degree they can be. The *Journal of Youth and Adolescence* is primarily a research periodical. Yet a review of the authors contributing to this journal reveals an illuminating fact—they are members of disciplines other than psychiatry.

Anthony (1975) has noted the discrepancy in child psychiatry between the large amount of clinical care provided and the small amount of research on which that clinical care is based. He states, "a review of the changes in child psychiatry . . . would suggest although some minor shifts in attitude and orientation have occurred, putting an emphasis on different issues, the practice has remained relatively unaffected, apart from the trial of different therapeutic maneuvers. The minimal research that has emerged . . . has had little impact on the establishment of a scientifically based body of knowledge" and further adds, "If we wish to enter the brotherhood of scientific professions, we must have more solid and verifiable underpinnings of knowledge than we currently possess." Although Anthony's complaint concerns only child psychiatry, that subdiscipline may in fact be better blessed with investigative work than is adolescent psychiatry. A review of all papers published in the *Journal of the American*

Academy of Child Psychiatry reveals a fair representation of research, and in the last several years more than 50 percent of the papers have been so based.

Note the similarity between Anthony's statement and the conclusion reached several years ago by authors in the field of adolescent psychiatry after they had tried to reconcile the conflicting conclusions on the adolescent developmental process presented in clinical vis-à-vis research publications. As Blotcky and Looney (1980) state,

> A final observation regarding the theoretical and research literature seems germane. One is struck by the relative paucity of research data available on adolescents when compared to the massive clinical efforts directed toward them, the latter being commonly reported in our literature. As clinicians, we do all kinds of things to help troubled youngsters, but, as noted, we infrequently involve ourselves in research-based efforts to understand the nature of normal adolescent growth and why some teenagers deviate from that progression, or to document the effectiveness of our clinical efforts. Our science is secondary to our art, and it behooves established clinicians to become involved in research to establish more solid scientific underpinnings of knowledge.

Although a five-year review of two general psychiatry journals, the *American Journal of Psychiatry* and the *Archives of General Psychiatry*, finds research articles on a wide variety of topics, research-based articles on adolescence are few. In the *American Journal of Psychiatry,* 1,670 papers were published during the years 1973–1978, but only thirty-nine (2 percent) concerned adolescence; furthermore, only seven of those thirty-nine papers (or 0.4 percent of the total contributions) were research based. A review of the *Archives of General Psychiatry* reveals a similar trend. These contributions seem inadequate when we consider that adolescents constitute a large segment of our population. The 1970 census (still the most recent for which we have accurate data) revealed that 16 percent of the population was adolescent and, furthermore, that those who were then becoming adolescent—that is, children younger than twelve—constituted 22 percent of the population (U.S. Bureau of the Census 1973). The paucity of research with adolescents does not match the high level of clinical involvement with them. An American Psychiatric Association survey reported by Arnhoff and Kumbar (1973) revealed that 65 percent of the respondents treated adolescents and that 35 percent spent more than ten hours per week doing so.

To continue accumulating evidence supporting the primary assumption of this report would become tedious and would in fact run the risk of demeaning ourselves. It is also not my intention to insist that everyone must do research or that writing data-based papers is something that must be done to document our clinical competence. Yet the point has been made that our science is weaker than our art. We need to ask why that is so. The answer, I think, is simple: lack of both personnel and training. There are few who select a career in research. For example, in a recent survey of younger psychiatrists from one to three years out of training, fewer than 5 percent spent five or more hours per week involved in research (Looney, Harding, Blotcky, and Marmer 1979); furthermore, these practitioners noted that, of all the things for which they were trained in residency, they were most poorly prepared for research.

Identifying the Researchers

The lack of an established cadre of well-trained researchers means that, if increased research is to be done, it will be done largely by people who have already established themselves as clinicians. To my mind, that state of affairs is good because meaningful and relevant clinical research is based on the wisdom garnered through treating patients. However, for established clinicians to become involved in research requires that they overcome certain internal as well as external resistances to it.

Internal resistances are several and serious. It is difficult to break out of an established clinical work routine and doing so may involve loss of income. Even with generous funding, every hour taken away from patient care reduces income. An even more villainous internal resistance may be a "quest for grandiosity." People often feel that, if they are to devote time to research, the project must be of grand design and have major impact. Such misconceptions are understandable when we consider that the research projects held up as examples throughout our medical training are indeed those of grand proportions; they were major breakthroughs, the Nobel Prize–winning accomplishments.

External impediments are easier to see. Many of us work for institutions, and institutions tend to categorize employees rather rigidly. A clinician is a clinician only, and a researcher is a researcher only. A question often asked of a clinician who would like to devote some time to a research venture is, "How will the research interfere with the work?" In fact, a limited research into specific aspects of one's clinical work often results in improved clinical care.

Defining Some Priorities

The title of this report concerns research priorities in adolescent psychiatry and has somewhat of a double meaning. First, in establishing priorities between clinical and research endeavors, we must hereafter give relatively more emphasis to research if the subdiscipline of adolescent psychiatry is to achieve the kind of scientific respectability it deserves. Second, it should be possible, based on our present knowledge, to begin to establish priorities for the different directions that this needed research might take. There are many interesting things that need to be done!

Although it is impossible to outline in detail all of the specific research projects that are needed, it is possible to define some areas of importance. One useful way of categorizing these areas would include (1) definition of the adolescent developmental process, (2) assessment of the etiology of psychopathological states in adolescence and of the effectiveness of currently used treatment modalities, and (3) special problem areas.

A. DEFINITION OF THE DEVELOPMENTAL PROCESS

A thorough and sound data-based knowledge of the process of adolescent development is essential for designing our clinical approaches, for designing public health recommendations fostering normative adolescent development, and for a study of the causes and optimal treatments of deviations from such normal development.

We do not suffer from a paucity of reports outlining what is normal development in teenagers. These reports first appeared around the turn of the century, beginning with the seminal work by Hall (1904), who used the term *Sturm und Drang* to describe the turmoil and upheaval he believed to be characteristic of this period of life. Many subsequent clinical theoreticians supported Hall's storm-and-stress view of adolescent development. In recent years, a small collection of research-based studies has challenged the idea that turmoil is an inevitable characteristic of adolescent development. Researchers such as Offer (1969), Weiner and Del Gaudio (1976), Looney and Gunderson (1978), Mead (1928, 1930), and others have collected data suggesting that although there is wide variability in adolescent behavior, the more modal teenager in the United

States (particularly the white, middle-class adolescent) progresses through this period of life with little of the behavioral storm predicted by the theories based on the study of patient populations. Oldham (1978) reviewed much of this literature and suggested that there is currently a continuum of ideas regarding what is normal in adolescence. At one end of this continuum is the storm-and-stress view, and at the other end is the view of the adolescent as progressing without turbulence, adapting to educational and vocational demands, and conforming to parental expectations and value systems. Clearly, a reconciliation of these conflicting ideas is needed. When Blotcky and Looney (1980) separated published reports on adolescent development into clinically derived and research-based papers, they found the clinically derived papers and the research-based papers to be primarily at the former and latter ends respectively of this continuum of conflicting ideas. As noted earlier, Blotcky and Looney plead for a relatively increased emphasis on research-based contributions.

One of the problems in studying the adolescent developmental process is the lack of a common definition of an adolescent. What is an adolescent? Is he or she the same in American and in other, markedly different cultures? If adolescence is defined by an age span, what is that span? Would an immature twenty-one-year-old who has failed to accomplish many tasks of adolescent development be an adolescent? A more adequate definition is needed that includes age parameters while also taking into account physiological changes, cognitive changes, changes in the social and sexual spheres, changing relationships to peers and nonparental adults, affiliation with the greater society, and the like. A simple illustration may be given to establish that age alone is not an adequate criterion. Consider an eighth-grade class picture. Even the most casual observation would document marked differences in the physiological development of these approximately contemporaneous youngsters.

What is needed, therefore, is a research design that teases apart and defines different aspects of the adolescent developmental process. A number of these different aspects are potentially rewarding, including (1) defining adolescent development in terms of physiological changes. The area of physiological development is particularly ripe for study because of our present ability to use sophisticated endocrinological, biochemical, and chronobiological investigatory techniques. (2) Defining adolescent development in terms of cognitive changes. The work of Piaget and his disciples offers us an approach for understanding the changes in cognitive development as they are related to concurrent changes in age, physiological development, and challenging educational environments. (3) Defining adolescence in terms of changes in moral development. Kohlberg's thorough preliminary studies document a changing basis of moral assessment throughout this phase of life. Again, these changes must be related to other, concurrent changes. (4) Defining adolescent development in terms of changes in sexual behavior. Differences in sexual behavior between boys and girls, between different ethnic groups, and between different socioeconomic groups need further investigation. (5) Defining adolescent development in terms of changes in social relationships, including consideration of (*a*) changes in patterns of relating to peers, parents, and the world of nonparental adults; (*b*) affiliation with the values and institutions of the greater society; and (*c*) a definition of those institutions—such as the family, school, legal system, and the like—that encourage or hinder this development. (Recent studies by Lewis and his colleagues allow for an assessment of competence in families along a continuum from severely disturbed to most competent. This ability to rate competence in families would allow for an assessment of the impact of families of differing levels of psychological health on the development of their adolescent offspring.) (6) Defining adolescent development in terms of increases in educational and vocational competency. (7) Defining adolescent development in terms of changes in self-concept, ideals, value systems, and identity.

From a procedural perspective, it would be ideal to develop collaborative research teams that could investigate how these various facets of adolescent development affect each other. Most studies of these developmental processes would properly be longitudinal in nature. As well, cross-sectional studies of subjects at various critical junctures—such as entry into junior high school and senior high school, graduation, emancipation from the family, and the like—could be conducted. It is likely that for all of these aspects of the developmental process there are differences among the sexes, among different ethnic groups, among different socioeconomic groups, and among such special youngsters as the exceedingly bright, the physically handicapped, and the mentally retarded.

B. ASSESSMENT AND TREATMENT

Once the normative process of adolescent development is better defined, both researchers and clinicians are in a much better position to assess and treat those youngsters who have deviated from the usual developmental route. Even at this time, before developmental studies have been completed, it is important to begin to assess both the number of troubled youngsters in our society and the types of disorders with which they are afflicted. To whatever degree it is possible, a search should begin for clues to the etiology of these disorders. Also important is the need to document the outcome of current types of treatment of disturbed adolescents. Three specific things are needed to accomplish this task. First, there must be large-scale epidemiological surveys to determine the nature of the psychiatric syndromes occurring in our adolescent population. Sexual, racial, regional, and socioeconomic differences must be taken into account in these estimates. Such surveys are extremely important in planning for rational and equitable distribution of limited treatment resources in the future and in documenting the need for increased clinical manpower.

Second, etiological studies continue to need refinement. To date, research into the etiology of such major syndromes as the affective disorders and the schizophrenias is very extensive. One problem with these studies (as will be outlined in a forthcoming report of the Committee on Research of the Group for Advancement of Psychiatry) is that researchers tend to remain isolated within their particular domains. That is, the geneticists, for example, study only genetic patterns, without taking into account the impact of variables from other systems, such as the family, the quality of the early developmental process, the impact of acquired psychophysiological aberrations, and the like. What is needed are studies having an integrated design that can assess the impact of variables from multiple systems, such as the genetic, the familial, the developmental, the biological, and the like.

Third, it is critical to design methods to assess treatment outcome. Currently, heterogeneous treatment modalities are employed with disturbed adolescents, including drug therapy, behavioral modification of many types, family therapy, individual therapy, group homes, foster homes, residential placement, short-term crisis hospitalization, long-term reconstructive hospitalization, training schools, and others. Gossett (1984) outlines how imperative it is to begin to assess the effectiveness of what we do as clinicians, outlines ideas for carrying out these assessments, and presents data showing the effectiveness of hospital treatment on extremely disturbed youngsters. These types of rigorous follow-up studies are extremely rare, and more of them will be needed to assess which treatment(s) is most effective for specific psychiatric disorders of differing severities. We also need to determine how optimistic we can be about the treatment we are currently able to offer. Certainly these assessment studies will offer us clues to new and innovative clinical approaches.

C. SPECIAL PROBLEM AREAS

The third general area includes a collection of research ideas on disparate issues. These are generally very specialized areas that need investigation because of their current significance. Included are such issues as (1) special developmental problems, treatment needs, and educational needs of adolescents with mental retardation and/or physical handicaps; (2) studies of substance abuse, particularly the suspected significant increase recently in the abuse of alcohol; (3) studies of the etiology, epidemiology, definition, treatment, and outcome of delinquency; (4) studies of the etiology, epidemiology, and prevention of suicide; (5) studies of the etiology, epidemiology, and prevention of accidents; (6) studies of the etiology, epidemiology, and outcome of early adolescent pregnancy; (7) studies of the etiology, epidemiology, treatment, and outcome of violent and murderous adolescents; and (8) studies of the effects of systematic mental health consultation in school systems for purposes of prevention and early identification of psychological problems in adolescents.

Conclusions

This brief report has attempted to document the assertion that increased emphasis needs to be given to research in the area of adolescent psychiatry. Because a well trained and sufficiently large cadre of reseachers is not available to move into the field of adolescent psychiatry, it is important that those psychiatrists interested in adolescents who currently function primarily in the clinical area become sensitized to the need for this increased research. Some of these clinicians may wish to refine their curiosity into hypotheses that can be tested through systematic investigation.

This report has also attempted to outline some general areas that I feel are potentially very rewarding areas for research. Certainly, this list can by no means be considered complete; with the passage of time, other important problems requiring investigation will emerge. The Committee on Research of the American Society for Adolescent Psychiatry, research committees of other professional societies acquainted with the needs of youth, the Committee on Research of the Group for the Advancement of Psychiatry, and governmental and privately funded centers of research will all add to and refine this list. What would be particularly helpful at this point would be a national survey to delineate which of these potential areas of research is/are currently being investigated. Since there is often a significant lag time between the inception of an ingenious project and publication of its results, such a survey would help prevent unnecessary duplication of effort and promote collaboration between researchers investigating the same or similar topics. Such a survey would also reveal which of the above listed or other research questions have not as yet been addressed.

NOTE

The ideas presented in this paper germinated from deliberations and previous presentations of the Committee on Research. I wish to acknowledge the assistance of Dr. Daniel Offer; of previous members of the committee, especially Drs. George H. Orvin, L. David Zinn, and John T. Gossett; and of the following professionals who were previously Fellows in Adolescent Research under Dr. Offer at Michael Reese Hospital: Drs. Shirley Maides, Jeffry Mitchell, and Ron Rosenthal. I also wish to acknowledge the editorial assistance of Ms. Susan B. Looney.

REFERENCES

Anthony, E. J. 1975. *Explorations in Child Psychiatry*. New York: Plenum.

Arnhoff, F. N., and Kumbar, A. H. 1973. *The Nation's Psychiatrists: 1970 Survey*. Washington, D.C.: American Psychiatric Association.

Blotcky, M. J., and Looney, J. G. 1980. Normal female and male adolescent psychological development: an overview of theory and research. *Adolescent Psychiatry* 8:184–199.

Hall, G. S. 1904. *Adolescence: Its Psychology and Its Relations to Physiology, Anthropology, Sociobiology, Sex, Crime, Religion and Education*. Vols. 1 and 2. New York: Appleton-Century-Crofts.

Looney, J. G.; Benedek, E.; Ellis, W.; and Showalter, J. 1984. Training in adolescent psychiatry for general psychiatry residents: a model curriculum. In this volume.

Looney, J. G., and Gunderson, E. K. E. 1978. Transient situation disorders: a longitudinal study in young men. *American Journal of Psychiatry* 135:660–663.

Looney, J. G.; Harding, R. K.; Blotcky, M. J.; and Marmer, S. 1979. Psychiatrists' transition from training to career: determination of career directions. Dallas: Timberlawn Psychiatric Research Foundation.

Mead, M. 1928. *Coming of Age in Samoa*. New York: Morrow.

Mead, M. 1930. Adolescence in primitive and modern society. In F. V. Calverton and S. D. Schmalhausen, eds. *The New Generation: A Symposium*. New York: Macauley.

Offer, D. 1969. *The Psychological World of the Teenager*. New York: Basic.

Oldham, D. 1978. Adolescent turmoil: a myth revisited. *Journal of Continuing Education in Psychiatry* 39:23–32.

U.S. Bureau of the Census. 1973. *Characteristics of the Population*. Washington, D.C.: Government Printing Office.

Weiner, I., and Del Gaudio, A. 1976. Psychopathology in adolescence. *Archives of General Psychiatry* 33:187–193.

PART II

DEVELOPMENTAL ISSUES: GROWTH AND LEARNING

EDITORS' INTRODUCTION

It is of the essence in work with adolescents that developmental and clinical issues are inseparable. All clinical judgments and decisions must be guided by developmental knowledge, while research on developmental trends and disorders will inevitably lead to questions of clinical application. Even studies of social institutions that serve normal developmental needs ultimately generate clinical implications, since all children, disordered as well as healthy, share these needs and require these institutions.

Aaron H. Esman discusses the techniques of psychotherapy with adolescents and believes that a developmental approach is in order. Recognition of the rapid and kaleidoscopic changes manifest in every sphere of adolescent life—physical, cognitive, affective, and social—demands correlation of therapeutic principles with developmental needs and tasks of the growing person. The author advises that the adolescent therapist's stance be one of openness, empathy, respect for the young person's autonomy, and flexibility without abandoning fundamental therapeutic principles.

John Toews, Robert Martin, and Harry Prosen continue their studies of the life cycle with a discussion of "death anxiety" as a manifestation of the transition from latency into adolescence. The authors explore the timing of death anxiety, the concept of review, preview, and explanation, and the developmental aspects of the concept of death. They conclude that an internalized life-cycle model is realized by adolescence and forms a fundamental part of identity: images of self and others are constantly being reworked as one examines one's life in reference to present attainments, recollections of one's past, and the image of the future.

Charles A. Burch describes a form of narcissistic disturbance during adolescence: identity foreclosure. Owing to a subtle developmental arrest, these adolescents are resistant to usual developmental changes and in a very real sense are locked into their identity. Burch draws on the theories of Kohut, Erikson, and Blos to construct a hypothesis that explains a psychological attempt to preserve narcissistic equilibrium while avoiding the central developmental tasks of adolescence—resulting in narcissistic impairments rather than intrapsychic conflicts. The author concludes that such identity foreclosure requires special therapeutic strategies.

Adolescent psychiatry and developmental research are making progress in synthesizing clinical and neuropsychological studies of learning theory and education in general. Achieving as complete an understanding as possible of each student rather than just reporting test scores can lead to greater understanding of adaptational problems. Irving H. Berkovitz observes that schooling and relationships in schools are a clinical influence second only to that of the adolescent's family. He describes clinical case management in schools and discusses adolescent anger, sexual energy, muscular energy, and intervention steps that can be recommended to the regular school milieu by the clinician. Berkovitz also discusses therapeutic school units and special education programs and insists that adolescents should remain involved in education while undergoing psychotherapy.

Jonathan Cohen explores the problems of the learning-disabled adolescent; those owing to the cognitive disability itself and those owing to psychological factors that are directly and/or indirectly related to being learning disabled. He discusses problems of work and learning, affective reactions (distrust and depression), the experience of experience and expectations of others, and personality development. Cohen concludes that the learning disabled as a group show characteristic difficulties: anxious concerns, low-level depression, impaired self-representations, and a sense of conflict, rigidity, and trauma.

Archie H. Silver and Rosa A. Hagin report their long-term study of occupational and academic outcome of children and adolescents with learning disability. In spite of adequate social and vocational adjustment in those who benefited from appropriate educational and environmental support, problems of spatial and temporal organization persist throughout adolescence and into adulthood. The authors found that, along with remediation, adolescents need assistance as they reach critical decision points during maturation.

9 A DEVELOPMENTAL APPROACH TO THE PSYCHOTHERAPY OF ADOLESCENTS

AARON H. ESMAN

As is well known, the first report of the psychoanalytic treatment of an adolescent was Freud's "Dora" case (1905). Freud's difficulty with the transference and countertransference issues in that case proved to be characteristic of the experience of many who have followed after him. His efforts to apply the psychoanalytic method to the treatment of adolescents were extended and applied in a more systematic, if highly modified, fashion by August Aichhorn (1935), who established a residential treatment program for "wayward youth" based on Freud's principles. Aichhorn served as teacher and model to a generation of psychoanalytically trained educators such as Anna Freud, Erik Erikson, Peter Blos, Fritz Redl, Rudolph Ekstein, and others, who brought with them the principles of analytically oriented psychotherapy with adolescents when they left Vienna. More recently, workers such as Bruch (1979), Laufer (1977), Masterson (1972), and others have expanded the range of adolescent psychotherapy to the borderline disorders, eating disorders, and "developmental breakdowns" that may characterize this phase. In addition, group (Berkovitz 1972), family (Williams 1973), and behavioral (Lehrer, Schiff, and Kris 1971) methods have been developed for special application to adolescent patients. I shall not consider these valuable methods here, for both lack of time and lack of expertise. I shall focus, rather, on ambulatory, individual, psychodynamically oriented psychotherapy—the kind of work which, I suspect, for most of us makes up the bulk of our professional activity with our youthful patients.

0-226-24058-4/85/0012-0029$01.00

Psychotherapy with Adolescents

Adolescence is, by definition, a transitional period. Its onset can, for most purposes, be arbitrarily defined as concurrent with puberty, but its end point is vague and indeterminate, shading off as it does into whatever a particular culture defines, by various criteria, as adulthood (Blos 1977). Rapid and kaleidoscopic change characterizes the period, manifest in every sphere of life—physical, cognitive, affective, and social. Accordingly, the techniques of psychotherapy must also vary as the adolescent progresses in the subphases of this protean and mercurial stage of growth. A developmental approach to the subject is, therefore, in order—one which correlates the therapeutic principles and the developmental needs and tasks of the growing person.

Blos (1962) has outlined some of the issues that apply here, emphasizing the intrapsychic factors that accompany these developmental shifts. This discussion will, in some respects, be an elaboration of his seminal contribution, but I shall, perhaps, paint with a broader brush. I shall attempt to delineate, not so much pathological variants, but the normally occurring expectable features of adolescent development that must affect our technical approaches to our patients.

INDICATIONS

A few words about the indications for the kind of treatment I am concerned with here. The adolescent who can, in principle at least, make use of ambulatory, psychoanalytically oriented psychotherapy is the nonpsychotic youngster whose symptoms and/or behavioral difficulties are not so severe as to preclude continuation of life in the community; the mildly to moderately depressed youngster who is actively experimenting with drugs but is not an addict; the academic underachiever who may or may not have a true learning disability but whose capacity to concentrate on his work is interfered with by anxiety or preoccupying thoughts; the anxious, socially inhibited adolescent; the adolescent whose behavioral difficulties—petty thievery, sexual promiscuity—seem on assessment to be derivatives of chronic, phase-related, intrapsychic conflict rather than manifestations of a sociopathic character disorder; the adolescent who is having difficulty in adapting to change in parental circumstances such as death or separation, divorce or remarriage. In addition, many adolescents whose rebelliousness, eating disorders, or overanxious behavior reveals them to be caught in the web of inextricably interwoven family conflicts may require and benefit from such individual therapy in addition to concurrent treatment focused on the family system itself.

EARLY ADOLESCENCE

I shall begin our developmental survey with a description of the sub-phase characteristics of the early adolescent, that is, the young person between the ages of about twelve and about fourteen. Persons in this age group are, at least in my experience, exceptionally difficult to engage in any individual exploratory psychotherapy. Some of the reasons for this difficulty are as follows:

1. The early adolescent is operating under intense drive pressure stimulated both by the pubertal activation of his endocrine system and by the sociocultural pressures attendant on the prevailing stereotypes of adolescent behavior as transmitted through the "media." This pressure is experienced with relation not only to sexual but to aggressive impulses and their derivatives as well. It is manifested behaviorally in a powerful action orientation; the early adolescent is not ordinarily disposed to deal with his internal tensions and conflicts by reflection or introspection but rather by action on and in his environment. Since psychoanalytic psychotherapy asks of its subjects the suspension of motor activity and the direction of attention toward internal mental processes, its demands are out of phase with the customary direction of early adolescent physical and psychological pressures.

2. A primary issue for the early adolescent is the protection of his nascent and still very tenuous sense of autonomy as he begins to break out of the relatively compliant position of normal latency and to test out his newfound strengths and competencies. The early adolescent rarely comes to treatment on his own initiative; he is usually brought by parents or sent by some authoritative institution such as the school or the court. In either case, he is likely to be mistrustful of those adults whom he sees as attempting to impinge upon or restrict his shaky sense of self-determination. In most circumstances he is likely to see the therapist as yet another such adult, an agent of his parents and/or the community institution that is attempting to impose itself upon him. He is likely, therefore, to relate initially to the therapist with suspicion and mistrust.

3. Offer (1969) and his associates, among others, have by now exploded the myth of "normal" adolescent turmoil. We know now that de-

spite the well-known stresses of this phase, the modal adolescent succeeds in passing through this developmental transition without major psychological disruption. It is still true, however, that in early adolescence some turmoil and rebelliousness normally occur if only with respect to minor issues bearing on personal autonomy such as length of hair, curfew hours, and so forth. Along with this transitory rebelliousness the early adolescent, in part because of his preoccupation with the changes that are occurring in his body and their psychic elaboration, is primarily self-oriented. Those persons relied on for interaction and emotional support are likely to be his peers rather than adults—that is, people whom he sees as like himself, sharing his concerns, and testing out the same issues. None of these—his rebelliousness, his narcissism, or his peer orientation—is likely to dispose him toward a relationship with a strange, intrusive adult.

4. One of the principal concerns—indeed, in the view of some, the principal concern—of the early adolescent is the mastery of his rising sexual fantasies and his conflicts around the pressure to masturbate. These are the natural and inevitable reactions to puberty and the awakening of genital sensations. In Laufer's (1977) view, it is precisely the ability to accept with comfort the "sexual body" and to permit guilt-free masturbation with full integration of pregenital and genital fantasy that is the essence of successful adolescent development. For most young adolescents, however, these impulses and fantasies are the source of intense feelings of shame and/or guilt despite the dissemination of factual information about the normality and inevitability of such feelings and wishes. It is difficult in the extreme for young adolescents to discuss these matters with anybody, even their peers. It is particularly difficult for them to discuss them with a strange adult, especially one of the opposite sex who may be seen as a surrogate for the parents who are the subject, consciously or unconsciously, of their forbidden fantasies.

5. The defensive structure of the early adolescent tends to be quite rigid, maintaining to a considerable degree the characteristic late latency reliance on denial and externalization as major defensive measures. This defensive rigidity is related, I believe, to the dominant cognitive mode characterizing most people in this age group. Although Piaget (1969) has placed the onset of formal operational thought in the twelve to fifteen age period, it is clear, as demonstrated by Dulit (1972), that many, if not most, adolescents, even among unusually intelligent and highly educated groups, do not achieve this cognitive pattern at least until mid adoles-

cence, if at all. Accordingly, the usual early adolescent remains somewhat concrete in his thinking and tends to be present oriented rather than capable of reflecting on his past and anticipating his future. Since psychoanalytic psychotherapy expects of its participants the ability to do both of these things, the capacity of those who remain fixed in the stage of concrete operational thought to engage in such therapy is limited.

These normal developmental aspects of early adolescence have significant implications for the technique of psychotherapy. Above all, they dictate a high degree of flexibility regarding procedural and technical arrangements with the pubertal and just postpubertal patient. These young people generally require of the therapist a degree of activity higher than that which is customary for older patients. Above all, they have an intense intolerance for silences, since these tend to throw them back on their own affectively charged fantasies and to leave them with the sense of being unsupported. It is incumbent on the therapist to be more present, or, if you will, "realer" than he is likely to be with his adult patients or, indeed, even with latency-age children. At times, the early adolescent who is uncomfortable with the relative passivity of the psychotherapeutic situation or is so guarded as to be unable to participate in verbal exchange may need to resort to child therapy techniques, such as game playing or model making, in order to preserve therapeutic contact.

A cautionary note should be introduced here, however. Many therapists of adolescents operate with the belief that, like some of those portrayed in films, they should relate to their adolescent patients as "pals," affecting casual dress, using adolescent lingo, and ostentatiously demonstrating their familiarity and comfort with adolescent folkways. In my view, this is a serious error and one likely to lead to unforeseen and unfortunate consequences. In the long run, the adolescent patient does not want his therapist to be a peer but a sympathetic and understanding adult. No one is more sensitive to inauthenticity than a young adolescent, and he is almost certain to identify such behavior on the therapist's part as spurious and seductive. I cannot, therefore, urge too strongly the maintenance by the therapist of his adult identity and the integrity of his professional status.

The establishment of the therapeutic alliance with the young adolescent is likely to take a long time. Most such patients are slow to trust and will require what Blos has referred to as a "preparatory phase" of uncertain duration before they can begin to understand the nature of psychotherapy and enter into a true therapeutic process. During this preparatory phase, the therapist must be prepared to meet his patient at the latter's own level.

This is likely to mean spending many hours listening to what the therapist may be inclined to regard as superficial chitchat about phase-typical preoccupations. Girls are likely to talk endlessly about the vicissitudes of their peer relationships and their newfound interest in clothes and make-up. Boys are likely to spend many hours talking about sports and the latest horror movies. The therapist who cannot under these conditions maintain an interest in his patient and a genuine awareness of the importance of these issues in the everyday life of the young adolescent is likely to have a difficult time engendering in him a sense of real empathy and shared concern.

The early adolescent is likely to be a very busy person. He is, as I noted earlier, primarily oriented toward action in a wide variety of spheres. In addition, particularly if he is of middle- or upper-class origin, his parents will have ambitions and concerns for him that transcend the therapeutic situation. Accordingly, he is likely to be involved with a wide range of activities that will make extensive demands on his time. Activities such as soccer games, track meets, piano lessons, appointments with the orthodontist, rehearsals for the school play, choral performances, preparation for Bar Mitzvah—all these will be of the most urgent importance in the young adolescent's life and will encroach on the time available for psychotherapy appointments. Together with the early adolescent's guardedness and reserve about the whole therapeutic procedure and his need to preserve his sense of autonomy and self-determination, these activities are likely to lead to frequent cancellations, demands for alternative appointments, and failures to appear at scheduled times. The therapist of the early adolescent must be prepared and must prepare the family for such eventualities. If he wishes to maintain his relationship with his patient he must, again, be prepared to be flexible about his time arrangements, be willing to change appointments and schedule makeups, and tolerate with reasonably good humor the inevitable cancellations and no-shows. On the other hand, it must be clear both to the patient and to the family that the therapist is entitled to compensation for his time and that the patient and the family must be responsible for scheduled sessions. In other words, the therapist must be flexible but not infinitely manipulable or masochistic with respect to the complicated and shifting scheduling requirements of his adolescent patient.

Above all, the therapist of the young adolescent is well advised to maintain a developmental orientation toward his therapeutic goals. Even when impelled by subjective distress, the young adolescent is likely to be interested in the therapeutic process only to the extent that it addresses itself to those particular problems interfering with his normal developmental progression. Once his symptoms or maladaptive behavioral difficulties have been resolved in the course of therapy, it is unlikely that he will have further interest in continuing therapeutic contact. Remember, he is likely, if he is a patient amenable to this therapeutic approach at all, to be a busy person with many competing interests. The therapist should, therefore, be prepared to accept limited objectives and to regard symptom relief as a legitimate therapeutic goal. Strategically, he should be agreeable to the notion of brief or interrupted episodes of therapy rather than striving for unrealizable goals of major personality transformation. A corollary of this is the likelihood that, except for the more passive patient, few early adolescents will be amenable to the extended and regression-inducing procedure of classical psychoanalytic therapy.

Finally, a note about the role of the therapist's sex. There are few circumstances in which I would regard the sex of the therapist to be a critical issue in the therapeutic process. In most situations, both maternal and paternal elements of transference paradigms can be experienced and worked with irrespective of the therapist's actual sex. The one exception to this view is that of the early adolescent patient. As indicated above, the critical phase-specific preoccupation of early adolescents with their nascent sexuality and their masturbatory conflicts is invested with feelings of shame and the potential for humiliation that make it difficult in the extreme for them to communicate with an adult of the opposite sex. Further, the proximity to consciousness of oedipal wishes and fantasies makes the opposite-sex therapist a potentially dangerous figure for many early adolescent patients. For these reasons I believe that, wherever possible, young adolescents are best treated by a therapist of the same sex. Where this is not feasible, of course, therapy should not wait on the unavailable therapist, but the process is more likely to proceed productively when such arrangements can be worked out.

MID ADOLESCENCE

So much for the problem of the young adolescent. What about the young person in the next subphase—that of mid adolescence, or, as Blos refers to it, "adolescence proper"—the period between about fifteen to about eighteen, that is, the high school years? Here again, subphase-specific characteristics will tend to shape ways in which the therapeutic interaction proceeds and the technical approach that the therapist brings to his work.

The healthy mid adolescent is likely to have arrived at some reasonable accommodation to his pubertal development. He is more comfortable with his body and more accustomed to the sensations and fantasies that his pubescence has generated. As a result, he is likely to be less rigidly narcissistic and better able to interact empathically with others than is his younger sibling. Although he is still relatively action oriented, he is under considerably less impulse pressure and is better able to engage in introspection and delay of gratification than he was at twelve or thirteen. Further, given the fact of his increased physical maturation and the likelihood under normal circumstances of his having been granted more opportunities for independent action, he is likely to be more secure about his developing autonomy and, therefore, less guarded and suspicious of the motives of adults. This being the case, he is less likely to employ rigid and relatively primitive defenses and, on the other hand, more likely to recognize and acknowledge subjective distress than is the younger adolescent. Although he is still deeply engaged in his peer culture, he is, as Ianni (1983) has recently demonstrated, more likely than he had been earlier to turn to adults for support and guidance in areas of value formation and the planning of his future. Indeed, it is during this period, as his cognitive development proceeds in the direction of formal operational thought and as his perception of reality becomes better consolidated, that he begins to think seriously about his future and about the potential consequences of his current behaviors. Serious consideration of vocational goals becomes a feature of this period and, along with the mid-adolescent preoccupation with values, ideals, and abstract philosophical concerns, may engender a need for the active support and guidance of valued and trusted adults.

Despite all these progressive developmental characteristics, however, it should be recognized that the normal mid adolescent may be prey to shifting moods and to a dysphoric diathesis as he steers his course through the gradual process of "object removal"—that is, the revision of his earlier intense attachment to his parents and the ultimate establishment of mature connections with nonincestuous love objects. Many will be exquisitely sensitive to rejections or losses that leave them feeling objectless and alone; under these circumstances, even the relatively healthy adolescent may experience depressive moments and entertain transient suicidal thoughts. Further, the normal mid adolescent is still capable of regressive movements that Blos believes are a necessary aspect of adolescent development. It is certainly true that premature consolidation of advanced developmental positions without the flexibility that allows for change, experimentation, and revision of identifications constitutes a significant restriction of the optimal unfolding of the personality. Still, one should be aware that even the most mature-appearing mid adolescent is capable of regressing from thoughtful introspection to frenetic activity, particularly where resistance can be rationalized as being adaptively appropriate. I recall, for instance, the case of an extraordinarily bright and gifted fifteen-year-old girl, the product of an enormously complex family of mixed racial origin and radical political orientation, who came to treatment in the throes of a moderately severe depression that was significantly interfering with her academic and social life. Consistent with her family background, she was deeply interested in the antinuclear movement and spent a considerable amount of time in treatment talking about her involvement with various aspects of the then current campaign against the development of nuclear reactors. She proceeded quite well in therapy, however, and was deeply engaged in examining her feelings about her relations with her parents and her profound sense of disappointment and disillusionment in them. When the Three Mile Island incident occurred, this girl was galvanized into activity. She became energized by the activation of the movement around this near disaster and profoundly immersed in a series of demonstrations, marches, and protests that came in its wake. Her depression lifted, and it became clear that she had no time in her busy schedule for the luxury of psychotherapy. She thanked me for my help and made it clear that life was now offering her more in terms of purpose and fulfillment than I was able to give her. That, in sum, was the end of her psychotherapy.

All of these developmental trends have influence on the principles of technique in our work with mid-adolescent patients. We are no longer likely to require the use of nonverbal child therapy devices to promote communication, although there may be special cases of withdrawn schizoid adolescents who may require and benefit from the use of such games as chess, as described forty years ago by Fleming and Strong (1943) as a means of establishing contact while maintaining a protective distance. Normally, the communicative process in the treatment of the mid adolescent will be essentially a conversational one, though still one that will require from the therapist more activity than he may be accustomed to employing with his adult patients. As indicated earlier, the mid adolescent is likely to be in quest of guidance and clarification around issues of values, morality, and ideals. The therapist may, therefore, have to express himself directly on such matters without attempting to impose his views on his patient. This may come up particularly around such matters as drug taking, sexual behavior, and the like. A due respect for the adolescent's autonomy and his phase-appropriate efforts to forge his own sense of identity will dictate both the therapeutic focus and the therapist's tactful, though frank, response.

Nonetheless, there may be occasions in the treatment of all adolescents—but particularly the mid adolescent—when active, limit-setting intervention on the therapist's part is not only advisable but essential. The mid adolescent's normative depressive propensity may, in a disturbed adolescent, advance to the point of active suicidal ideation or behavior; his normal experimental tendency may carry him so far as to involve him in behaviors that threaten his health or even his survival. In such instances, the therapist must be prepared to act decisively and appropriately to protect his patient from the consequences of the miscarried extremity of his phase-related dispositions and his still imperfectly developed impulse control.

The mid adolescent probably poses the greatest challenge of any patient to the therapist's ability to monitor and regulate his countertransference responses. Anthony (1969) has written convincingly about the reactions of adults to adolescents and their tendency to stereotype adolescent behavior in response to the anxieties that it arouses in them. In this respect the therapist is not likely to be different from other adults. He must constantly be on guard against the danger of being seduced into recapitulating with the adolescent behaviors to which the latter is accustomed in his transactions with people in his everyday life. This applies to both sexual and aggressive responses. Two polar positions may be assumed by an unwary therapist in reaction to such seductions, either of which can have disastrous consequences. The first is that of overidentification with the adolescent and concomitant hostility toward parents and other authoritative figures whom the patient and then the therapist see as oppressing him. This would be equivalent to the parental stance that "I was like that when I was a kid and I turned out all right." The second is overidentification with parents and authority figures and concomitant hostility to the adolescent himself. This would be the corollary of the parental position that "I couldn't get away with that stuff when I was his age and I don't see any reason why he should either." In either case, the therapist is likely to be responding not so much to the realities of the patient's situation and behavior but to unresolved adolescent conflicts of his own that the patient's behavior reactivates. Constant self-scrutiny, therefore, is a necessary condition for psychotherapeutic work with adolescents at all stages—but particularly during this crucial mid-adolescent period.

LATE ADOLESCENCE

About the older adolescent, the eighteen- to twenty-one-year-old college-age youth, there is less specifically to be said. He is fully matured physically, frequently well advanced into higher-level cognitive functioning, and at least potentially capable of self-observation and introspection. The college-age adolescent who is otherwise suitable for psychoanalytically oriented psychotherapy can be treated, from a technical standpoint, very much in the manner of an adult. At this age, classical psychoanalytic technique can more frequently be employed, and the therapist may assume a less active, more observant stance than he is likely to be able to use with the younger adolescent. Special circumstances will arise here again, related to phase-appropriate developmental needs where considerations of going away to college or graduate education conflict with continuing in or initiating therapy in a particular geographic locale. In such instances, therapeutic needs must be carefully balanced against appropriate developmental advances, but the ultimate decision should, except in emergency situations, be left after appropriate reflection to the maturing adolescent himself. In most cases, alternative therapeutic arrangements can be made even in what seem relatively remote settings. One does not wish to present the adolescent with a situation in which he must view leaving as an act of rebellion or staying as an act of submission (although, of course, in the transference he may well do so).

I want to emphasize again what you all know—that all adolescents are likely to be provocative and constantly to test the therapist's commitment and his neutrality. The therapist must respond with, in Trilling's (1972) terms, "sincerity and authenticity" if he is to engender credibility with adolescent patients. The therapist must be prepared for the fact that only in rare instances can he anticipate anything resembling a full resolution of the transference in his therapeutic work with adolescents. Indeed, recent studies by Firestein (1978), Pfeffer (1974), and others seriously question the possibility of such full transference resolution in even the most intensive analytic work with adults. But certainly in work with adolescents, one has to be prepared to do "pieces" of therapy addressed to specific and limited conflictual areas, making knowing use of positive transference configurations and recognizing that, in many instances, the exploration of negative transference issues and the ultimate resolution of those negative oedipal residues that Blos (1977) regards as crucial for the attainment of true adult status must await more intensive and systematic exploration at a later time. Certain fundamental therapeutic dicta apply particularly to work with all adolescents, particularly that dictum which prescribes interpretive work directed primarily at maladaptive defenses rather than, or at least considerably prior to, attempts at unearthing pathogenic instinctual conflicts.

THE ROLE OF THE FAMILY

Finally, a few words about the role of parents. I believe that in any work with an adolescent, at least one who is either physically or financially dependent on parents, the latter should be seen initially with, of course, the permission of the patient, and with or without his or her presence, as he or she chooses. Not only is valuable information to be obtained from such meetings, but I believe that parents have the right to see the person to whom they are entrusting the care of their child and to whom they are paying what is usually a substantial fee. On the other hand, for mid and late adolescents, I prefer to see the patient first, whenever possible, in order to emphasize my position that I am there to take care of him rather than to deal with his parents' complaints. Similarly, I discourage parents from making appointment arrangements for their adolescents; I prefer to make such arrangements directly with the patient as a way of recognizing the real demands that they have on their schedules and their growing self-regulation. Although family therapy is frequently useful as a mode of treatment for adolescents, in the kind of treatment I am discussing parents are not regularly or systematically included in the treatment process. I do, however, find that it is useful in specific circumstances to arrange family meetings where clarification of obscure issues and resolution of specific situational conflicts are frequently possible. I am very protective, however, of the confidentiality of my patients' communications and make it clear from the outset that whatever they tell me remains with us, whereas whatever their parents tell me is not so protected. I feel free to communicate to the adolescent anything that his parents have told me so as to make it clear that no collusion exists between them and me and that he has a right to know whatever concerns him. Finally, and as a matter of course, it appears to me that where parents need sustained work either as a couple or individually, or where family therapy is indicated, I should make no effort to conduct such treatment myself but refer them to others. I believe that my ability to focus my attention on the adolescent himself, and his ability to see me as his working collaborator, would be compromised were I to attempt to be everyone's therapist at once.

In considering these comments about family involvement, I have come to realize that I am speaking from a special and perhaps unusual perspective—the perspective of one who practices in the center of a great metropolis richly endowed with public transit facilities that make it possible for even early adolescents to make and keep appointments on their own. For those in other, less favored communities where the adolescent, at least until driving age, is dependent on parents for transportation to and from his sessions, the situation will be quite different and, I believe, less desirable. There one does not enjoy the prerogative of choice as to whether the patient comes alone to his initial session; one may not even be able to schedule such an appointment—or any appointment at all—without considering the complexities of parental schedules, and, if both parents work, these may be complicated indeed. And, as one colleague put it, "as often as not it is the parents who cancel the kid's appointment because they're sick or have something else to do." Having largely been spared these problems, I can say little about their management except to underscore both the inevitable need for flexibility and the inherent limitations that such circumstances impose on the therapeutic process in work with younger adolescents. Certainly the goal that many of us set—the promotion of the adolescent's functioning and his sense of a truly autonomous self—is not favored by such practical reinforcements of his dependent status.

Conclusions

Let me, in concluding, then, state what I regard as the essential elements of the climate of the therapeutic encounter in work with adolescents. I believe that the therapist's stance should be one of openness without inauthentic self-exposure, of empathy without overidentification or loss of appropriate distance, of respect for the patient's autonomy without affective detachment, and, finally, of flexibility without abandoning fundamental therapeutic principles. A lightness of touch need not conflict with, but should not subvert, a seriousness of purpose—that purpose being the restoration to the adolescent of his normal, phase-appropriate development and function. In a climate such as this, I believe the adolescent can grow, can resolve crippling inhibitions and revise maladaptive defenses, and can, where his basic psychic organization permits, return to a healthy developmental track. Psychotherapy cannot insure against later difficulties, nor can it undo the corrosive effects of social disorganization and deprivation. As physicians and psychiatrists, however, we have the means to alleviate needless suffering for many troubled adolescents and their families if we but use it wisely and well.

REFERENCES

Aichhorn, A. 1935. *Wayward Youth*. New York: Viking, 1948.

Anthony, E. J. 1969. The reactions of adults to adolescents and their behavior. In A. H. Esman, ed. *The Psychology of Adolescence*. New York: International Universities Press, 1975.

Berkovitz, I. 1972. *Adolescents Grow in Groups*. New York: Brunner/Mazel.

Blos, P. 1962. Intensive psychotherapy in relation to the various phases of the adolescent period. *American Journal of Orthopsychiatry* 32:901–910.

Blos, P. 1976. When and how does adolescence end? *Adolescent Psychiatry* 5:5–17.

Bruch, H. 1979. Island in the river: the anorexic adolescent in treatment. *Adolescent Psychiatry* 7:26–40.

Dulit, E. 1972. Adolescent thinking a la Piaget: the formal stage. *Journal of Youth and Adolescence* 1:281–301.

Firestein, S. 1978. *Termination in Psychoanalysis*. New York: International Universities Press.

Fleming, J., and Strong, D. 1943. Observation on the use of chess in the treatment of an adolescent boy. *Psychoanalytic Review* 30:399–416.

Freud, S. 1905. Fragment of the analysis of a case of hysteria. *Standard Edition* 7:7–122. London: Hogarth, 1953.

Ianni, F. 1983. *Home, School and Community in Adolescent Education*. Washington: U.S. Department of Education.

Laufer, M. 1975. Preventive intervention in adolescence. *Psychoanalytic Study of the Child* 30:511–528.

Laufer, M. 1977. A view of adolescent pathology. *Adolescent Psychiatry* 5:243–256.

Lehrer, P.; Schiff, L.; and Kris, A. 1971. Operant conditioning in a comprehensive treatment program for adolescents. *Archives of General Psychiatry* 25:515–521.

Masterson, J. 1972. *Treatment of the Borderline Adolescent: A Developmental Approach*. New York: Wiley.

Offer, D. 1969. *The Psychological World of the Teen-Ager: A Study of Normal Adolescent Development*. New York: Basic.

Piaget, J. 1969. The intellectual development of the adolescent. In A. H. Esman, ed. *The Psychology of Adolescence*. New York: International Universities Press, 1975.

Pfeffer, A. 1974. The fate of the transference neurosis after analysis. *Journal of the American Psychoanalytic Association* 22:895–903.

Trilling, L. 1972. *Sincerity and Authenticity*. Cambridge, Mass.: Harvard University Press.

Williams, F. 1973. Family therapy: its role in adolescent psychiatry. *Adolescent Psychiatry* 2:324–329.

10 DEATH ANXIETY: THE PRELUDE TO ADOLESCENCE

JOHN TOEWS, ROBERT MARTIN, AND HARRY PROSEN

Anxiety about death is evident in various forms throughout life and is characteristic of preadolescent children. During this stage of development, children often experience diffuse anxiety over a period of time and refer to concerns about their own death or the death of others without the anxiety reaching pathological proportions. It comes to clinical attention when it presents symptomatically—for example, through a severe phobic reaction. We believe that experiencing "death anxiety" is evidence of the child's coming to a major life-cycle transition, at the completion of which the self can finally be viewed as mortal.

Although death anxiety at this age is probably universal, it has not received a great deal of attention in the literature. This chapter will explore, from a life-cycle perspective, death anxiety in preadolescent children. The following example will be used to illustrate many of the issues to be considered.

Case Example

Paul made his first trip alone to visit his grandparents in a nearby city at age nine. He had often expressed the wish to make such a visit, but previously had always been told that he was too young. When given permission to go, he showed elation and acted very grown-up as he left his parents and boarded the bus. The bus ride was a direct one to the city in which his grandparents lived, and he was met at the end of the ride by relatives. Immediately on returning home, he excitedly recounted the visit,

0-226-24058-4/85/0012-0063$01.00

which he felt had gone very well. He described sleeping in his father's old bedroom and visiting his father's grandparents, who were in their mid-eighties and lived nearby. Paul's father casually asked him whether the great-grandfather had recognized Paul. On hearing this question, Paul seemed momentarily confused and then asked why his father wanted to know. The father replied that sometimes when people become very old they have difficulty with their memory and that the great-grandfather tended to become confused these days. Paul then said, "The old grandpa gets confused. Grandpa might get confused, too. Dad, when you grow old, will you get confused as well?" After posing this question, he suddenly stopped and did not seem to want to permit an answer. He then said, "The old grandpa is going to die soon. Grandpa will die sometime. Then, Dad, you are going to die." He stopped again for a short time and started to cry, exclaiming that he too would die some day. He said, "I can't let myself die. I can't let myself be buried and have people throw dirt on me. Dad, what is it like to die? I am afraid." This conversation was highly pressured and condensed, and the entire interchange lasted no more than two or three minutes. At bedtime Paul returned to the subject, repeating his anxieties in an almost identical fashion. He expressed fear of dying and asked, "Dad, do you get scared of dying?" For the next few days he was somewhat more pensive, cried more readily than usual, and would occasionally ask questions about death. After this, he appeared to become composed, and the subject no longer seemed to be prominent in his mind.

The Timing of Death Anxiety

In this example, experience of death anxiety occurs at the age of nine. This is in keeping with the generally accepted observation that such anxiety occurs during the preadolescent years. Cognitive-development theorists point to the fact that the child's concept of death develops in conjunction with cognitive development and only at this age begins to approach the adult understanding of death's universality, inevitability, and irreversibility (Hostler 1978). In earlier stages of development, death is experienced as reversible and akin to going away. The younger child believes that a return from death is possible. The four- to six-year-old may see death as a malevolent force that removes people against their will, as suggested by the child's fears of monsters, bogeymen, and ghosts. The seven- to ten-year-old sees death as universal and irreversible. Childers and Wimmer (1971) documented this realization in seventy-five normal children, noting that at age six only 22 percent of the sample fully realized that death was universal. By the age of nine, however, 100 percent of their sample recognized the universality of death. White, Elsom, and Prawat (1978) studied the development of the concept of death during the Piagetian stage of concrete operations and suggested that the universality rather than the irreversibility of death is the key concept for the child to grasp. Some children, as well as some adults, may continue to believe in the reversibility of death, particularly those whose religious beliefs teach that there is a life after death.

Studies of fatally ill children have also indicated a maturation in the child's concept of death during childhood. For some time it was thought that fatally ill children under the age of ten feared pain and mutilation more than they did death (Natterson and Knudson 1966). Therefore, it was taught that in many clinical settings fatally ill children need not be told about the imminence of death. It was held that children could not appreciate their own demise until adolescence. Spinetta and Maloney (1975) refuted this belief by demonstrating that latency-aged children suffering from a potentially fatal illness respond with a qualitatively different anxiety—that is, one focused specifically on death—than that felt by children suffering from chronic nonfatal illness. Both groups experienced the same separation from parents, similar invasive medical tests and treatment, and a similar quality of pain and discomfort (Spinetta 1974; Spinetta, Rigler, and Karon 1973).

The literature on this subject deals primarily with cognitive development of the appreciation of death in fatally ill children but generally does not discuss what the realization of death as one's own personal fate means to the child. Paul was cognitively and maturationally ready for the realization of death and was at the age when this experience usually occurs.

Review, Preview, and Explanation

During Paul's visit to his grandparents, he had a series of encounters with both grandparents and great-grandparents that appeared to reinforce for him the fact that all people—himself included—grow old and eventually die. Reconstructions of what probably happened in these encounters enable identification of a number of themes in the preadolescent development of one's conception of one's internalized life cycle. During the visit, Paul experienced many reminders of his father's childhood. He lived in the same house and slept in the same room that his father had occupied as a child. He dealt with his father's parents just as he might have imagined his father had related to them as a child. One might imagine a certain sense of dissonance in this experience, however, since concomitantly with the reminders and images of his father as a young boy and his grandparent's reminiscences on his father's youth, Paul also had to acknowledge that in reality his father and grandparents were now considerably older than they had been during the days being recollected.

The intensity of the experience was probably heightened by his father's absence. This lack of a stimulus to structure and bind his observations freed Paul to fantasize on his father's youth at the very time that his father occupied the same position in relation to Paul that Paul's grandparents had once occupied in relation to Paul's father.

This collage of images of significant people who were now older but had once been younger parents or children propelled Paul to undertake his own life-cycle work. Through a process of identification—primarily with his father but also with his grandparents and great-grandparents—he resolved his feeling of dissonance by recognizing his own future in the basic life process of aging and the shifting of generational positions. In effect, the lives of his older relatives now became images of his own future.

The view of one's life as a dynamic process that is bounded by birth and death and is an evolving entity appears to arise in part from a process in which one scans backward in time to review experiences and forward to preview anticipated events (Toews, Martin, and Prosen 1981). Memories depend on many variables, including age, level of intellectual and emotional development, and the presence of repression. They include views both of oneself and of one's parents at different ages. Images of the future depend not only on anticipation of the future but on actual consideration of older family members and others as images of one's own possible future outcomes or experiences and also on stories about parents and grandparents that carry a strong statement about one's own identity and what one's own future might be. Although age disparities between family members allow one to delay the consideration of one's own death, it is not possible to escape the fact that as generations proceed and as time progresses so one's own remaining life is shortened. On the other hand, one sees in those younger than oneself, particularly in one's children and grandchildren, images and reflections of one's own past. All of these internalized images of the past and future are arranged sequentially and projected temporally along a course that encompasses the life span from birth to death. Thus, this arrangement of images, memories, and anticipations of one's life from birth to death represents a vital component of the internalized life span as it has been lived, is lived, and is projected into the future.

This ordering of life images is a fundamental aspect of the development of one's own internalized life cycle. Younger children tend to think categorically, that is, children, parents, and grandparents are viewed as separate, discontinuous categories. However, in the cognitive developments occurring during preadolescence, this categorical thinking becomes less pronounced. It is then possible for the child to develop a sense of continuity through time that is essential in an appreciation of the aging process. Instead of considering children, parents, and grandparents as separate classes of beings, the child now sees them as persons who have progressed through their own life stages in a continuous process of aging just as children progress through their own lives eventually to become old.

This view of one's participation in the dimension of time provides a framework from which life can be viewed. This framework contains elements of the figure ground reversal in that one can shift between a narrow-frame or cross-sectional view, such as the life experience at a specific age or stage of life, and a broad-frame or longitudinal view of life, such as one's continuity through time. As with the figure ground perception, this multidimensional view, once recognized, continues to organize the observation of life. Even when not part of conscious thought, it still has influence. Because of the way it organizes and directs observations, this framework of one's life cycle both gives and derives meaning and structure from life events. In his attempts to grapple with his experience while concomitantly acknowledging the inevitability of his own aging, Paul participated in and finally perceived the significance of this framing process in his own life.

It is apparent that one's location along this internalized lifeline is determined to some extent by actual age. The subjective sense of where one is in one's life course comes about as a result of scanning, that is, of reviewing images of one's past and of observing those family members who represent selfobjects that are both younger and older than oneself. This scanning process appears to be a rapidly oscillating cycle that combines both review and preview (Toews et al. 1981). We hypothesize that it is this process that makes it possible for individuals to gain a personal sense of the unity of their own life cycle and of the point they have reached in their own life in relation to both their sense of personal time and the lives of others.

We hypothesize further that one's place on the internalized life span determines whether the basic scanning process is predominantly one of review or preview, that children (like Paul) would probably preview their lives, anticipating a full future, while the elderly would be more likely to review their lives. Neugarten (1970) asserts that at the midpoint of life, life is seen as time left to live rather than as time lived. In relation to this scanning process, the significance of middle age may also be seen as the realization that one has reached the midpoint of life, at which the scanning process is balanced between review and preview. Butler (1963) emphasizes the importance of the life review in the aging person; however, this is surely a special instance of this basic life-cycle scanning process, since the older person dwells in memories not only in order to remember better times and deal with losses but also because there is more room to scan backward over the past than there is to scan forward into a contracting and often somewhat bleak future.

It is evident from the preceding discussion that Paul was probably not alone in life-cycle scanning during his visit. While he previewed his life, his grandparents and great-grandparents probably actively participated in a process of life review, remembering their own childhoods through the images that Paul evoked and remembering when they were parents through the stimulus of their responsibility for Paul.

The Concept of Death

As far as we know, this was Paul's first real affective encounter with the concept of his own death. On the surface, it seems that one question from his father, "Did the old grandfather recognize you?" was sufficient to precipitate his acknowledgment of his own death. The question touched on a whole range of associations and issues, both personal and generational, that had urgent meaning for Paul. His father's question touched on stages in the process of aging. It also questioned the meaning of Paul's experience in his relationship with the great-grandparents. The failure to realize the significance of his own ultimate death could no longer protect Paul. The realization that he had been struggling with throughout the visit finally broke through in Paul's recognition both of his own mortality and of his participation, along with his parents and grandparents, in the sequence of generations. It was as if Paul, with the cognitive abilities of the child in the stage of concrete operations, was finally able to understand the classic syllogism: "All men are mortal, Socrates is a man; therefore, Socrates is mortal"—or, in Paul's terms, "All men are mortal, I am a man (like my father and grandfather); therefore, I am mortal."

This realization was possible because Paul was cognitively capable of the realization, was sensitized by his own life-cycle observations during the visit, and was stimulated in a way that made the realization conscious. The experience illustrated by this example is not unique; there has been extensive discussion in the literature of how the concept of death is understood by a child. Nagy's (1959) study, one of the oldest and still relevant, notes that before the age of five children see death as reversible, as an altered state of being. To a child of this age, death seems to be a transformation of life to another state and is not perceived as being a definite end of life. During latency, that is, from the ages of five to nine, children personify death as a being forcibly removing people from life. Death becomes something done to one by an outside, often sinister force. Only after the age of eight or nine does Nagy note the development of a more adult concept of death. Developmental theorists consider the Piagetian stage of concrete operations to be the stage at which the child eventually becomes capable of understanding the concept of death in a full, adult sense.

During this stage the concept of reversibility/irreversibility develops, so that the child is now capable of perceiving death as final and inevitable. Kastenbaum (1959) has pointed out that in 85 percent of the adolescents he studied, the concept of a personal death is removed from among the major organizing life themes of the adolescent. The eternal present and emphasis on the immediate future that characterize adolescence take precedence over fears about death; consideration of death is left to older age, where it is thought to more appropriately belong.

However, that death anxiety experienced in preadolescence continues as an active force throughout adolescence can be seen in the anxiety of teenagers as they respond to images that evoke the knowledge or realization of one's mortality. Many view fearfully the possibility of disease, wars, disasters—almost anything that might in some sense interfere with the completion of their anticipated life. Many approach death almost counterphobically, although the popularity of horror shows among adolescent moviegoers demonstrates the great fascination that death imagery holds for them. Death anxiety may also be seen in the reactions of the adolescent to the future. Adolescent suicide may well result from a feeling of being unable to face the future, a feeling that in turn derives from either feelings of personal inadequacy or the feeling that one is bound to recapitulate the failures that one sees in those models, either parents or others, who represent the future to the adolescent.

Since it assumes that each developmental period has its own characteristic conflicts, stage theory is often presented to restrict the consideration of these conflicts exclusively to a particular period of human life. Death anxiety can be used as an example in tracing the notion that these conflicts persist throughout life. We have suggested that death anxiety becomes a major developmental issue in the latter part of latency, largely as a result of the individual's achieving a level of cognitive development that permits the realization of death as both a universal and personal event. Some degree of death anxiety precedes this stage in the guise of various kinds of childhood imagery. Once the realization of one's mortality has developed, death anxiety will remain an active and molding force throughout life. It is often transformed into a constructive and vital involvement in the process of living, reaching consciousness when some consideration produces a realization of the frailty of individual life. This transformation is noted frequently in adolescence, although it often thinly veils pervasive anxiety about death. There seems to be another major period of ascendancy of death anxiety in middle age, occurring with one's realization that one has passed the midpoint in life and with the awareness of the progressive constriction in time left to live. We have referred elsewhere to ways of dealing with this mid-age transition and with the concerns about death that develop during and continue after this stage (Prosen, Toews, and Martin 1978). As parents age and die, individuals become aware that they are the oldest generation and the next to face death. In addition to the ultimate experience of it in old age, death anxiety may be uncovered in any period of life as a result of various types of trauma, physical threats, and the premature loss of significant others.

The Internalized Life-Cycle Model

It is against this developmental dynamic that successive steps in the formation within the child of a life-cycle model must be viewed. The significance of Paul's realization of his own mortality rests in part on the fact that he henceforth saw his life bounded—it could no longer be seen as endless or limitless. Certain aspects of Paul's experience also draw attention to preceding maturational tasks and conflicts that serve to structure the individual life span. First, it is unlikely that Paul would have experienced death anxiety with this intensity and in this compressed form if he had not been separated from his parents and in a relatively strange environment. The separation anxiety experienced by Paul during his visit underscored a basic developmental theme first expressed in the separation anxiety of the infant—that is, even though one is enclosed within the milieu of the family, one is still separate and distinct from others and, in effect, vulnerable.

Paul was exposed to a second, related anxiety because of the strange environment, even though it was safe and somewhat familiar. Stranger anxiety, as experienced by the infant, seems predicated on an identification of those whom one can trust and expect to meet certain needs; through it, the child develops a family/friend-versus-stranger differentiation. During his visit, Paul had to deal with a strange environment, be dependent on people whom he knew but whom he could not expect to know and meet his needs in the way that his parents could at home. In a life-cycle sense, this stranger anxiety is evidence of the child placing himself securely within a family matrix within which to mature.

The third major developmental conflict that was evident in Paul's visit was a generational conflict brought about by the absence from his parents and the fact that all of Paul's interactions were with people two or three generations older. In a sense, the basic structuring of life along generational lines is the task of the oedipal period of development, during which the child realizes not only the existence of generational boundaries but also the sense of order in the progression of generations. The absence of the intervening generation appears to have been a significant feature of Paul's experience. The ordering of generations during the oedipal period of development also aids the child in (1) obtaining a sense of his own future in the models that the parents present and (2) being willing to wait to be like the parents. In Paul's experience, this sense of a personal future was further heightened by identification with his father's boyhood and by the images of the future presented by his grandparents.

Paul's experience, in a life-cycle sense, was of the need to put boundaries on the sense of personal time. Children are able to comprehend birth as a boundary to life at an earlier age, since they are exposed to it much more frequently than they are to either death or the concept of death. They may note, often by the beginning of school age, the beginning of a life and extrapolate to when they themselves were infants. Death, however, is generally more remote, is in fact even hidden from children. Only the later death anxiety experienced by Paul and noted as being characteristic of his age-group gives evidence of the sense of another sort of boundary to one's life.

Paul's experience has been used to demonstrate and develop a model of the life cycle that contains both structural and dynamic components. The onset of puberty and the realization of the reproductive potential of the individual allows the child the chance to participate fully in the cyclical progression of the life cycle through various generations by producing offspring. Sexuality is one of the motive forces throughout adolescence, and at this stage the youth is obligated to synthesize aspects of an identity by taking into account various ambitions and motivations.

Frequently, adolescents are bothered by thoughts about their life and react to images of the future (derived both from childhood and from seeing older people) as if those images are statements of the details of their own future instead of being engaged in determining how one should live and function. This raises the question of the modification of one's internalized life cycle throughout the passage through life. It must be recognized that, except for its broad structural components, this internalized life cycle is mutable. It forms a fundamental part of identity; the images of self and others are constantly being reworked as one examines one's life in reference to present attainments, recollections of one's past, and images of the future. The realization of the need for such mutability is essential to the child's and adolescent's striving for identity and ability to escape the restrictions of a static and truncated view of who he or she is and yet may be.

Conclusions

That death anxiety remains a motive force throughout life has been pointed out by Becker (1973) in his contention that many adult activities and dreams are also denials of the fact of an eventual and inescapable death. The importance of death anxiety during preadolescence is that it is the first major statement of a theme that continues throughout life; the realization of one's own mortality structures the internalized life cycle and introduces the idea of finite time. A latency-aged child's experience of this anxiety has been used to illustrate the development of an internalized life cycle and to highlight the importance of this major but often unrecognized life-cycle transition.

REFERENCES

Becker, E. 1973. *Denial of Death*. New York: Free Press.

Butler, R. N. 1963. The life review: an interpretation of reminiscence in the aged. *Psychiatry* 26:65–76.

Childers, P., and Wimmer, M. 1971. The concept of death in early childhood. *Child Development* 42:1301–1449.

Hostler, S. 1978. The development of the child's concept of death. In O. J. Sahler, ed. *The Child and Death*. St. Louis: Mosby.

Kastenbaum, R. 1959. Time and death in adolescence. In H. Feifel, ed. *The Fear of Death*. New York: McGraw-Hill.

Nagy, M. H. 1959. The child's view of death. In H. Feifel, ed. *The Fear of Death*. New York: McGraw-Hill.

Natterson, J., and Knudson, A. 1966. Observations concerning fear of death in fatally ill children and their mothers. *Psychosomatic Medicine* 22:456–465.

Neugarten, E. 1970. Dynamics of transition of middle age to old age. *Journal of Geriatric Psychiatry* 4:71–87.

Prosen, H.; Toews, J.; and Martin, R. 1978. Is middle age a state of mind? *Canada's Mental Health* 26(4):22–25.

Spinetta, J. J. 1974. The dying child's awareness of death: a review. *Psychological Bulletin* 81(4):256–260.

Spinetta, J. J., and Maloney, L. J. 1975. Death anxiety in the outpatient leukemic child. *Pediatrics* 56(6):1034–1037.

Spinetta, J. J.; Rigler, D. R.; and Karon, M. 1973. Anxiety in the dying child. *Pediatrics* 52:841–845.

Toews, J.; Martin, R.; and Prosen, H. 1981. The life cycle of the family: perspectives on psychotherapy with adolescents. *Adolescent Psychiatry* 9:189–198.

White, E.; Elsom, B.; and Prawat, R. 1978. Children's conception of death. *Child Development* 49:307–310.

11 IDENTITY FORECLOSURE IN EARLY ADOLESCENCE: A PROBLEM OF NARCISSISTIC EQUILIBRIUM

CHARLES A. BURCH

To call attention to narcissism among adolescents thirteen to fifteen years old would at first glance appear to be merely emphasizing the obvious. Clinical experience and the theoretical assumptions which support our work have demonstrated that the narcissism so evident in this age group is often phase specific and an indication of developmental process. However, I have observed in some young adolescents a form of narcissistic disturbance which I believe represents something quite different from normal adolescent narcissism.

The adolescents I wish to discuss in this theoretical essay are frequently an enigma to parents, teachers, and clinicians. They appear to be mature, and yet the level at which they function in their daily lives does not parallel their supposed maturity and sophistication. They are often of superior intelligence, as revealed in objective measures of intelligence and achievement, but they do poorly or marginally well or are identified as underachievers scholastically. They seem to prefer and seek out the company of older peers whom they perceive as being more like themselves in their manner and interests than their age-mates. They also do well in the company of adults, especially in social situations in which conversation or sharing in a mutually enjoyed activity provides considerable gratification. Yet these adolescents are also viewed by their parents as overly manipulative and demanding, even though at other times they are perceived as the enjoyable and agreeable companions they can be. Often these youngsters come to our attention because one or both parents have

0-226-24058-4/85/0012-0006$01.00

become alarmed over some marked slippage in school performance, increased moodiness, or an almost phobic avoidance of age-appropriate contact with peers. Although at first parents tend to explain away or rationalize these difficulties, they now begin to become concerned that these children have not met their expectations in any consistent way in their social and scholastic roles.

The adolescents I am discussing present clinical pictures which closely parallel the kinds of narcissistic disturbances discussed extensively by Kohut (1968, 1972, 1977) and others (Goldberg 1980; Kernberg 1975; Modell 1976). They appear to have carried forward into adolescence precocious identity components derived during much earlier phases of development. In brief, they have more or less committed themselves in early adolescence to a personality configuration that comprises defensive and compensatory structures (Kohut 1977) that are only minimally open and available for further modification and revision during later adolescent development. This is not normal adolescent narcissism but, rather, a subtle developmental arrest. I have chosen to call this form of early adolescent narcissistic disturbance "identity foreclosure." Resistance to reformulation and resistance to revision of personality components and conflicts differentiate these youngsters from their adolescent peers who may appear, to the casual observer, equally self-centered in their fluctuating moods, unpredictable behavior, and rebellious, callous attitudes. The normal adolescent, however, who oscillates between adult and infantile modes is actually developing a more integrated, elaborated identity with which to commence adult life. Adolescents who have foreclosed are in a very real sense locked into their identity. They firmly resist efforts by parents, therapists, and others to change.

Identity Formation and the Self

For Kohut (1977), a crucial sequence of emotional and behavioral interactions exists between the infant or young child and the mother (nurturant figure). This sequence includes the following steps: disturbances in the child's psychophysiological equilibrium result in tension states that eventually are expressed behaviorally in distress cues or signals. In response, the mothering person first calms or soothes the child; second, determines through empathic understanding what is specifically needed by the child; and, finally, provides need-satisfying actions. "The selfobject, equipped with a mature psychological organization that can realistically assess the child's need and what is to be done about it, will include the child into its own psychological organization and will remedy the child's homeostatic imbalance through actions" (Kohut 1977).

In this way the mother enables the child to merge with her empathically, and in so doing the child learns to respond to affect as a signal rather than becoming entrenched in a psychological state in which the experience of affect spreads to the point of panic—a state described by Freud long ago as primary or traumatic anxiety, which overwhelms the immature psychological structures of the child. Inevitably, there are empathic failures or shortcomings on the part of the mother, and Kohut asserts that *these failures provide an important impetus for the developing child to form his own set of psychological structures through the process of transmuting internalization* (emphasis mine). In this process, the child identifies with the selfobject's methods of coping with tensions and anxiety and, therefore, is eventually able to employ self-soothing or other means of reducing tension and preventing the spread of affect to panic states. Gradually, through the process of transmuting internalization and through the parents' becoming increasingly selective in their mirroring responses to the child, he is able to relinquish his adherence to the grandiose self and the need for an idealized selfobject while moving toward realistic self-esteem, ambitions, and ideals.

Kohut maintains that the sequence of empathic responses I outlined is developmentally essential as a basis for adult mental health. What is often overlooked in his formulation, however, is the idea of normal parental failures. Optimal frustration is also crucial for the development of psychological structures. It is my assertion that empathic failure on the part of the parents of the adolescents under discussion here contributes to the unique clinical features observed in their children in early adolescence. Specifically, it is hypothesized that the parents of these children remain overly enmeshed in trying to attune to their child's needs beyond age-appropriate demands. Stated differently, it is hypothesized that the parents' attempt to maintain a level of understanding of the child's emotional needs is excessive. As a result, the child does not adequately internalize the ability either to tolerate frustration and delay or to recognize and accept the concomitant affect states which emerge when narcissistic needs are not gratified. In short, the youngsters reveal considerable difficulty in responding to affect as a signal. Instead they remain especially vulnerable to the spread of affect. This is most apparent in relation to narcissistically derived rage. If the formulations above are accurate, there exists in the adolescents I am discussing a distortion in personality development that is derived from a specific breakdown in parental empathy early in the child's life. This breakdown very likely takes the form of the inability on the part of the parents to fail in ways that would have benefited internalization of the selfobject functions. Moreover, these parents, especially the mothers, are likely to be overinvolved in mirroring responses which have the effect of reinforcing the archaic, grandiose self-image. The fathers are likely not to have been available by virtue of being too passive and withdrawn, too intimidating or overly narcissistic themselves, for the "second chance" (Kohut 1977) to occur, wherein the child can identify with an idealized figure in order to stabilize a core self-experience. When a child from this emotional matrix comes to adolescence, the stage is set for identity foreclosure, a premature occlusion of self-development and elaboration.

From Kohut's work, therefore, emerge two ideas pertinent to my discussion: (1) a trajectory toward excessive and unmodified infantile, grandiose narcissism deriving from the parents' being unable to fail optimally in ways that promote development and (2) parental inadequacy at providing increasingly selective mirroring responses tailored to the child's shifting developmental needs. It is hypothesized that they also contribute to the inability of the child to modify the grandiose nuclear self in the direction of realistic ambitions and ideals. I would add that in my experience these parental failures are in no discernible way conscious efforts; rather, these parents appear to me as overly devoted to their children. They may also maintain the illusion of the "perfect" child much longer than other parents.

Erik Erikson's familiar and subtly complex ideas with respect to identity formation also bear a relationship to the ideas I am setting forth in this chapter. For Erikson (1968), ego identity is "an enduring psychological structure which is subjectively experienced as a sense of psychosocial well-being. Its most obvious concomitants are a feeling of being at home in one's body, a sense of knowing where one is going and an inner assuredness of anticipated recognition from those who count." Time and again, Erikson makes the point that identity is established through an active and reciprocal exchange between the individual and the psychosocial matrix in which he lives. The multiple exchanges between the adolescent and his peer group, family, and others imply something which everyone who lives or works with adolescents knows very well, namely, that the adolescent, under normal circumstances, experiments (behaviorally and in fantasy) with relationships and roles. The adolescents with whom I am concerned appear all too willing to forgo the actual, behavioral experimentation, or it is abruptly suspended after some disappointment which disrupts their narcissistic equilibrium. They appear indifferent to the idea of new ventures, quite unconcerned about their social isolation, and often more interested in psychological play as expressed in elaborate fantasies which may often have a decidedly grandiose quality. In my experience these fantasies become a primary source of comfort and gratification. Actual interpersonal relationships with peers and others outside the family become secondary sources of gratification. Such withdrawal into fantasy is one facet of an overall movement toward the solipsistic orientation that Modell (1976) has described as a psychological "cocoon." The cocoon provides an effective shield against threats to these adolescents' narcissistic balance and thus becomes much like a closed system. Therefore, instead of accomplishing a more or less stable sense of ego identity achieved gradually over the several years of adolescence, these narcissistically orbited adolescents leap toward a crystallized identity in the early adolescent period. In this way they short-circuit the demands of a developmental process that poses too great a threat to their tentatively maintained narcissistic balance. Thus, the foundation for further elaborations of the self in adulthood is a rigid, albeit mostly stable, psychological structure rather than a flexible one.

Although the ideas of Kohut and Erikson provide a general theoretical framework for my discussion, Blos (1967) has written extensively on issues that bear directly on the idea of identity foreclosure.

Blos (1979) described the syndrome of "the overappreciated child" who is impaired developmentally as a result of early parent-child experiences in which the child was "inordinately praised and admired, while shortcomings and inadequacies were ignored unduly long or excused by the parents." Although Blos addressed himself to the late-adolescent or young-adult patient, he recognized that the developmental defect becomes apparent over the whole course of adolescence. Blos makes a crucial point with respect to the upbringing of these children. Not only were they overvalued by the parents, but also these youngsters were allowed from an early age to make decisions or independent judgments. Blos (1979) terms this a form of "premature overexpectation" that I believe is integral to understanding the notion of identity foreclosure. That is, one of the precursors for the leap forward toward a crystallized, narcissistically based identity is having been allowed to make independent decisions as if one were adequately equipped to do so. The young adolescent I am discussing is, in a very real sense, doing what comes naturally in expressing a sense of entitlement with respect to adult prerogatives while the parents become increasingly frustrated and chagrined that their offspring expects to be treated as a peer.

The difference between my assertion and Blos's is that I believe one can observe the process of identity foreclosure in early adolescence and that the disturbance closely parallels its counterpart in adults, narcissistic personality formation. These adolescents deal with adolescence by not dealing with it and instead become caricatures of adults. In this respect they very likely avoid much of the typical adolescent distress, but they do suffer, as Blos (1979) reports, a "desolate, empty, dark and frightening" existence. Young adolescents who have prematurely committed themselves to their ego identity in order to preserve their narcissistic equilibrium present to themselves and their social environment a "false self" (Winnicott 1965) which aids in maintaining the illusion of maturity.

I will illustrate some of my ideas through the following case example and discussion.

Case of Bryan R.

REFERRAL INFORMATION AND FAMILY BACKGROUND

Bryan R. was fourteen years old at the time of referral. I was called by his mother who expressed parental concern over Bryan's very poor performance scholastically since entering high school. Mrs. R. also commented on her son's being "depressed and listless" at home; he appeared to be quite uninterested in anything.

At the time I began working with Bryan there were four people living in the home: Mr. R., aged fifty-two, self-employed in his own photographic business; Mrs. R., aged fifty, who was at home but did the bookkeeping for her husband's business; Herb, aged twenty; and Bryan. Two other siblings, both male, were living in their own homes within the same metropolitan area.

It was evident from the outset that Mr. and Mrs. R. had a marital relationship riddled with conflicts and strains that included many disagreements over Bryan's rearing. Mrs. R., a plump, superficially congenial woman, made clear almost immediately that Bryan was "special" to her, her "baby," which among other factors made it nearly impossible for her to carry out appropriate parental discipline. Instead, she had for many years succeeded in placing Mr. R. in the position of the enforcing parent, a role he accepted. However, the demands also produced thinly veiled, intense hostility toward his wife. For example, Mr. R. was sarcastically critical of his wife's ineffectiveness as a mother and disciplinarian, as well as of the pervasive, clinging dependency on him that had characterized this relationship. Throughout my contacts with the parents, Mr. R. maintained his highly controlled, weary manner, which was interrupted by occasional expressions of genuine concern, humor, and subdued warmth. In rearing the three older children, Mr. R. used harsh physical punishment meted out when he came home in the evening. Up to the time of my involvement with the family, however, Mr. R. had never "laid a hand on Bryan." For her part, Mrs. R. presented the conflicting message to her husband of expecting him to do the actual punishing and yet criticizing him for his harshness, rigidity, and affectional and material parsimony. However, despite these marital conflicts, including child-rearing disagreements, Mr. and Mrs. R. were committed to continuing their marriage.

With this parental context as a background, I turn now to Bryan's somewhat limited personal history as obtained from Mr. and Mrs. R., who were poor historians.

The mother described him as a child who was "wanted but not planned." When she learned she was pregnant, she initially wanted a girl but at the time of treatment expressed being "glad he is not" because of the family situation, on which she would not elaborate.

At age eleven months Bryan was diagnosed as having celiac disease, which required that Mrs. R. be especially devoted to his dietary needs until he was eighteen months old. The life event of the disease appeared crucial in terms of solidifying the mother's already watchful devotion. Both parents, however, emphasized that Bryan never did well socially. By this they explained that as a young child—as early as age three—Bryan seemed more concerned over his possessions remaining in perfect order than in playing with other children. As a result, play with other children both in and out of the home began to diminish considerably, until at the time of referral Bryan neither sought out nor was approached by other youngsters except, from his report, in school.

Bryan was described as a good student until the eighth grade. In the second half of the year his performance began to deteriorate in two classes, and this appeared to be very much a function of his dislike for his two teachers. Bryan expressed his resentment and dislike by choosing not to do required assignments; in the latter part of the academic year he marshaled himself sufficiently to pass all of his courses.

Mr. and Mrs. R. also discussed some of the protracted difficulties they had with brother Herb. From the data obtained during the evaluation, from subsequent counseling sessions, and from Bryan, it appeared that Herb was at best a marginally adjusted young man who periodically would terrorize and torment Bryan both physically and verbally. Moreover, neither parent was for several years able effectively to control Herb, nor could they get him to move out on his own. When Bryan would complain about being mistreated by Herb, the parents would tend mostly to blame Bryan for provoking his brother or would tell him he had to learn to defend himself. Thus, the parents, while acknowledging that Herb was a major problem to them and Bryan, disclaimed responsibility for managing his overtly aggressive and inappropriate behavior.

SUMMARY OF THE PSYCHOTHERAPY

From the outset, Bryan presented himself in a composed way, with little evidence of the anxiety frequently observed in children when they are brought for a consultation. He spoke in an affectively flattened way most of the time. He was usually pleasant and appropriate; only occasionally did he display the kind of lively animation typical of adolescents. These instances usually involved his plans or thoughts about something he wanted to obtain. He would also express some emotions of anger and frustration when discussing his father's restrictions, the denial of his requests, or his mother's frustrating manner. In all of these, the expression of affect was muted and constricted, which resulted in Bryan conveying a lifeless quality. The depressive undercurrent was evident, revealing more an aspect of emptiness rather than sadness, guilt, and diminished self-esteem.

From the initial session and until he discontinued therapy nine months later, Bryan identified his difficulties as arising from external sources, namely, his father's restrictive, punitive manner; Herb's sadistic behavior; and mother's "craziness," meaning her multiple and chronic phobic fears. Bryan also discussed the other major sector of his life—school—from a similar standpoint of the many ways in which his curriculum, the teachers, and other students were not right for him.

The therapeutic relationship and transference reactions replicated much of the patterns above in that Bryan's favorable attitude toward treatment and me appeared linked with an unconscious perception of me as an idealized, perhaps omnipotent, object. For example, in one session near the end of my experience with him, Bryan expressed much gratitude for my being able to change things in the family so that his parents were not on his back all the time. The message was one of my joining him in his perception that what needed modification in his life were problematic aspects external to himself that intruded on his comfort, his world. I was perceived, I believe, as someone powerful enough to influence his parents and help Bryan get what he wanted. It was when I eventually attempted to move the therapeutic relationship in the direction of introspection and self-examination that Bryan decided to discontinue therapy.

Bryan expressed much rage toward his father, which centered on his experience of the father as a restrictive and punitive person. It became clear, however, that Bryan was usually successful in getting what he wanted, despite Mr. R.'s persistent no, by first approaching Mrs. R. with a request. For example, Bryan, with brother Herb's support, was able to "borrow" several thousand dollars from his mother to purchase highly sophisticated stereophonic components. The equipment was installed before Mr. R. knew about the purchase; he did not insist on its return. Thus, although Bryan was greatly intimidated by his father, he usually was successful in manipulating or maneuvering both his parents. In characteristic fashion, Bryan lost interest in the stereo equipment within six to eight weeks.

Bryan's difficulties in school with respect to peer relations hinged on an incident early in the school year when he was serving as freshman class representative to the student council. He was in charge of the construction of the class float for the homecoming parade. Bryan became very angry when the other students would not follow his directions exactly and when they mischievously modified and then eventually destroyed the float. Bryan withdrew completely from the project and resigned his class office.

His involvement with peers outside the home or school setting narrowed to a limited involvement in a culturally affiliated youth group. Most of the members were two to four years older than he, which he found quite comfortable. Other than these weekly meetings, however, Bryan spent virtually all his free time in the house. There he occupied himself with listening to music, caring for his tropical fish, and watching television. About three months after therapy began he tentatively revealed his feelings about peers in school, stating he did not want to be with them because they were reckless, silly, immature, or frankly dangerous. He said he considered himself more mature and was comfortable in his state of being alone most of the time.

In a family counseling session, Mr. R. reported that Bryan expected and required perfection from all around him; he described him as being intolerant of any mistakes in others. Moreover, he seemed to want others to know what he wanted without having to express his wishes verbally. This was revealed in the therapeutic relationship when he became quite angry with me for not understanding implicitly how upset he felt over his parents' predicting he would not be able to finish high school.

Bryan denied having any fantasies and after six months of treatment admitted that he really had little or no interest in anything.[1]

Perhaps one last vignette will best illustrate the manner in which Bryan approached life when I knew him. He had his bicycle stolen some time before treatment began. In the course of our work he decided it was time for a new bike, and what he especially wanted was a Moped-style one. Mr. R. predictably said no to this request; Bryan then settled for his second choice, a rather expensive twelve-speed bike carefully selected as to color and specifications. However, he did not ride the bike in the time I knew him because it did not have the special kind of seat he wanted, and he could not find time nor would he solicit his parents' assistance to get the proper saddle. The new bike remained in his room unused, with Bryan appearing quite indifferent to it.

The material presented above is, of course, a partial report of the clinical data, which I end now in order to discuss the implications of these data in light of my theoretical notion of identity foreclosure.

Discussion

The examination of the clinical material results in a diagnostic conundrum. There are aspects of Bryan's presentation which would support a diagnosis of an obsessional personality with phobic and depressive trends. For example, his insistence on having just the right equipment, his mother's remarks about his wanting everything perfect, the attempts to control the parents, his constricted affective style, all of these features would support a view that Bryan was relying on obsessional mechanisms to cope with strong and unacceptable impulses and feelings both of an aggressive and sexual nature. Moreover, if one chose to follow the categorization of DSM III (1980), a plausible argument could be advanced for a diagnosis of avoidant disorder of adolescence or even for schizoid disorder of adolescence in view of Bryan's isolative and uninterested position regarding social interactions with peers.

Although the clinical data are available to support these diagnostic assertions, they would also miss the mark in explaining Bryan's underlying personality structure, which I believe was organized around excessive and pathologically infiltrated narcissism. He was clearly an "overappreciated child" as discussed by Blos (1979) in that the maintenance of his self-esteem appeared linked to the mirroring experiences provided by his mother. Utilizing the theoretical vantage point of excessive narcissism, therefore, enables one to explain Bryan's behavior and manner in a way different from an emphasis on symptom, defenses, and impulses. Though the aspects of conflict were evident and were attended to in the therapeutic work, I viewed the conflictional problems as being embedded in a larger matrix of disturbances in self-development.

The pubertal surge of early adolescence and the concomitant societal demands for increased independence posed a serious problem for Bryan because he appeared unable to allow for exposure to the experimentation and socialization typical of adolescents. His fragile sense of self-esteem could not tolerate the teasing, ridicule, and challenging that constitutes so much of early adolescent peer relationships. He was, instead, thrown back on his family, in a sense an equally unsatisfactory solution since it would result in a regressive pull that was difficult for Bryan to accept as there was some forward developmental thrust evident in his functioning. His psychic solution, therefore, was a "flight forward" (Blos 1979), with the implied expectation that he would be treated as an adult. This is the process that I term identity foreclosure, which, to these narcissistically vulnerable adolescents, represents the best possible solution between the regressive pull toward childhood relations and current developmental demands to further their individuation through peer relationships and other social and intellectual endeavors beyond the family.

One of the problems I faced in trying to understand Bryan was formulating a suitable explanation for the depression which precipitated his referral. His frustrating experiences with peers early in the school year appeared to represent a narcissistic injury that precipitated a rapid lowering of self-esteem. Bryan's withdrawal from the class office position and from any further contact with the other youngsters was a behavioral response by which he was protecting himself from further narcissistic wounds. In a conventional dynamic formulation, aggression in the form of angry, rageful feelings directed originally toward the peers would be withdrawn, along with other connections to the objects, and redirected unconsciously toward the self, resulting in a depressed state. This explanation, although reasonable enough, is, I believe, insufficient. On a deeper and more pervasive psychological level, Bryan yearned for a continuation of the mirroring experiences provided by his mother, in which his primitive grandiose self was reinforced. Since his peers not only did not provide the mirroring but in fact behaved in ways which directly challenged his grandiosity, Bryan was left with returning to or intensifying his dependence on his parents. This solution, as discussed, was unacceptable owing to the developmental thrust of adolescence; Bryan instead became more immobilized. However, an additional factor—one which I suspect was integral to Bryan's depression—was that his mother was no longer willing to function as a mirroring selfobject for him. Although Mrs. R. made it clear that Bryan continued as her special child, she was increasingly angry and exasperated with him. Her rageful feelings, I believe, stemmed from two primary sources. First, Bryan was not moving his life in the direction of her fantasy of the ideal child. Instead of living out the mother's wishes to have an adolescent who was highly successful both in school and in social relations, Bryan was becoming a clear disappointment to her. Second, she was quite afraid that Bryan would, in a few years, repeat the unfortunate pattern of his brother Herb, who remained an unresolved and serious problem for the parents. The mother's withdrawal of the mirroring responses was perhaps the final and most important element in Bryan's becoming depressed, as it resulted in his feeling abandoned and bereft of the external sources of self-esteem.

My theoretical speculations about Bryan's psychological status hinge, therefore, on several interlocking factors. First, it was clear that Mrs. R. provided many opportunities for Bryan to merge empathetically with her early in life; these mergings were expressed in the mother's mirroring activities, which conveyed her valuing him as a special child. Second, it appears that Mrs. R. was unable or unwilling to provide the optimal frustration experiences described by Kohut and others that facilitate the building of psychic structures. Third, Mr. R. was not available either physically or psychically to offer Bryan the "second chance" for developing appropriate self-esteem by serving as the idealized selfobject, nor could the father serve as a buffer between the mother and son to modulate the mirroring of Bryan's grandiose self. Mr. R. was so angry with both of them that he remained effectively detached and withdrawn, only occasionally revealing some expression of his emotional involvement, which mostly took the form of heavy-handed discipline. Fourth, Bryan became addicted, as Blos put it, to the narcissistic gratification issuing from his mother's mirroring responses. Fifth, his inability to deal with the frustrations and conflicts inherent in adolescent peer relations and his mother's substantial withdrawal of the mirroring responses left him feeling lost and depressed. His psychic resolution, at least for the time I knew him, was to consolidate himself through a forward leap which resulted in the illusion of self-sufficiency (Modell 1976).

I want to stress once again that Bryan in particular and more generally the group of adolescents around whom I have built my hypothesis began the task of the leap forward to a consolidated but rigid identity long before adolescence. As mentioned earlier, these are children who appeared, in many respects, mature, but whose demandingness and other developmental impairments could be safely concealed within the family matrix. Although the primary developmental fixations occur in early childhood experiences, the claims of adolescence are pivotal in moving these narcissistically centered youngsters to crystallize prematurely the identity formation process. The outcome is a pseudo-adult personality structure which closely resembles narcissistic personality disorders of adulthood.

One way in which my hypothesis regarding premature foreclosure on personality development is vulnerable to criticism is that I am reporting on a phenomenon with insufficient follow-up either to substantiate or to refute my assertions. Those who work clinically with adolescents know full well that the therapeutic relationship with them is a highly "fragile alliance" (Meeks 1971). Many adolescent patients, whether or not they are overly narcissistic, discontinue treatment before it is advisable they do so, and therapists are left to speculate about the eventual outcome of both the developmental period and the therapeutic effort. It is precisely because I do not know the adult outcome for Bryan or other young adolescents from whom I developed the ideas set forth in this chapter that I regard my notion as a hypothesis requiring further and more rigorous study, particularly long-term follow-up to provide data regarding adult adjustment.

I also did not address myself to the pervasive problems of aggression evident in this family. The multiple phobias of Mrs. R. and the violent outbursts of Herb and Mr. R. are all indices of poorly managed and unintegrated aggression. In this family environment, separation-individuation also was not adequately fostered, in part because the aggression could not be used in service of differentiation. Thus, Bryan's solution to not deal with his adolescence appears both understandable and, for him, the best available alternative. The long-term problem with his solution, however, was that his centripetal pull toward narcissism appeared too laden with defensive and conflictual elements to provide him with a permanent, adaptive resolution for his personality, one in which ideals and ambitions could be successfully integrated.

I also did not address the issue of treatment. Although nonintensive, analytically oriented psychotherapy utilized with Bryan was effective for the amelioration of the depressive symptoms and the modification of some family interactional patterns, it is clear that no basic personality changes occurred. The question of the type of treatment most suitable for the adolescents I am considering here remains an open one for me, since it was not my purpose in this chapter to discuss the form and structure of the treatment.

Despite these qualifications, I contend that young adolescents such as Bryan are encountered regularly in practice settings and that diagnostic understanding of them is impaired if the theoretical focus is on the nature of the intrapsychic conflicts. In my view the problem is chiefly one of a developmental distortion or failure in the area of the self-experience, with the result being a primary disturbance of the self strikingly similar to Kohut's (1977) description of the narcissistic personality disorder. Moreover, although I have emphasized the early adolescent period as the one in which the developmental distortion of identity foreclosure is manifested, similar outcomes may also occur in childhood, since the essential fixations are rooted in the first years of life.

Conclusions

In this chapter I have presented some theoretical ideas with respect to a concept of identity foreclosure evident in certain young adolescents. Drawing on the works of Kohut, Erikson, Blos, and others, I have asserted that these problematic youngsters reveal a form of psychological disturbance that is best understood as a developmental impairment. This impairment is rooted in early childhood experiences but may become evident in the early adolescent period when the demands for progressive development in the midst of concurrent regressive pulls are high. Despite a good superficial adaptation, these youngsters reveal their prior developmental difficulties in a variety of emotional and behavioral contexts.

These include poor self-esteem regulation, social isolation and withdrawal, poor school performance, a high degree of demandingness and manipulative behavior, poor frustration tolerance, and a generalized inability to utilize affect experiences to further the development of psychological functions.

I hypothesized that the developmental impairment resulted from empathic failures on the part of parents. These failures included an extension of the mirroring responses of the child's infantile grandiosity beyond what may have been helpful, an inability to impose optimal frustration, and the persistence of an illusion, namely, of the child representing an actualization of the perfect child. In other words, I hypothesized that these parents were too involved in providing for the gratification of narcissistic needs in these children. Thus, when a different developmental phase emerged, the parental responses were not likely to promote development of increasingly internalized and differentiated psychological functions in their children.

The youngsters then arrive at adolescence with increased vulnerability to interpersonal and intrapsychic difficulties. They appear to resolve the multiple pressures exerted on them through a maneuver I have termed identity foreclosure, a psychological attempt to preserve narcissistic equilibrium while avoiding the central developmental tasks of adolescence. I illustrated my concept with clinical material and discussed the ways in which the case of Bryan can be understood, arguing that the central issue appeared to be narcissistic impairments rather than intrapsychic conflicts.

The limitations of the clinical material were discussed as these refer to the concept of identity foreclosure. It is clear that long-term follow-up is needed to verify the outcome of youngsters who reveal this type of developmental disturbance. In addition, more systematic study of the presence of the phenomenon would serve to validate the utility of the concept. I believe one of the chief values of the concept of identity foreclosure is that many therapeutic efforts may currently be directed at conflict resolution rather than at the already present narcissistic problems which require different therapeutic strategies.

NOTE

1. As mentioned in the theoretical portion of the chapter, most of the adolescents I have seen who reveal identity foreclosure appear to value their fantasy life more highly than actual peer relationships. Although

Bryan claimed he had no fantasies or dreams, his assertion was made in a defensive way. I believe that my attempts to elicit the fantasies he may have had were technical errors that blocked his being able to share his fantasy life at that time, or that his fantasy life remained repressed. In any event, Bryan was not able to let me know what his fantasies were during the time we worked together. Other youngsters I have seen who reveal identity foreclosure described active, highly elaborated fantasies stimulated by comic books or science fiction novels. Although the process of indulging in fantasy in adolescents is usual enough, what is different in the youngsters I am discussing is the amount of time devoted to it and the function it serves of primary gratification and defensive avoidance of real relationships.

REFERENCES

American Psychiatric Association. 1980. *Diagnostic and Statistical Manual of Mental Disorders*. 3d ed. Washington, D.C.: APA.

Blos, P. 1967. The second individuation of adolescence. *Psychoanalytic Study of the Child* 22:162–186.

Blos, P. 1979. The overappreciated child. In *The Adolescent Passage*. New York: International Universities Press.

Erikson, E. 1968. *Identity, Youth and Crisis*. New York: Norton.

Goldberg, A. 1980. *Advances in Self Psychology*. New York: International Universities Press.

Kernberg, O. 1970. Factors in the psychoanalytic treatment of narcissistic personalities. *Journal of the American Psychoanalytic Association* 18:51–85.

Kernberg, O. 1975. *Borderline Conditions and Pathological Narcissism*. New York: Aronson.

Kohut, H. 1968. The psychoanalytic treatment of narcissistic personality disorder: outline of a systematic approach. *Psychoanalytic Study of the Child* 23:86–113.

Kohut, H. 1972. Thoughts on narcissism and narcissistic rage. *Psychoanalytic Study of the Child* 27:360–400.

Kohut, H. 1977. *The Restoration of the Self*. New York: International Universities Press.

Meeks, J. 1971. *The Fragile Alliance*. Melbourne, Fla.: Krieger.

Modell, A. 1976. The "holding environment" and the therapeutic action of psychoanalysis. *Journal of the American Psychoanalytic Association* 24(2):285–307.

Winnicott, D. W. 1965. The true and the false self. In *The Maturational Processes and the Facilitating Environment*. New York: International Universities Press.

12 THE ADOLESCENT, SCHOOLS, AND SCHOOLING

IRVING H. BERKOVITZ

Schooling and relationships in schools are a crucial influence in the growth and development of young people, second only to the influence of the family. In all, more than 15,000 hours of a person's lifetime are spent in the twelve grades of early school experience.

In the United States, the adolescent years (from age eleven) are spent in junior high school (grades six to nine), senior high school (grades nine through twelve), and college. By junior high school, however, many attitudes toward family, school authorities, and self have been formed but, fortunately, not entirely foreclosed. Significant positive changes can still occur, even in disturbed adolescents and their families. Ameliorating influences can be provided by interested and caring school personnel, resulting in new feelings of mastery and self-esteem from success in learning, new friends made in school, and pride in the development of new skills.

A psychotherapist who is aware of the potentials of the school experience can help a troubled young person and his or her family to optimize the constructive contribution of school to development. There are many skilled, conscientious, caring educators in the public and private schools who can be enlisted to help in the growth and even the therapy of young people through a supportive, facilitating relationship with the therapist (Ekstein and Motto 1960; Rutter 1975). In this chapter I shall describe some of the steps families and therapists may be able to take to assist young people in schools—whether they are in therapy or not. A vast literature is available on mental health consultation techniques and ex-

0-226-24058-4/85/0012-0033$01.00

periences with school personnel (Berkovitz 1980b; Berlin 1974; Caplan 1970). Some of these concepts will be a part of the discussions here.

In school, children learn to form satisfying and ego-enhancing relationships with nurturant adults who are not parents or otherwise related. Children also learn to relate to a new and larger group of peers, expanding and strengthening skills in interpersonal relating such as trust, sharing, reciprocating, accepting disappointment, and making new friends. Most schools deemphasize or ignore the affective part of child development and school experience. Understandably and appropriately, school personnel place a major emphasis on encouragement of cognitive acquisition of basic information and development of learning skills and work habits (Berkovitz 1980b).

Many professionals feel that one of the contributants to current adolescent difficulty in Western civilization is the loss of the extended family. Miller (1970) states that "disruption of a relationship with parents results also in the disruption with other significant adults. In this hiatus, school systems especially, but not exclusively, are organizations of society that could provide adolescents with contexts in which they could continue to grow."

Many would argue that schools are places to learn the three R's and that placing importance on relationships distracts from that goal. Nonetheless, young people learn about relationships in school from the informal curriculum, namely, from the way the teacher and other personnel treat them (and vice versa) and the ways that peers treat each other. Some attempts have been made to include consideration of relationships in the formal curriculum or even to allow ad hoc discussions during class time. Some teachers are able to tolerate periods of free discussion in the classroom without loss of control or lessened attention to curriculum subject matter. The younger adolescent in junior high school, for example, especially appreciates discussion with peers. Rarely does a curriculum or crowded school day provide an opportunity. Most adults regard this kind of open discussion by young teenagers as silly, a waste of time, and unnecessary. However, this is the context in which the young teenager learns and practices many interpersonal techniques. Hours spent on the telephone with peers, for example, are important to such development.

Very often, skilled teachers can engage students in animated, involved discussion of historical events, poetry, drama, science, and art. This can mobilize the young person's emotions in such a way that catharsis, sublimation, insight, and rearrangement of constricted, distorted emotional patterns can improve future development. Some secondary schools provide a curriculum where males especially can engage in child care in affiliated nursery schools or take cooking classes. These activities have been thought to help reduce some violent, aggressive directions for these males.

Some schools provide community opportunities in city council offices, veterinary hospitals, museums, and so forth, where the high school student can begin to test career choices as well as entry into community responsibilities and increased self-respect. The discomfort with self, peers, and adults is acute in the young teenager. Action and movement are frequent forms of expression and defense. Clubs, special-interest groups, athletic activities, visits to community facilities, and recreation can absorb some of the energy and facilitate development in 70–80 percent of adolescents in schools. The other 20–30 percent (Offer and Offer 1975) will need special support and facilities. The junior high school postpubertal years are crucial to many youngsters. The difficulties in these years may be presaged even in fifth and sixth grades, ages ten to twelve, or earlier.

Clinical Case Management in Schools

Certainly all of the DSM III clinical syndromes can be found in students in junior and senior high school classes. However, three behavioral descriptive categories—the aggressive, defiant adolescent, the depressive and/or apathetic adolescent, and the learning-disordered adolescent—will be considered. Aggressive, defiant adolescents are among the most difficult for educators (and, indeed, mental health professionals) to help. These are the young persons identified in most longitudinal studies as most at risk for adult psychopathology (Robins 1966). However, adolescents usually do not intend serious defiance but can be testing new assertive skills, fighting against depression or personality disorganization, currying favor with peers, or serving other developmental purposes. It is difficult, at times, for teachers to distinguish these motivations, and, in addition, the need for control in the classroom often outweighs diagnostic considerations. Some educator reactions can at times reinforce aggressive patterns. I do not mean to overlook the fact that some teenagers have familial problems and can be seriously disturbed, possibly even dangerous. But sometimes a teacher is oversensitive in reacting to some less serious aggression from a student. Control techniques are often necessary, and teachers do not receive sufficient training in these. In recent years consultants have been employed more often by school districts to teach classroom management skills (Canter 1976; Jones and Eimers 1975).

ADOLESCENT ANGER

At times, aggression is provoked, knowingly or unknowingly, by subtle or overt negative remarks and attitudes from teachers who are having normal crises. Unfortunately, there are some teachers who are disgruntled or disillusioned. Occasionally an outburst by an impulsive teenager can precipitate an overreaction from a tense school person. For example, the following occurred in one school:

> Gail comes storming down the hall in school yelling that someone has stolen her Parker pen. The language is unbearable. A teacher stops her and starts to shout at her about her language. They both yell at each other for a short period of time. Students gather. The teacher grabs the student by the arm to take her to the office. Gail resists, calling the teacher names. In fact she attempts to hit the teacher and finally does. Other teachers join in and they take the girl to the office. The principal, hearing the story, suspends the girl because of her language and because she struck the teacher. Parents, teachers union, civil rights leaders, etc., enter the situation until finally she (the student) is reinstated. [DeCecco and Richards 1974, p. 118]

If one is treating an angry young person who has problems of aggression that manifest themselves in the school situation, collaboration or at least contact with the school personnel may be desirable and helpful to reduce retaliatory reactions. The level of violence in some secondary schools, especially in the inner city, has been of concern to many educators, law enforcement authorities, parents, and teenagers. Security guards, locked campuses, and alarm systems constitute a regular component of many schools. Learning is often rendered more difficult, teachers are too tense, student trust of each other is reduced, and racial tensions are exacerbated. However, some administrators and staffs have been able to maintain a more open and peaceful atmosphere than others under such conditions, suggesting that it is more than the student body alone that contributes to this campus condition. A study of twelve high schools in London determined that an "ethos" created by conscientious attention to the educational task and respect for the students could improve the educational achievements of high school students (Rutter, Maughan, Mortimore, and Ouston 1979).

SEXUAL ENERGY

Aggressive potential is a threat often felt by adults dealing with teenagers. Equally threatening is the new sexual energy. The adolescent sexual awakening presses the need for a comfortable and confident integration of these new abilities into self-identity. Unfortunately, the need for more education and frank open discussion of these events with the chance to receive helpful information is not always fulfilled in the public and private schools. School boards often fear criticism from more moralistic parts of the community, although some health classes in junior and senior high schools do provide open, useful discussion opportunities.

The rise in the number of adolescent pregnancies and the level of venereal disease make this need imperative. In one rural high school of only 250 students, it was impressive to see how mental health professionals from a nearby community mental health center were allowed to teach a full year's course in preventive mental health. The course stressed communication skills felt to be essential to establish a healthy family atmosphere and problem-solving techniques for dealing with predictable life challenges in adult life, such as marriage, birth, and death; debilitating physical or mental illness; and threats to the ability to provide adequately the material needs of a family (Dunlap and Porter 1978). This model can be duplicated readily, and school personnel could teach it if given freedom and support to do so.

MUSCULAR ENERGY

Physical activity, especially in sports, is very important to adolescents as a discharge of hormonal and muscular energy, for development of feelings of control and command of the body, and for other interpersonal aspects of peer relations, such as self-esteem, peer approval, and competitive pleasure. Schools offer opportunities to fulfill these needs in physical education classes and team competition.

The young person's relations with coaches or physical education teachers can be a source of positive self-image building or adding to negative identity. Coaches can be helpful mentors to some. Unfortunately, some are overburdened with the need to produce a winning team rather than to provide a constructive experience for the individual students. The team experience has also been identified as a model for later skills in group activities in business and industry, especially for men, but it has been less available to women (Sheehy 1976).

The school spirit and enthusiasm involved in athletic programs are described by some as distracting from necessary academic emphasis. Yet this group participation can be seen to represent as well a progression from individual narcissism to group narcissism, reducing feelings of alienation for many young persons. Each school, it is hoped, will be providing equal opportunity and appreciation for academic excellence through theatrical productions, newspaper and magazine publications, debating clubs, and school government. Thus, a balanced set of options can be available for students with varying needs and skills. Valuable growth experiences can occur in each of these activities even for very conflicted young people trying to heal themselves or find a respected identity.

In the consideration of the therapy for an angry defiant youth, close communication between the therapist and school personnel is desirable to avoid possible countertherapeutic disciplinary action, suspension, or angry conflict. The average large secondary school, with thirty to fifty students per classroom and five to six periods per day, may be inappropriate for and damaging to some disturbed young persons. Most young people can meet the challenge and even be strengthened by it, but some with serious pathology cannot. For these students, there are remedial units in most school systems—or a therapeutic program may be necessary.

INTERVENTION STEPS

Before considering remedial efforts, one should consider the steps that can be taken in the regular school milieu when the child is showing disturbance and enters therapy. There are a variety of helpful relationships that often can be arranged with teachers, counselors, school psychologists, nurses, and/or principals if these personnel are receptive and if the therapist is knowledgeable in working with school personnel. Occasionally, parents can be informants for the therapist about the skill and sensitivity of particular school personnel. However, parental reports need to be accepted with caution since an adversarial relationship may have already become entrenched between the parents and the teachers, with each blaming the other for the young person's problems and failures in school.

Communication difficulties between clinical and school personnel are frequent. "The report of the clinic is often couched in psychiatric jargon and it is extremely difficult for the teacher to understand its implications for the educational setting. In addition, the same term may have a different meaning for clinic and school when applied to a specific child. For example, the clinic's recommendation for 'individualized attention' may mean an approach to the child that takes into account any special problems and vulnerabilities. The school, however, may have referred this child to begin with because he was demanding 'excessive' individualized attention from the teacher" (Chess and Hassibi 1978).

A face-to-face discussion with the involved school personnel is preferable to a letter or a phone conversation, but this may not always be possible. Some parents, and even some insurance companies, are willing to pay for such meetings as a part of the proper treatment of the young person. In such a meeting, one must be careful to reveal only necessary data, since educators may not receive the same training about the need for confidentiality as do mental health professionals. Hearing from school personnel about the student's behavior can be valuable, since the data are not always communicated fully by the adolescent. Of course, the adolescent has to be willing that the meeting occur, since many fear that everyone in the school will soon know that they are "weird and seeing a shrink." Occasionally these fears do have some justification, but, more often, they are part of the shame the adolescent feels in needing therapy. At times, seemingly deviant behavior does contain creative, innovative energies, and parental or school demand for compliance has to be examined from a neutral, unbiased point of view.

Talking with the teacher can effect some change in the teacher, encouraging a greater sympathy for, acceptance of, tolerance of, or interest in a particular student. Occasionally, but less often, there may be stigmatizing, oversolicitousness, or even hostility created by the intervention of a therapist. It is often hard to predict which of these reactions is likely to occur. In secondary schools, the young person has many teachers. Possibly a nurse, a counselor, or a homeroom teacher does become a more available, dependable key relation. Discussion with one or all of these personnel could be helpful at times but may be difficult to arrange. A cooperative administrator can be useful in bringing this about. The principal (or at times a vice-principal) is the key figure in the school who can exert significant influence. This administrator may be very willing to facilitate helpful relationships for the therapist. When cooperation at the school is lacking, there are times when the parents or even the therapist may be able to complain at the central office of the school district. Such intercession can be for the purpose of changing attitudes or transferring the student to a more receptive class or school. This is rarely necessary, but it is a last resort.

One of the helpful modalities available in some schools is group counseling, especially if this is being conducted sensitively by a knowledgeable school person (Berkovitz 1975). It is hard to predict the value of any particular group in a particular school unless one knows that school and group, has visited it, or has a reliable informant who is aware of what is going on there. Occasionally one may talk with the counselor or other person conducting the group and in that way make some assessment of the possible value of the group. This type of group dialogue between adolescents and adults usually allows for the maturing influence of input from a sensitive, trusted adult.

Evaluation of twenty counseling groups in junior and senior high schools showed a 58–61 percent improvement, rising to 84 percent with more frequent attendance. The most difficult problem area proved to be acting-out, impulse-ridden, and/or antisocial behavior. Surprisingly, 71.8 percent of the students were judged improved in family problems as well as in school-centered problems (Kaplan 1975). Clinicians should be aware of school groups, especially if teenagers they are treating are involved in group programs. Often this involvement may obviate the need for therapy in some or assist ongoing therapy in others.

As therapy progresses, and significant anxieties or conflicts with parents are modified, parts of the conflict displaced to school personnel may be eased as well. Sometimes this conflict is too far advanced to be modified in the therapy. For example, Mike, a thirteen-year-old eighth grader, was finishing his first year in a private, academically oriented junior-senior high school. He had been defiant, belligerent, and oppositional at home and in school for two years prior to and for a period after entering therapy. By May he had begun to limit his provocative behavior, improve his academic performance, and form long-range goals. Most of his teachers noted the progress and felt he should continue in the school. Unfortunately, the principal was less positive and insisted on his dismissal. The therapist had not intervened at the school directly but did counsel the parents to speak up for their son. Subsequent work in therapy was needed to reduce this boy's feelings of failure, anger, and sadness.

Therapeutic School Units

The array of therapeutic modalities used in any particular school system may vary in different school districts. For example, many schools have a weekly case conference called by various names, such as guidance committee or student assessment team (S.A.T.). In this particular meeting, there can be a discussion of an individual student's problems and needs. Usually the teacher, the school psychologist, and sometimes the nurse, the principal, the vice-principal, or the counselor attends these meetings. When there is also a mental health consultant from outside the school system participating regularly in this conference, it seems to encourage more effective functioning. In this meeting, decisions are often made for referrals, additional tests, special programs, and so forth.

For students who are recommended for placement in special education classes, especially under Public Law 94-142 (1975), an individualized education plan (I.E.P.) emerges. The I.E.P. describes the educational and behavioral goals for that particular student for the school year. By law, assessment of progress has to be repeated at the end of the year. Usually the I.E.P. has to be signed by the parents as well as by the school personnel. The parent is allowed to bring a mental health professional or other expert to the meeting. If there is a controversy about whether the school can provide the kind of milieu and education that the particular student needs, there can be a fair hearing where it will be decided whether the school is required to pay for outside schooling.

Most schools will resist the pressure to pay for the adolescent's attending a nonpublic school, since this has become a serious burden in many school budgets. As a result of this pressure, many school systems have created special classes for smaller groups of pupils within the schools in order to work with these more disturbed students.

There are other school programs which may assist students having difficulties. Peer-counseling programs exist in some secondary schools. In these programs, a trained older student, possibly in grade eleven or twelve, will be available to counsel younger students in grades six to ten. This is more than simply a "buddy" system, since the peer counselor has been taught interview techniques, some knowledge of symptomatology, and referral opportunities. The peer counselors themselves often receive a valuable therapeutic experience from this particular role and the training they have taken. Many go on into careers in mental health.

In some secondary schools, especially high schools, suicide prevention has been taught in health classes by mental health professionals from a suicide prevention center (Ross 1983).[1] It has been interesting to learn from some of these classes that 63 percent of students knew someone who threatened to attempted suicide and 10–15 percent had themselves attempted suicide. Several students confided suicidal plans and were able to accept help. The opportunity to discuss suicidal feelings and thoughts seemed to be of great value to most of the students. Postvention programs often are also useful to reduce survivor guilt and to avoid the contagion effect that may occur after a suicide.

In 1983, a pioneer piece of legislation was passed in California mandating that the Department of Education encourage suicide prevention programs in the secondary schools—in collaboration with local suicide prevention centers, where possible.

Besides the teacher, counselor, school psychologist, and principal available to intervene for better mental health of adolescents, there is also the nurse. Fiscal stringencies are causing schools to reduce the numbers of nurses, but many are still present—and overworked. "The nurse can work with the administration and teachers in integrating mental health concepts into the curriculum. The nurse can emphasize to teachers their role as observers, listeners, and promoters of health in children through classroom activities" (Blomquist 1974) and perform individual and group counseling (Elkin 1975).

Another level of secondary school structure where depressed, apathetic, or at times aggressive defiant young persons can be helped is the continuation high school. Here the students work individually or in small groups. They attend school for a shorter day and meet in a building near but usually separate from the large high school. In California, there are about 100,000 students in continuation high schools, about 2 percent of the school population. These students may not have adjusted to large high school classes. They often do better in the smaller continuation setting where there may be only one or two teachers and only ten to fifteen students per class (Berkovitz 1984). Some students also attend because they wish or need to be employed rather than attend school a full day.

Some continuation high schools include group counseling and family counseling (Evans, Johnson, and Thomson 1975). There is an attempt to reconnect these isolated, failure-oriented, disruptive, or apathetic students and develop better verbal communication with teachers, peers, and parents. Some schools, unfortunately, simply keep students to the legal age and do not strive for improved communication. Other schools strive ingeniously to reestablish family-school–young person communication. For many students, these schools represent the last contact with any kind of organized assistance or, for that matter, hopefulness about their futures. The better schools do convey an attitude that there is hope and that there is a good chance to reverse a previously negative pattern of behavior or thinking (Berkovitz 1984).

Yet another continuation-type school unit showing the efforts of a school district to provide a therapeutic milieu especially for the aggressive, defiant student is called a community-centered classroom (Tri-C) (1980). This is for students expelled from regular classes because of illegal actions. Classes usually contain eight to ten students and may be located in a church, synagogue, boys' club, or other appropriate community location. Teacher, aide, part-time counselor, and nurse provide individualized education, group counseling, and family intervention.

Education for pregnant adolescents is provided in many districts in special classes or schools apart from the other students. In 1970 only one-third of the school systems in the United States provided continuing education for school-age pregnant women. This number has probably increased. In many districts which provide continuing education of pregnant women, the quality of the education and the benefits of a small group experience are greater during the pregnancy period than after delivery ("Pregnant Teenagers" 1970). Some districts provide infant care and parenting education for adolescent mothers so that they can continue their education.

The effect of schools on the development of the female adolescent deserves special mention. Schools have usually reinforced the narrow role stereotypes for women prevalent in the larger society. In the United States, the Higher Education Act, Title IX of 1972, prompted many districts to change materials and programs relating to stereotypes and practices affecting female students. Since the passage of that act, for example, more adolescent girls are allowed to take industrial arts classes and shop rather than only home economics. However, restrictive stereotypes still occur in peer group and faculty attitudes, textbooks, tests, and counseling assistance. These stereotypes often involve a view of the female as passive, submissive, less assertive, less competitive, pleasing others more than self, less active physically, often less capable than males generally but especially in math, science, and technical subjects. In addition, vocationally, women are often depicted as mothers, nurses, secretaries, and teachers rather than in a wider range of occupations. Often some of these stereotypes are related to and reinforced by what seems required to obtain a man's regard and companionship (Berkovitz 1979).

It is important to consider the role of the school for adolescents exposed to divorce in their families. With many a teenager, school was useful because it provided structure at a time when the major structure of his life, the family, was crumbling. Going to school daily, being required to perform certain tasks in and out of school, and having routine social contacts assist a child in his adaptations to divorce. Wallerstein and Kelly (1980) found that school served as a good support system, particularly for those children who were of above average intelligence and psychologically healthy. Although this was not necessarily dependent on the teacher's being a supportive figure, a good relationship was helpful. Some older boys no longer seeing their fathers turned to extended family, a teacher, or school as a source of support.

Some schools provide programs to reduce alcohol, drug abuse, and cigarette smoking in students. Mental health professionals, even as volunteers, can be very helpful. It is becoming apparent that such programs—especially for drug abuse—need to start earlier in the child's school career, perhaps in the earliest grades.

Special Education

Other remedial units and personnel in secondary schools provide services in resource specialist programs, classes for the educationally handicapped, learning handicapped, and severely emotionally disturbed. In most school districts, about 10 percent of the student body require special education facilities. This group has various problems, including deafness or impaired hearing, blindness or partial sightedness, cerebral palsy, autism, orthopedic handicaps, mental retardation, emotional disturbance, and psychosomatic illnesses such as asthma, anorexia, or obesity.

When treating a disabled adolescent, the therapist will often find a group of trained and dedicated school personnel in well-equipped remedial schools and classes. The higher adult-to-student ratio can usually allow for more responsive collaboration with the therapist as well. Work with families is also often a part of the school's program.

Smaller school districts (fewer than twenty schools) often form a group with other districts to share facilities and expenses for educating the disabled. In many districts, a student can continue in the school program until age twenty-one if necessary. Occupational centers and, recently, some colleges have programs for learning-disabled students. In urban school districts, the larger numbers of disabled allow special schools for each of the problems. Recent efforts at mainstreaming have led to a greater return of some handicapped students to regular classes. While this has helped many to feel less isolated from nonhandicapped peers, in some cases it has removed a necessary protective milieu. Teachers in regular classes do not always receive the extra assistance needed for optimum mainstreaming of students.

Space does not permit description of the various programs and classes for adolescents with special needs. Two programs, however, do deserve mention since they are new with P.L. 94-142. One is the resource specialist and his or her classroom. This is usually a special education teacher assisted by an aide and a school psychologist. They function as a special team, with a room to which handicapped students, including the emotionally disturbed, may be assigned for part of the day, returning to their other classes for the rest of the day. In this resource room, help with certain subjects may be given, as well as individual and group counseling. The student, thus, is provided with a more supportive base of operations in school.

Another new program is the class for severely emotionally disturbed students (S.E.D.). Some of these students are those who formerly would have been placed in nonpublic facilities at school district expense. These classes may contain only six to eight students, a teacher, an aide, and occasionally a psychiatric or psychological consultant. In this smaller unit, education in a therapeutic socializing setting may be more possible than in other units described. Not all teachers are able to use the group potentials equally but concentrate instead on the individual goals. The clinician can often provide useful support and intervention for patients in these classes, and a cooperative relationship can be established with school personnel.

Conclusions

Knowledge of various special programs and options in the school setting can be valuable to therapists in their work with adolescents. One may be better able to negotiate with school personnel, make suggestions to parents, and, in some cases, avoid the necessity for private-school placement. It is very important that adolescents remain involved in education while undergoing psychotherapy. In some districts, home teachers are available for those adolescents who need to remain at home and are unable to attend school for a period of time. Most hospital programs for teenagers have school units available as part of the program.

This brief overview of an important part of an adolescent's life and development emphasizes that the quality of self-esteem, hope for the future, coping abilities, and peer relations are significantly enhanced or diminished by relations with peers and adults in the years of schooling.

NOTE

This chapter is based on "The Adolescent and the Schools" from the series *Clinical Update of Adolescent Psychiatry* (Princeton, N.J.: Nassau Publications, 1983–1984), which is sponsored by the American Society for Adolescent Psychiatry.

1. M. Peck, "Youth Suicide: The Role of School Consultation" (unpublished).

REFERENCES

Berkovitz, I. H., ed. 1975. *When Schools Care: Creative Use of Groups in Secondary Schools.* New York: Brunner/Mazel.

Berkovitz, I. H. 1979. Effects of secondary school experiences on adolescent female development. In M. Sugar, ed. *Female Adolescent Development.* New York: Brunner/Mazel.

Berkovitz, I. H. 1980a. Improving the relevance of secondary education for adolescent developmental tasks. In M. Sugar, ed. *Responding to Adolescent Needs.* New York: Spectrum.

Berkovitz, I. H. 1980b. School interventions: case management and school mental health consultation. In G. P. Sholevar, R. M. Benson, B. J. Blinder, eds. *Treatment of Emotional Disorders in Children and Adolescents.* New York: Medical and Scientific Books.

Berkovitz, I. H. 1984. The role of schools in child, adolescent and youth suicide prevention. *Adolescent Suicide.* M. Peck, N. Farberow, and R. E. Litman, eds. New York: Springer.

Berlin, I. N. 1974. Mental health programs in the schools. In S. Arieti, ed. *American Handbook of Psychiatry.* 2d ed. New York: Basic.

Blomquist, K. R. 1974. Nurse, I need help. *Journal of Psychiatric Nursing and Mental Health Services,* pp. 22–26.

Canter, L. 1976. *Assertive Discipline.* Los Angeles: Lee Canter.

Caplan, G. 1970. *The Theory and Practice of Mental Healthy Consultation.* New York: Basic.

Chess, S., and M. Hassibi. 1978. *Principles and Practices of Child Psychiatry.* New York and London: Plenum.

Community Centered Classroom Program. 1980. Publication No. 382. Research and Evaluation Branch, Los Angeles Unified School District, October.

De Cecco, J. P., and Richards, A. K. 1974. *Growing Pains, Uses of School Conflict*. New York: Aberdeen.

Dunlap, D. A., and Porter, D. 1978. *The School Consultant as Teacher*. Presented at the Fifty-fifth Annual Meeting, American Orthopsychiatric Association, San Francisco.

Ekstein, R., and Motto, R. L. 1960. The borderline child in the school situation. In M. G. Guttsegen and G. B. Guttsegen, eds. *Professional School Psychology*. New York and London: Grune & Stratton.

Elkin, M. 1975. The school nurse organizes a group counseling program in a high school. In Berkovitz 1975.

Evans, A.; Johnson, M. A.; and Thomson, M. 1975. An administrator team as group counselors to an opportunity class. In Berkovitz 1975.

Jones, F. H., and Eimers, R. C. 1975. Role playing to train elementary teachers to use a classroom management "skill package." *Journal of Applied Behavior Analysis* 8:421–433.

Kaplan, C. 1975. Evaluation: twenty-seven agency-school counseling groups in junior and senior high schools. In Berkovitz 1975.

Kellam, S. G.; Branch, J. D.; Brown, C. H.; and Russell, G. 1981. Why teenagers come for treatment. *Journal of the American Academy of Child Psychiatry* 20:477–495.

Miller, D. 1970. Adolescents and the high school system. *Community Mental Health Journal* 6:483–491.

Offer, D., and Offer, J. D. 1975. *From Teenage to Young Manhood*. New York: Basic.

Pregnant Teenagers. 1970. *Today's Education* 59(7):26–29.

Public Law 94-142. 1975. Education of all handicapped.

Robins, L. N. 1966. *Deviant Children Grown Up*. Baltimore: Williams & Wilkins.

Ross, C. P. 1983, Teaching children the facts of life and death: suicide prevention in the schools." In H. Sudak, ed. *Suicide in Children and Adolescents*. London: Wright (in press).

Rutter, M. 1975. *Helping Troubled Children*. New York and London: Plenum.

Rutter, M.; Maughan, B.; Mortimore, P.; and Ouston, J. 1979. *Fifteen Thousand Hours*. Cambridge, Mass.: Harvard University Press.

Sheehy, G. 1976. *Passages*. New York: Dutton.

Wallerstein, J. S., and Kelly, J. B. 1980. *Surviving the Breakup*. New York: Basic.

13 LEARNING DISABILITIES AND ADOLESCENCE: DEVELOPMENTAL CONSIDERATIONS

JONATHAN COHEN

Clinicians and educators have long been concerned about the psychodynamic causes for and implications of learning problems. This has been a productive exploration, revealing that psychogenic factors often inhibit ego functioning and the process of learning. Many children and adolescents, however, have difficulty learning owing to specific cognitive deficits. These learning disabilities are neuropsychologically based deficits that interfere with reception (e.g., perception), integration (e.g., sensory processing and synthesis), remembering (e.g., memory), and/or expression of information. They are considered bodily rooted events that adversely affect the operation of one or more aspects of autonomous ego functioning.

Perhaps 10 percent to 15 percent of the school population are learning disabled (Brown 1978). Ochroch (1981) noted that learning-disabled children are more vulnerable to emotional disturbances. Although there are many children with learning problems who are not learning disabled, there are virtually no learning-disabled children or adolescents who do not evidence significant psychological conflicts and concerns.

Learning and the process of adaptation involve a reciprocal relationship among constitutional givens, ego functioning, and the environment. Although Hartmann (1939) suggested that the examination of specific maturationally or biologically based ego deficits provides a useful opportunity to further understand ego development, psychoanalytic investigations

0-226-24058-4/85/0012-0025$01.00

have tended to focus on how conflict alone interferes with the learning process. Comprehensive studies that seek to understand the developmental interrelationships between psychological and neuropsychological factors in learning-disabled children have been rare (Blanchard 1946; DeHirsch 1975; Liss 1955; Pearson 1952; Rothstein 1982; Silver 1974; Weil 1970, 1971, 1977, 1978), with virtually no investigations in learning-disabled adolescents.

Historically, it was believed that high achievers could not be learning disabled. Even when there was a history of learning disabilities, it was assumed that they would not significantly affect secondary and postsecondary learning or work. Recently, however, Bellak (1979), Clark (1981), Cruickshank, Morse, and Johns (1980), Kline and Kline (1975), Rudel (1981), and Rutter (1978) reported that specific cognitive deficits usually do not disappear with age. In fact, they affect learning and psychological development during adolescence and beyond.

Past discussions about psychological ramifications of being learning disabled in adolescence have tended to emphasize reactive change in the adolescents' self-concept and self-esteem. Learning disabilities induce frustration and failure that in turn contribute to a poor self-image and low self-esteem (Palombo 1979; Rome 1971). However, I believe this is a limited and limiting perspective.

The experience of being learning disabled inevitably becomes interwoven with other concerns, conflicts, interests, strengths, weaknesses, wishes, and adaptive strategies. Over time, it becomes more and more difficult to distinguish the neuropsychological from the psychological and the reactive aspects of the person from the characterological.

Methods of Study

The present report is based on fifteen high school and college students who ranged in age from sixteen to twenty-one years. Twelve were male, three were female. All were of at least average intelligence; eleven were in the high average or superior range of intellectual functioning.

Eleven students received comprehensive neuropsychological diagnostic evaluations (Cohen 1983) during the study. The other four students had a history strongly suggestive of learning disabilities; three had been tested and diagnosed in childhood.

I worked in psychotherapy with six Columbia College students (ranging in time from briefly to an extended period). Four of the other students were seen in consultation and later received neuropsychological evaluations. I treated the other five psychotherapeutically for from three months to four years. Seven students had no idea that they were learning disabled.

In my evaluations and reevaluations of these students, I have attempted to compare them with a roughly similar group of fifteen non-learning-disabled middle and late adolescents I have seen who were struggling with roughly comparable types of work, learning, or social difficulties. I have done this to aid my attempt to understand, clinically and systematically, the unique developmental ramifications of learning disabilities. However, the present investigation is certainly not a controlled experiment but, rather, an analysis designed to generate a series of hypotheses or proposals.

PROBLEMS OF WORK AND LEARNING

The nature of work and learning becomes more complex and demanding, academically and psychologically, for the middle and late adolescent. More work is assigned, and pressure to do it well increases concomitantly as a result of competitive concerns about getting into college and developing a work identity. In addition, students are required increasingly to work without close supervision and support from parents and teachers.

The learning-disabled adolescents showed two particular configurations of problems with work and learning: (1) problems owing to the cognitive disability itself and (2) problems owing to psychological factors that are directly and/or indirectly related to being learning disabled.

There are many subtle and striking ways in which learning disabilities interfere with learning and work in the middle and late adolescent student. Depending on the type of disability, reading speed may be significantly slowed and result in students' having to spend two or three times as much time on home reading assignments. Reading comprehension may be adversely affected, again slowing the reading process. Learning new languages (whether foreign, computer, or science) can be an onerous task for learning-disabled adolescents. The same cognitive disability that interfered with learning to read in childhood may interfere with learning to read French. And writing or mathematical work may be significantly complicated by cognitive deficits in adolescence (see Cohen [1983] for a more comprehensive review of these issues).

The psychological implications of being learning disabled adversely affect the following work-related processes: (1) working in an increasingly independent manner; (2) defining what they (rather than what parents or teachers) want to study; and (3) being able to compete without undue anxiety.

Long-standing and frequently hidden concerns about being inadequate were accentuated by working alone and with less external support. The fact that these concerns were usually hidden only exacerbated the students' anxiety, for they feared that now they would be "found out to be a dummy and damaged." Commonly, these concerns joined with the more central developmental task of defining and coming to terms with one's strengths and weaknesses. All learning-disabled students attempt to discover and use strategies that allow them to circumvent the area of disability. A surprisingly high number of the students studied attempted to compensate by utilizing avoidance strategies (including plagiarism).

Self-doubts about academic capabilities typically resulted in considerable confusion about intellectual and career aspirations. This question becomes particularly important in college and constitutes a central psychosocial task. To answer this question successfully a student must have begun to realistically assess his or her strengths and weaknesses and develop a belief that one can be competent, effective, and an active agent.

In the following discussion of the more internal, and often unconscious, experience of being a learning-disabled adolescent, it will be seen how concerns about themselves and others interfere with a realistic assessment of strengths, weaknesses, and interests. Often their emotional lives and experiences of self-doubt also inhibit adolescents in the naturally competitive arena of school. This is potentially debilitating because adolescents need to clarify what they want to study and then be able to produce and compete academically (Medalie 1981).

AFFECTS: DISTRESS AND DEPRESSION

The learning-disabled adolescents evidenced two major affective configurations: (1) an unusually high propensity to experience distress and anxiety; and (2) a low-level, chronic depression. These affective characteristics were uniquely interwoven into the larger fabric of each adolescent's personality.

The learning-disabled adolescents showed a great tendency to experience distress and anxiety. These feelings of suffering and the unpleasant anticipation of calamity were related both to internal concerns alone and to a combination of internal and external concerns. The majority of their concerns related to feeling "not good enough" and "damaged." These concerns were sometimes projected onto the external world, for example, as fears about what others would think of them. Many adolescents imagined that if others knew how "inadequate and damaged" they were, they would lose their love. Performance, academic and otherwise, was typically perceived as a danger situation—one in which they would humiliate themselves, fail, and be helpless. However, their high propensity to become distressed and anxious extended beyond performance situations. This experience may very well reinforce the belief that avoidance is a necessary anxiety-reducing strategy, despite the fact that it is usually a non-adaptive psychosocial strategy in the long run.

Learning disabilities result, to a greater or lesser extent, in moments of helplessness and confusion and feelings of humiliation and failure. These moments are repeated but cannot be predicted or anticipated because of the intermittent nature[1] of most mild to moderately severe learning disabilities. Their unpredictable nature can only underscore the person's experience of helplessness and, as a result, suffering and the anxious anticipation of failure and humiliation.

Virtually all of the learning-disabled adolescents also evidenced a chronic, low-level depression. Sad feelings related to loss seemed to be an integral and long-standing aspect of their characteristic ways of thinking about themselves. Specifically, their sense of loss was related to the feeling that they had lost a valued part of themselves. Often (but not always) this sense of loss was related to part of their "head/brain."

Although almost all the learning-disabled adolescents experienced a somewhat depressing conscious sense that their expectations of themselves were higher than their actual achievement (a sense of low self-esteem), these feelings, to a large extent, characterized both the learning-disabled and non-learning-disabled adolescents studied. For these students, adolescence is a period of turmoil and of often painful evaluation of oneself (expectations, wishes, dreams, and actual performance). The sad feelings that there is a discrepancy between what one "is" and what one "ought" to be were not unique to the learning-disabled adolescents. However, a low-level, chronic depression and the fantasy that they had lost a valued part of themselves were common.

It was initially assumed that this fantasy of having lost a valued part of self would be related to castration anxiety. Several adolescents did evidence castration anxiety and/or a related sense of loss in their dreams, in slips of the tongue, and on projective test material. In addition, a number of the adolescents evidenced narcissistic concerns about genital potency, which is often related to castration anxiety (Deutsch 1967). For the learning-disabled adolescents who showed significant concerns about castration anxiety, their concerns, conflicts, and fantasies about the experience of being learning disabled became intertwined. For example, concerns about intellectual adequacy constituted, in part, a displacement upward of more fundamental concerns related to castration. However, the low-level, chronic depression that was evidenced by the learning-disabled adolescents did not seem to be consistently linked to castration and oedipal related concerns.

It is unclear how this depression or a sad sense of having lost part of oneself is related to learning disabilities. The learning disabilities were lifelong: the adolescents never had the ability to lose. However, their experience may have been that they could not do what they sometimes could. Again, the intermittent nature of mild to moderately severe learning disabilities may contribute importantly to various psychological ramifications.

Low-level, chronic depression seems to be a psychological response to the experience of being learning disabled. Recent research is beginning to show that there may be a link between learning disabilities and biologically based depressive illness (Brumback and Staton 1983). Whatever the specific etiology, this finding has important clinical implications. A learning-disabled person usually does not seek help because of chronic depression, which has been a part of his usual self; rather, he comes for counseling or psychotherapy because something new or unusual has occurred. Thus, the person presents with a problem superimposed on an underlying chronic depression that is not recognized. When this occurs, it may have important consequences for recovery rates and relapses (Keller and Shapiro 1982).

THE EXPERIENCE OF SELF

The learning-disabled adolescent's conscious experience of self was commonly and consistently marked by feelings of incompetence, inadequacy, and the anxious anticipation of failure. However, the non-learning-disabled adolescents (who presented with various work or learning problems) often evidenced the same types of conscious concerns. These findings may be in accord with a recent study that found learning-disabled adolescents' conscious self-concept comparable with that of a non-learning-disabled, normal adolescent control group (Silverman and Zigmond 1983). In the present investigation, the learning-disabled adolescents did present a much wider range and intensity of conscious negative feelings about self, but there were no consistent findings that would indicate a significant difference between the two groups.

The learning-disabled adolescents did tend to evidence a low sense of self-esteem: they tended to set unrealistically high and/or inappropriate goals for themselves (academic and otherwise); they had difficulty achieving these goals; and they tended to feel dissatisfied and incompetent regardless of whether or not they had achieved their conscious aim. However, a great number of the normal adolescents also showed these characteristics. It seems that learning disabilities may have an adverse effect on adolescent self-esteem, but impairment of self-esteem is not unique to learning-disabled adolescents.

What begins as a reaction to periodic failure and frustration becomes a core aspect of character by adolescence. The learning-disabled adolescent's unconscious representation of self does seem to be significantly different from the non-learning-disabled adolescent's. A consistent and core aspect of their self-representation was that of being painfully damaged, inadequate, dumb, and vulnerable. As noted in my discussion of their affective life, many of the learning-disabled adolescents believed that there was something damaged "in their head."

In a study of ten learning-disabled children (Cohen 1984), it appears that these negatively colored, disparaging internal self-representations are becoming a crystallized and integral aspect of the child's character by the mid-juvenile years (seven to eight years of age).

This self-experience of being "dumb, damaged, and inadequate" was typically unintegrated with other self-perceptions. Most of the learning-disabled adolescents typically oscillated between feeling bad about themselves, on the one hand, and had any number of other self-representations, on the other. For example, one adolescent said, "I'm just not good enough, I feel there's something wrong . . . but other times I feel good, I feel real smart—it's confusing 'cause all these feelings aren't together."

Almost all of the adolescents did not understand exactly what their specific cognitive disability was and how it had affected their experience in general and learning in particular. None understood how his psychological concerns and conflicts exacerbated his disability. This internal lack of integration may also be due to the discrepancies and accelerated development that learning-disabled students often show. By definition, learning disabilities contribute to uneven cognitive development and a discrepancy between achievement and intelligence (Rudel 1980). In recent years, authors have noted that many dyslexics have precocious and superior talents in a number of nonverbal skills, such as art, architecture, engineering, and athletics (Geschwind 1983; Porac and Coren 1981). This disparate and uneven experience may contribute to the striking lack of integration in self-representation.

The central developmental task of middle and late adolescence is to establish a stable identity. This necessarily involves questioning of values that produces varying degrees of conflict with parents, rebellion, anger, separation from the family, and the development of individuality (Freud 1971). To a large extent, it is impossible to say that being learning disabled has a particular effect on the identity formation process. This process is one of the more complex and multidetermined transitions in the life cycle. However, being learning disabled seems to color this transition in important ways. An examination and reexamination of "who am I?" is a central aspect of identity formation. This commonly involves a painful, often excruciating, and confusing exploration of those aspects of self-experience.

In the learning-disabled adolescent, the process of identity formation is made more painful and confusing than it normally is because many learning-disabled adolescents do not know that they are still affected by their learning disabilities, and because it involves thinking about oneself as a "damaged, dumb, and inadequate" person. It is often hard for these adolescents to realistically assess the extent of their actual disability and differentiate it from the psychological meanings they have given it.

Another important component of the "adolescent passage" is the formation of the "dream" (Levinson, Darrow, Klein, Levinson, and McKee 1978) or one's image of oneself in the adult world. What kind of person will I be when I grow up? What kind of life structure do I want to create? Naturally, the adolescent's emerging experience of self, both conscious and unconscious, will importantly influence and even determine his image of himself in the future. Although not in any consistent form, the belief that one is a damaged, inadequate, and dumb person certainly influenced the learning-disabled adolescents' dreams in one of two ways: either by limiting aspirations or by setting unrealistically high expectations and as a result feeling relentlessly driven to achieve them.

Another significant and perhaps organizing aspect of self-experience was the learning-disabled adolescents' pronounced and consistent tendency to set unrealistically high standards and ideals and to self-condemnation. This pattern of inner controls or superego functioning may importantly organize the self-representations, depression, and object representations and rigidity.

EXPERIENCE AND EXPECTATIONS OF OTHERS

A number of clinicians and other investigators have described and underscored the importance of understanding the learning-disabled child's experience with family members, peers, and teachers (Blanchard 1946; Buxbaum 1964; Liss 1955; Pearson 1952). There is no question that others' response to the learning-disabled person—be it empathic support or critical, humiliating, demanding insensitivity—plays a central role in his psychological development.

One of the most surprising findings, however, was that, regardless of how parents and teachers responded to the child and the child's difficulties, the adolescents studied showed similar difficulties, anxious concerns, low-level depression, impaired self-representations, and a sense of conflict, rigidity, and trauma. Certainly, the adolescent who grew up in environments where parents and teachers knew about the child's disability and seemed to respond in a supportive and empathic fashion had significantly less difficulty than those who did not. It was surprising to discover, however, that, even in optimal situations, the learning-disabled adolescent was still plagued by the psychological concerns and struggles discussed.

The learning-disabled adolescents' expectations of how they are likely to be treated seemed importantly related to how they remembered, imagined, and fantasized that they were treated as young learners. How these adolescents imagined they would be received, judged, loved, punished, gratified, and controlled varied widely. During in-depth psychotherapy, it emerged most clearly that how they imagined and remembered others responding to their trials and tribulations during the learning process powerfully affected the development of internal representations of others. This is probably always the case, but because learning disabilities seem so often to result in frustrating, confusing, humiliating, and anxiety-provoking moments, how others respond seems to have a great effect on the development of learning-disabled adolescents' expectations of how others will now see and treat them. Again, this is but one element in the larger, ongoing process. Internal representations and expectations of others always have profound consequence for two interpersonal processes that are important parts of normal adolescent development: learning how to collaborate and developing the capacity for intimacy.

Learning Disabilities and Personality Development

The relationship between learning disabilities and psychological development is a complex and ongoing intrapsychic and psychosocial process. It is interwoven with the concerns, conflicts, strengths, weaknesses, coping strategies, dreams, wishes, and various psychosocial factors of each developmental stage. However, being learning disabled is an element that seems to organize psychological development in a subtle but significant fashion and is experienced as an ongoing strain. In fact, the experience of being learning disabled is akin to what has been called a strain trauma (Kris 1956) or a cumulative trauma (Khan 1963).

LEARNING DISABILITIES AND CUMULATIVE TRAUMA

The relatively intermittent nature of mild to moderately severe learning disabilities seems to contribute to the belief that frustration and failure are unpredictable and uncontrollable. These repeated moments of frustration, failure, and helplessness seem to be accompanied by a painful lowering of self-esteem and negative self-representations. Gradually, these repeated moments (and the anxious anticipation of them) seem to result in trauma.

The notion of trauma usually refers to a wound produced by sudden physical injury or an emotional shock that creates substantial and lasting damage. Being learning disabled is not a shock in this sense. In fact, the effects of a learning disability are rarely acute or sudden. Rather, in the adolescents studied, the experience of being learning disabled was characteristically subtle and ongoing. But their self-esteem and sense of stability were stressed repeatedly throughout childhood and adolescence. These repeated moments of helplessness come to be associated with painful feelings of distress, anxiety, humiliation, and loss.

Usually parents and teachers attempt to buffer the child from repeated experiences of helplessness. When a child—for whatever reason—is not protected from repeated moments of helplessness, the cumulative result is a feeling of trauma (Khan 1963). It was quite striking to discover that, even in the best of situations (i.e., where the child seemed to have been empathically raised and supported at home and school), none of the adolescents studied completely escaped these repeated moments of helplessness and a sense of stress and trauma.

This experience of feeling emotionally injured resulting from repeated moments of helplessness, inadequacy, and pain does not seem to be an immediate response in childhood. I have not observed it in most learning-disabled children under the ages of seven or eight (Cohen 1984). Rather, it seems to be a much more gradual and subtle process that does not manifest itself until the mid-latency years or later. As such, it is perhaps similar to the psychological concomitants of other physical handicaps (Burlingham 1961; Sandler 1963) or constitutional sensitivities (Escalona 1953) that make it impossible for the parents (and later, teachers) to protect the child from the repeated and frightening experience of helplessness.

It is not clear from the present investigation how this cumulative trauma interacts with the various developmental tasks of childhood. In the continuation of examining psychological development and the experience of being learning disabled, this will be an important area of study.

LEARNING DISABILITIES AS AN ORGANIZER OF DEVELOPMENT

One of the important, although perhaps not surprising, findings that emerged was that learning disabilities are an organizer of the adolescents' sense of identity. A developmental organizer is a notion that has referred to a biobehavioral event (e.g., the smiling response) that reflects the culmination of previous maturational and developmental processes (Spitz 1965). Being learning disabled is not an event at one point in time. Rather, the ongoing effect of the disability itself and the meanings attributed to it is a biopsychosocial process that organizes experience by being a determinant of strengths, interests, weaknesses, and the development of adaptive strategies.

Learning disabilities are cognitive weaknesses. Weaknesses are always a determinant in the person's unfolding sense of self and identity. We learn through experience, and when a given process or task is difficult, we tend to react in one of two ways: either we avoid (and in a related fashion come to feel that we are "bad" at) it, or we do the opposite—we expend a tremendous amount of energy and time on becoming "very good" at what was initially a difficult task. A common example of the latter response is the dyslexic child who becomes an avid reader. In either case, the weakness shapes behavior and our experience of self. This is particularly true when a given weakness interferes with an ongoing process (e.g., the learning process) that has powerful emotional as well as practical consequences.

Learning disabilities potentially contribute to the person's repertoire of strengths. Characteristically, if the learning disability is not too severe, and if teachers and/or parents empathically support the child, difficulty in learning tends to become a challenge to be met and overcome. Although this does not make the disability go away, it does tend to make the person feel effective and competent and provides a foundation for achievement.

Learning disabilities often seem to contribute to accelerated or precocious development in other psychological abilities and interests. As noted, a number of studies have shown that many dyslexics have superior talents in a number of nonverbal (right hemisphere) areas, such as art, architecture, engineering, and athletics (Geschwind 1982, 1983; Porac and Coren 1981). Geschwind (1982) has suggested that there is a genetic basis to this that may be evolutionarily advantageous. Recent neurological research shows that, if there is damage or delayed development in one hemisphere, there is compensating growth during fetal life of the corresponding region on the opposite side (Goldman 1978). In a series of recent anatomical studies, it has been shown that the brains of dyslexics reveal cortical disturbances in one of the major left hemisphere language areas (Galaburda 1983; Galaburda and Eidelberg 1982; Galaburda and Kemper 1979). Apparently, in addition to the disadvantage of being learning disabled, there are significant advantages (i.e., superior talents in certain other areas) for the dyslexic. In addition, unaffected relatives who share the same genetic predisposition often have high talents in the absence of serious difficulty with language acquisition (Geschwind 1983). Although unrelated to linguistics, these talents are clearly advantageous to society as a whole.

This accelerated development may also represent a psychological compensatory response to being disabled. The experience of inadequacy, helplessness, strain, and failure usually gives rise to the wish to become very competent and accomplished. In fact, a great number of the learning-disabled adolescents were characteristically somewhat grandiose. In any case, accelerated development in other areas (i.e., nonverbal) characteristically leads to individual strengths which, like a weakness, are virtually always a personality determinant. We become interested in and like to do what we do well, and hence we usually do that more often. This further reinforces and supports the development of that skill. The precocious development of one ego function, however, may lead to excessive narcissistic gratification in that area and make the person susceptible to narcissistic injury in other less developed areas (Newman, Dember, and Krug 1973). This may further contribute to the learning-disabled adolescent's experience of being narcissistically damaged.

LEARNING DISABILITIES, THE COMPENSATORY PROCESS, AND ADAPTATION

The ways that the adolescents compensate for their learning disabilities seem to be directly related to important aspects of their self-representation in general, their work identity in particular, and various concerns and conflicts. It is well known that the experience of being learning disabled characteristically results in the child's developing compensatory strategies. Compensatory strategies involve the discovery and use of coping strategies that allow the student to circumvent the area of disability. A child who confuses *b* and *d* will read slowly, to check and recheck the letters or discover that a *b* looks like his left hand, thumb up, fingers closed into a hitchhiking sign. Children adapt to their disabilities automatically with compensatory maneuvers, and teachers often instruct learning-disabled children to do just this. In the adolescents studied, these compensatory strategies seem to become generalized or characteristic adaptive patterns. And how we cope or adapt to difficulty always directly and/or indirectly affects our sense of identity; in fact, it is a psychologically central trait.

For example, a number of students I studied worked quite slowly as one important adaptive maneuver. In fact, this was an educationally adaptive strategy, for, when they read or performed mathematics very quickly (e.g., because of external time pressure or anxiety), they were much more likely to manifest their disability. Working slowly seemed to allow adaptive, hypervigilant checking and rechecking. This process of checking and rechecking occurs automatically and outside of the adolescent's awareness. However, being "slow" was more than adaptive in that task. It also had become an important aspect of his sense of self and identity as a worker and a person. On projective tests and in psychotherapeutic explorations of learning-disabled adolescents' experience, negative feelings of being "slow," not being "quick enough," and related anxious concerns about what others would think about them in this regard emerged repeatedly. Furthermore, these adolescents evidenced painful conflicted feelings about this.

A large number of the students manifested a much less adaptive strategy to compensate for their disability: avoidance. Again, feelings of being an "avoider," a "manipulator," "not being what one appears to be" loomed large in these youngsters' images of themselves. In addition, avoidance was a characteristic psychological defense. For example, instead of writing a paper to the best of their ability, they would plagiarize. Or, when hurt and angry at a friend, they would withdraw.

It seems that compensatory strategies and psychological defenses became significantly interrelated. From the present investigation, it is unclear whether the compensatory strategy serves as a model for the development and use of related defenses or vice versa. However, it was striking to observe repeatedly that the compensatory strategies seemed to predict psychologically central characteristics in the learning-disabled students studied.

That psychological conflicts and organic disabilities may simultaneously use the same channel of expression has been noted before (Betheim and Hartmann 1924; Rapaport 1958; Sarvis 1960). And Pine (1980) has described how specific cognitive disabilities can become nodal points for psychological symptom formation. The experience of the disability (e.g., the dyslexic child's utter confusion when trying to read) may provide an analogue or model for what happens when he experiences psychological difficulty. In a somewhat similar fashion, the development of compensatory strategies may also create a model for a variety of other types of defensive and adaptive patterns.

RIGIDITY

One of the most striking and consistent findings that emerged from the present investigation was that the adolescents' defensive and coping strategies were employed in a relatively rigid fashion. They tended to rely on a limited number of defensive operations that were utilized with little regard for the actual situation. However, acting rigidly also seemed to be an important aspect of their character. That is, they tended to show an exaggerated and tense deliberateness of behavior. Their purposiveness often became intense and did not allow for deviation, distraction, or spontaneity. Such a continuously deliberate, purposive, and tense self-direction involves a special kind of self-consciousness (Shapiro 1981). This rigidity was not a manifestation of any one character structure (e.g., obsessive-compulsive): it was an important aspect of functioning regardless of character type.

The learning-disabled adolescents seemed to need to continuously reinforce a sense of mastery. In fact, they felt (again, to varying degrees) that they were engaged in a special kind of battle to achieve a sense of mastery and avoid the experience of losing control, of being inadequate and helpless. Rigidity seems to be the outcome of this battle and the solution to the struggle.

Being learning disabled contributes to the individual's doubting his ability to be in control and avoid the repeated experience of helplessness. Acting in a rigid manner in the ways described may help these youngsters feel more in control. In addition, it is possible that, as learning-disabled children anxiously struggle and then gradually learn what helps them to compensate for the disability and defend against the experience of helplessness, distress, and depression, they then tenaciously and rigidly maintain these coping strategies. In any case, to the extent that this rigidity is a generalized finding among learning-disabled adolescents, it is an important one, because rigidity always significantly interferes with development—educational and psychological. Being rigid, by definition, is limiting and maladaptive. In fact, this rigidity is commonly a major therapeutic obstacle and needs to be a focus for clinical work. It is not uncommon for therapeutic gains to be made with these adolescents. But if the rigidity is not identified and worked with, it will undermine integration and development.

Conclusions

The presence of a learning disability sets in motion a series of ongoing psychological processes that become interrelated with various aspects of ego functioning and development. Not only does the cognitive deficit directly and adversely affect autonomous aspects of the ego apparatus (e.g., perception or memory); these aspects, in part, seem to organize the adolescents' ego interests, strengths, weaknesses, identity, experience of self, and rigidity. In the learning-disabled adolescents studied, there is a complex interaction between the cognitive deficit itself, the actual frustration and failure that it engenders, conscious and unconscious interpretations and anticipations of events, self-experiences, and affectively related repercussions. These events and responses are often mutually reinforcing and become interwoven into the character and evolving identity of the person.

Unless learning disabilities are diagnosed and treatment is undertaken, these bewildered children are at risk for emotional problems. The present investigation suggests that learning-disabled adolescents are at risk even when they seem to have been helpfully and comprehensively diagnosed and treated. These cognitive disabilities and the adolescents' interpretation of them inhibits adaptation, learning, and a realistic appraisal of self. Learning disabilities inhibit the experience of being a successful maker, doer, and effective initiator of change. The high anxiety, low-level depression and the sense that one is a vulnerable, damaged, traumatized, "dumb," helpless person contribute to the development of narcissistic vulnerabilities, nonadaptive coping strategies, and ego rigidity.

NOTE

1. Specific cognitive deficits vary in terms of frequency: intermittent versus constant. Although rarely discussed, mild to moderately severe learning disabilities (e.g., a visual processing disability) interfere with functioning (e.g., reversal and rotation of percepts) in an intermittent manner. The process of assessing the severity of learning disabilities in childhood and adolescence is complex and inexact. However, the frequency of a disability in conjunction with the extent to which the disability interferes with learning (delimited versus total), extent of discrepancy between achievement and intelligence, overall IQ (Verbal and Performance), and psychological factors all need to be evaluated and synthesized to determine severity.

REFERENCES

Bellak, L. 1979. Psychiatric aspects of minimal brain dysfunction in adults: their ego function assessment. In L. Bellak, ed. *Psychiatric Aspects of Minimal Brain Dysfunction in Adults*. New York: Grune & Stratton.

Betheim, S., and Hartmann, H. 1924. On parapraxes in the Korsakow psychosis. In D. Rapaport, ed. *Organization and Pathology of Thought*. New York: Columbia University Press, 1951.

Blanchard, P. 1946. Psychoanalytic contributions to the problems of reading disabilities. *Psychoanalytic Study of the Child* 2:163–187.

Brown, B. S. 1978. Foreward. In A. L. Benton and D. Pearl, eds. *Dyslexia: An Appraisal of Current Knowledge*. New York: Oxford University Press.

Brumback, R. A., and Staton, R. D. 1983. Learning disability and childhood depression. *American Journal of Orthopsychiatry* 53(2):262–263.

Burlingham, D. 1961. Some notes on the development of the blind. *Psychoanalytic Study of the Child* 16:121–145.

Buxbaum, E. 1964. The parents' role in the etiology of learning disabilities. *Psychoanalytic Study of the Child* 19:421–447.

Clark, F. 1981. *Major Research Findings of the University of Kansas Institute for Research in Learning Disabilities*. Research Report no. 31. Lawrence: Institute for Research in Learning Disabilities, University of Kansas.

Cohen, J. 1983. Learning disabilities and the college student: identification and diagnosis. *Adolescent Psychiatry* 11:177–198.

Cohen, J. 1984. Learning disabilities and childhood: psychological and developmental implications. Paper presented at the New York Orton–Dyslexia Society Meeting, March 23, 1984.

Cruickshank, W. M.; Morse, W. C.; and Johns, J. S. 1980. *Learning Disabilities: The Struggle from Adolescence toward Adulthood*. Syracuse, N.Y.: Syracuse University Press.

DeHirsch, K. 1975. Language deficits in children with developmental lags. *Psychoanalytic Study of the Child* 30:95–126.

Deutsch, H. 1967. *Selected Problems of Adolescence*. New York: International Universities Press.

Dinklage, K. T. 1971. Inability to learn a foreign language. In G. Blaine and G. C. McArthur, eds. *Emotional Problems of the Student*. 2d ed. New York: Appleton-Century-Crofts.

Escalona, S. 1953. Emotional development in the first year of life. In M. J. E. Senn, ed. *Problems of Infancy and Childhood*. New York: Josiah Macy, Jr., Foundation.

Freud, A. 1971. *The Writings of Anna Freud*. Vol. 7. New York: International Universities Press.

Galaburda, A. 1983. Developmental dyslexia: current anatomical research. *Annals of Dyslexia* 33:41–53.

Galaburda, A., and Eidelberg, D. 1982. Symmetry and asymmetry in the human posterior thalamus. II. Thalamic lesions in a case of developmental dyslexia. *Archives of Neurology* 39:333–336.

Galaburda, A., and Kemper, T. C. 1979. Cytoarachitecnoic abnormalities in developmental dyslexia: a case study. *Annals of Neurology* 6:94–100.

Geschwind, N. 1982. Why Orton was right. *Annals of Dyslexia* 32:13–30.

Geschwind, N. 1983. Biological associations of left-handedness. *Annals of Dyslexia* 33:29–40.

Goldman, P. S. 1978. Neuronal plasticity in primate telencephalon: anomalous projections induced by prenatal removal of frontal cortex. *Science* 202:768–770.

Goldstein, K. 1939. *The Organism*. New York: American Book Co.

Hartmann, H. 1939. *Ego Psychology and the Problem of Adaptation*. New York: International Universities Press, 1958.

Keller, M. B., and Shapiro, R. W. 1982. Double depression: superimposition of acute depressive episodes on chronic depressive disorders. *American Journal of Psychiatry* 139(4):438–442.

Khan, M. M. 1963. The concept of cumulative trauma. *Psychoanalytic Study of the Child* 18:286–306.

Kline, C. C., and Kline, C. L. 1975. Follow-up study of 216 dyslexic children. *Bulletin of the Orton Society* 25:125–44.

Kris, E. 1956. The recoveries of childhood memories in psychoanalysis. *Psychoanalytic Study of the Child* 11:54–88.

Levinson, D.; Darrow, C. N.; Klein, E. B.; Levinson, M. H.; and McKee, B. 1978. *Seasons of a Man's Life*. New York: Ballantine.

Liss, E. 1955. Motivation in learning. *Psychoanalytic Study of the Child* 10:100–116.

Medalie, J. 1981. The college years as a mini-life cycle: developmental tasks and adaptive options. *Journal of the American College Health Association* 30:154–158.

Newman, C. J.; Dember, C. F.; and Krug, O. 1973. He can but he won't; a psychodynamic study of so-called gifted underachievers. *Psychoanalytic Study of the Child* 28:83–129.

Ochroch, R. 1981. A review of the minimal brain dysfunction syndrome. In R. Ochroch, ed. *The Diagnosis and Treatment of Minimal Brain Dysfunction in Children*. New York: Human Sciences.

Palombo, J. 1979. Perceptual deficits and self-esteem in adolescence. *Clinical Social Work Journal* 7(1):34–60.

Pearson, G. H. J. 1952. A survey of learning difficulties in children. *Psychoanalytic Study of the Child* 7:322–386.

Pine, F. 1980. On phase-characteristic pathology of the school-age child: disturbances of personality development and organization (borderline conditions), of learning, and of behavior. In S. E. Greenspan and G. H. Pollack, eds. *The Course of Life: Psychoanalytic Contributions toward Understanding Personality Development.* Vol. 2. Washington, D.C.: Government Printing Office.

Porac, C., and Coren, S. 1981. *Lateral Preferences and Human Behavior*. New York: Springer.

Rapaport, D. 1958. The theory of the ego autonomy. *Bulletin of the Menninger Clinic* 22:13–35.

Ritvo, S. 1971. Late adolescence. *Psychoanalytic Study of the Child* 26:241–263.

Rome, H. D. 1971. The psychiatric aspects of dyslexia. *Bulletin of the Orton Society*. Vol. 21.

Rothstein, A. 1982. An integrative perspective on the diagnosis of learning disorders. *Journal of the American Academy of Child Psychiatry* 21(4):420–426.

Rudel, R. 1980. Learning disability: diagnosis by exclusion and discrepancy. *Journal of the American Academy of Child Psychiatry* 19:547–569.

Rudel, R. G. 1981. Residual effects of childhood reading disabilities. *Bulletin of the Orton Society* 31:89–100.

Rutter, M. 1978. Prevalence and types of dyslexia. In A. L. Benton and D. Pearl, eds. *Dyslexia: An Appraisal of Current Knowledge*. New York: Oxford University Press.

Sandler, A. M. 1963. Aspects of passivity and ego development in the blind infant. *Psychoanalytic Study of the Child* 18:343–360.

Sarvis, M. A. 1960. Psychiatric implications of temporal lobe damage. *Psychoanalytic Study of the Child* 15:454–481.

Shapiro, D. 1981. *Autonomy and Rigid Character*. New York: Basic.

Silver, L. 1974. Emotional and social problems of children with developmental disabilities. In R. E. Weber, ed. *Handbook on Learning Disabilities*. Englewood Cliffs, N.J.: Prentice-Hall.

Silverman, R., and Zigmond, N. 1983. Self-concept in learning disabled adolescents. *Journal of Learning Disabilities* 16:8–14.

Spitz, R. A. 1965. *The First Year of Life*. New York: International Universities Press.

Weil, A. P. 1970. The basic core. *Psychoanalytic Study of the Child* 25:422–460.

Weil, A. P. 1971. Children with minimal brain dysfunction. *Psychosocial Process* 1:80–97.

Weil, A. P. 1977. Learning disturbances with special consideration of dyslexia. *Issues in Child Mental Health* 5:52–66.

Weil, A. P. 1978. Maturational variations and genetic-dynamic issues. *Journal of the American Psychoanalytic Association* 26:461–491.

White, R. 1963. Ego and reality in psychoanalytic theory. *Psychological Issues Monograph* 2, 3:3.

14 OUTCOMES OF LEARNING DISABILITIES IN ADOLESCENCE

ARCHIE A. SILVER AND ROSA A. HAGIN

For an individual with a learning disability, the outcome in academic, social, vocational, and psychological adjustment is the result of many factors: the causes, extent, and severity of the learning disability; the presence of complicating attentional deficits, hyperactivity, and neurological signs; the cognitive and biological substrate with which the child comes into the world; the psychological defenses he has established; and, most important, the adequacy and appropriateness of the environmental and educational support he has received.

With this complex interplay of forces, it is not surprising that long-term reviews of the outcomes of children with learning disabilities report inconsistency in outcome. For example, Schonhaut and Satz (1983) describe four studies reporting favorable outcomes, twelve with unfavorable outcomes, and two with mixed outcomes. So many variables influence outcome that, from study to study, the results may not be comparable. Methodological considerations, such as comparability of subjects, nature and intensity of treatment, and follow-up variables, must be considered if one is to compare outcome studies. The focus of outcome studies may also vary, with some emphasizing academic or vocational status, or social adjustment, or neuropsychological maturation, or psychological status. Few studies to date have attempted to evaluate all these areas. Even those that assess similar outcome variables differ as far as methodology and subjects are concerned.

For example, in one favorable outcome study, Rawson (1968) studied only occupational and educational outcomes. Her sample, however, was

0-226-24058-4/85/0012-0013$01.00

drawn from a private school with high socioeconomic level, with the sample mean Stanford-Binet IQ 130, and with every educational support available. Satz, Taylor, Friel, and Fletcher (1978), on the other hand, studied the entire white male population (*N* = 426) of a public school system in rural Florida in which IQ scores were not specified. They found that of forty-nine children who were severely retarded readers at the end of second grade, only 6 percent were rated as average or above-average readers by the end of fifth grade. Of sixty-two children considered mildly retarded readers at the end of second grade, only 17 percent were rated average or above by the end of fifth grade. Rawson's sample presumably was treated with an Orton-Gillingham approach; Satz does not specify the teaching approach used with his sample. Thus, with two different populations with presumably different intervention systems and with different outcome measures, Rawson and Satz et al. came to different conclusions.

Spreen (1978), in a ten-year follow-up of a sample from a neuropsychological clinic, found that "in most aspects of educational, occupational, and social and psychological adjustment, the outcome of learning disabled children was worse than that of a control group." Spreen, moreover, found that, with the learning-disabled group, children with neurological signs had a poorer prognosis than those without them. With few exceptions, population samples from public schools and from clinics tended to have poor academic achievement on follow-up, while children in the higher socioeconomic groups, who had the benefit of excellent educational support and remedial help, tended to have a greater measure of occupational and academic success.

Our initial follow-up studies (Silver and Hagin 1964) of children with learning disabilities focused on academic achievement and on neuropsychological maturation. The emphasis was on the perceptual variables of orientation in space and in organization in time, functions which we believe to be basic to learning, reading, and the language arts. These functions were assessed through measures of visual discrimination, recall of asymmetric figures, visual figure ground discrimination, visual motor control, auditory sequencing and immediate auditory recall, and right-left discrimination, praxis, and fingergnosis.

A group of forty-one children with learning disabilities, originally referred to the Bellevue Hospital Mental Health Clinic at ages eight to ten years for behavior problems, were studied for ten years after initial contact. A control group of thirty children, also originally referred to the Bellevue clinic for behavior problems and matched with the learning-disability group for age, sex, and socioeconomic status, was also identified. The groups differed in academic achievement and in the presence of the neuropsychological problems in temporal and spatial organization.

At the time of the follow-up, it was possible to obtain information on all but five of the original learning-disabled group and to examine twenty-four. Of those who were located but unavailable for examination, six had moved from the metropolitan area, two were in correctional institutions, one was in a state psychiatric hospital, and three were in the armed forces. Of the original control group, eleven were available for individual study. On follow-up examination, the learning-disability group was composed of twenty-one boys and three girls with median age of nineteen years. Wechsler Adult Intelligence Full-Scale IQ of the group ranged from 78 to 118, with a median IQ of 105. Controls consisted of eight boys and three girls with median age at follow-up of twenty years; IQ for the control group ranged from 94 to 124, median at 112. As children, the distribution of IQ scores did not differ significantly between reading-disability and control groups. As adults, however, the IQs of controls were significantly higher ($P < .01$) than those of the reading-disability group.

When the neuropsychological maturations of learning-disabled and control groups were compared on follow-up, both groups could distinguish right and left in themselves, and there was some maturation in visual motor function. However, some of the primitive verticalization seen in learning-disabled children did not entirely disappear. Angulation problems on the Bender Visual-Motor Gestalt Test were singularly tenacious. Visual figure ground problems, tactile figure ground errors, difficulty with auditory figure ground, and persistent fingergnosis immaturity were seen in the learning-disabled adults. It seemed reasonable to conclude that, in spite of the children's maturation in some areas, the neuropsychological problems in spatial and temporal organization which were seen in the children with learning disabilities do not disappear but persist into adulthood.

With the twenty-four children with reading disability examined in the follow-up study, there were five children who, in addition to the basic perceptual deviations in spatial and temporal organization, had complicating findings on neurological examination. These findings include hyperactivity, marked choreoform motility, or poor gross or fine motor coordination. These children are designated as a subgroup we have termed "organic." It is recognized, however, that structural defect of the central nervous system may not be demonstrated in them, and they may actually represent a more severe form of the learning-disability syndrome. The findings on neurological examination are important, however, when we compare adequacy of educational outcomes within the subgroups.

Adequate readers were defined as those individuals whose reading scores obtained on the Wide-Range Achievement Test did not fall more than ten points below the adult IQs as obtained on the Wechsler Adult Intelligence Scale. By this criterion, fifteen of the reading-disability group were found to be adequate readers as adults, while nine were inadequate. Our data (table 1) showed that adequate readers (1) tended to come from the developmental rather than the organic group ($P < .025$); (2) tended to have been less severely retarded in reading when tutoring was initiated ($P < .005$); (3) tended to show a rise in IQ as adults, although there was no significant difference as children ($P < .05$); and (4) tended to have fewer figure background problems in visual perception ($P < .05$). On the other hand, the less adequate readers were found to have greater perceptual problems in all areas as adults ($P < .025$). No specific pattern of perceptual defects characterizes the group. The more adequate readers as adults, although relatively free of perceptual problems compared with the inadequate readers, still persisted with the body image and laterality problems they had demonstrated as children (figs. 1, 2, and 3).

The data lead to the conclusion that basic neuropsychological problems which plague these individuals as children do not simply disappear but persist into adolescence and early adult life. Furthermore, the presence of complicating "organic" factors should alert the clinician to a more guarded outcome and suggest the need in those children for modification of the usual compensatory remedial teaching.

The children of the initial follow-up study came from the Bellevue Hospital Clinic population, the poor of the Lower East Side of New York

TABLE 1

CHARACTERISTICS OF ADEQUATE AND INADEQUATE READERS

Characteristic	Percentage Adequate Group	Percentage Inadequate Group	*P*
Diagnosis: organic	27	78	<.25
Diagnosis: developmental	73	22	<.25
Initial reading quotient below median for group	8	89	<.005
Initial IQ below median for group	46	50	NS
Rise in IQ as adults	77	25	<.05
Perceptual anomalies below median for group	53	0	<.025

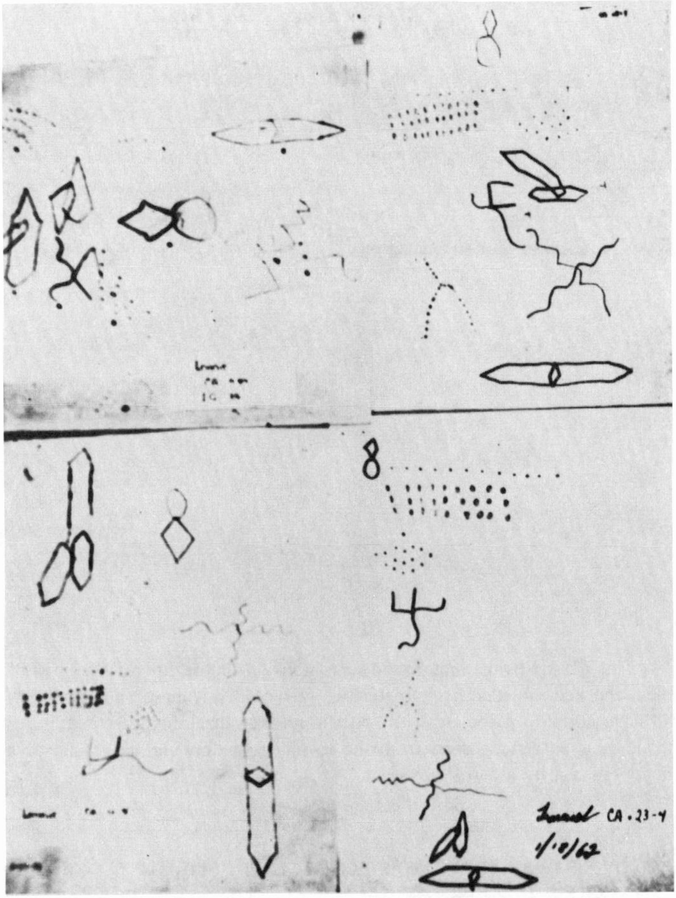

FIG. 1.—This illustrates the persistence of visual-motor problems in a boy of average intelligence who had marked choreoform motility and gross intention tremor when seen at age eight. The upper left drawing illustrates the disorganized placement of the Gestalt figures together with gross rotations and angulation difficulty. The upper right drawing was done one year later with significant improvement in organization but with a dramatic 90-degree rotation of Figure A. The lower left drawing, done at age twelve, and the lower right drawing, done at twenty-three, reveal the same primitive verticalization.

City. By contrast, this report will describe a second follow-up: the occupational and academic outcome in seventy-nine patients with learning disabilities, studied and treated in a private practice of psychiatry and psychology during 1956–1976. In contrast to the Bellevue group, the private practice patients were drawn from middle and upper income families. There were eighteen girls and sixty-one boys. The ages at which

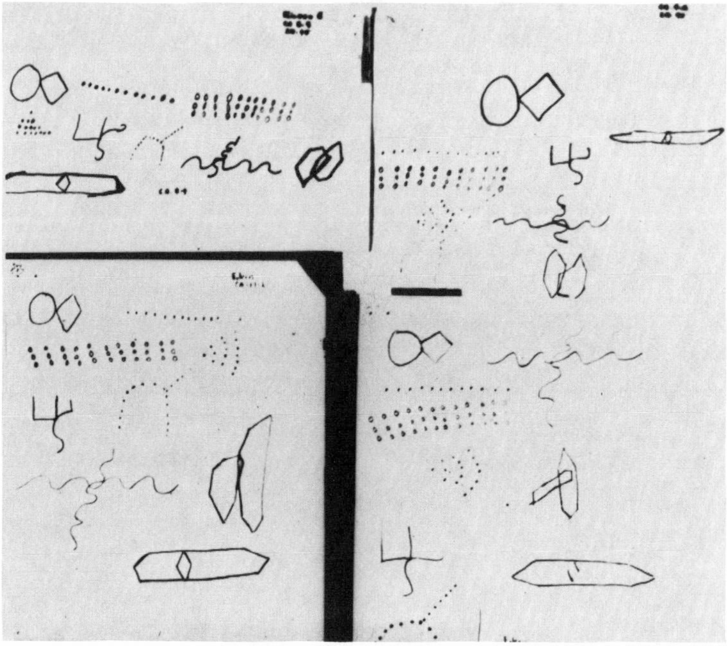

FIG. 2.—This illustrates the maturation seen in visual-motor function in a girl of average intelligence who had the specific immaturities in spatial orientation and temporal organization we have come to associate with specific reading disability. Her reading improved in treatment, but, as can be seen from the lower right drawing, remnants of her early visual-motor immaturity are still apparent.

treatment by us was begun spanned a range, with five children seven years or younger; forty-six (more than half) between ages of eight and ten years, fifteen between eleven and thirteen years, ten between fourteen and sixteen years, and three seventeen years of age.

Diagnostically, the cause of their learning disabilities varied. Our diagnostic criteria for learning disability had both inclusionary and exclusionary features. In addition to significant discrepancy between educational expectancy and achievement in reading and the language arts, to be designated as having a specific learning disability the child had to demonstrate immaturity in spatial orientation and temporal organization as evidenced in visual discrimination and recall of asymmetric figures, in visual figure ground, in visual motor function, in auditory rote sequencing, immediate auditory recall, and in body image, including right-left discrimination, praxis, and fingergnosis. These immaturities might

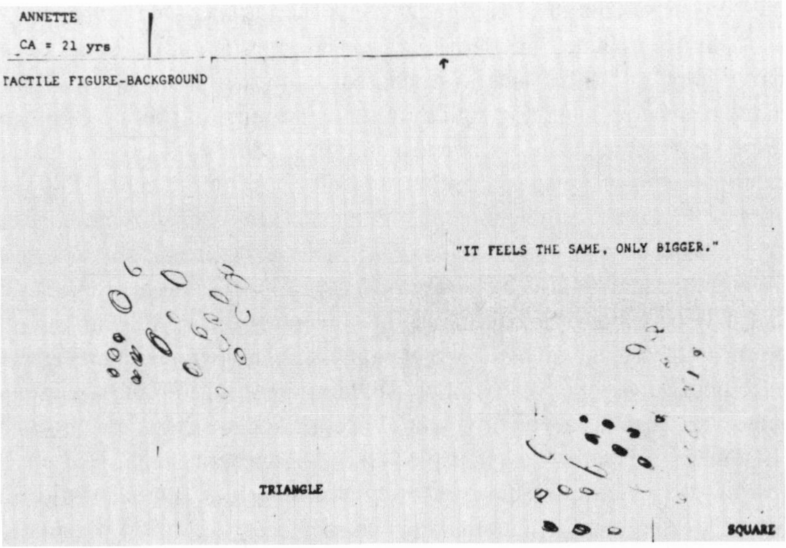

FIG. 3.—This is a tactile figure ground test in which the patient is asked, with her eyes closed, to identify a simple geometric figure of raised rubber-capped thumbtacks in a field of smooth thumbtacks. The figures to be identified are triangle and a square. Even as an adult, Annette could not perform this task. She was first seen at age ten; she was anxious and depressed and had significant immaturities in all perceptual areas. In addition, gross and fine-motor coordination was poor. At age twelve, her WISC, full scale, was 87 (V.89, P.87). At age eighteen, her verbal IQ increased to 105, but her performance IQ was at 80. At age twenty-one, her verbal IQ on the WAIS was 110. She refused to do the performance subtests. Her reading improved only to a sixth-grade level.

appear in any combination and/or degree of severity. The degree of immaturity was estimated from the normative performance expected of the child's chronological age. As exclusionary criteria, children with Full-Scale IQ on the WISC below 80, those with severe emotional handicaps, and those with organic signs were not considered to have specific learning disabilities.

Criteria for the diagnosis of organicity included not only the presence of one or more deviations in the classical neurological examination of cranial nerves, muscle tone, power and synergy, deep and superficial reflexes, and gross sensory evaluation, but also the finding of so-called soft neurological signs. Soft signs have been considered as (1) minimal deviations in the classical neurological examination in which there are none of the signs of a localizing lesion, and (2) as immaturity in the normative aspects of development, as a developmental lag in the maturation of central nervous system function (Shaffer, O'Connor, Shafer, and Prupis 1983). As such, we include immaturity in fine and gross motor coordination, in motor impulse control such as in choreoform motility and in synkinesis, in motor synergy including equilibrium, the presence of primitive postural response such as persistent neck-righting response, evidence for lack of clear-cut hemisphere specialization, sensory immaturity such as the presence of the extinction phenomenon on bilateral simultaneous stimulation, or the displacement of sensory stimuli. It is recognized, of course, that the specific learning-disability category may itself be a heterogeneous group and may be subgrouped into areas of perceptual difficulty. Further, the presence of organic signs does not imply similarity in etiology but may encompass a variety of conditions including prematurity, anoxia, injury, infections, genetic deviations, and idiopathic seizure disorders.

With these criteria, however, fifty-six of our seventy-nine children fitted into the specific learning-disability category, nineteen had "organic" learning disabilities, one child was considered as suffering from schizophrenia, and one child was functioning at a retarded cognitive level and was diagnosed as having Noonan's syndrome. In addition, two children were separately categorized as attention deficit disorders.

All children were evaluated with a comprehensive study that included neuropsychiatric examination, psychological testing, educational evaluation, and survey of the reality pressures at home and at school. All children received educational intervention. This training, done by the second author, was based on the three principles: (1) that accurate spatial orientation and temporal organization are necessary for progress in learning reading and the language arts; (2) that deficits in these neuropsychological functions may be remedied by specific perceptual stimulation of the deficit areas; and (3) when these foundation skills are in place, code-based instruction in reading and the language arts should proceed until the individual's skills are appropriate to expectancy. Remediation accordingly differed from the conventional remediation, concentrating first on stimulation of the deficit areas and then providing intensive code-based instruction until the individual was achieving appropriately.

Of the seventy-nine children, forty-seven were considered as having emotional problems already internalized—some a reaction to the frustration of failure, the confusion of their perceptual distortions, and the reality pressures at home and at school. These children received psychotherapeutic help in addition to the educational training. The remaining thirty-two children received educational help without formal psychotherapy, but in these children, also, educational support in the form of necessary school adjustments and parent counseling was provided. It must be remembered that this was not a controlled study of treatment effect but an attempt to offer optimal treatment to families in a private practice setting.

In 1983, occupational and academic data were obtained on seventy-two of the seventy-nine children originally seen during the years 1956–1976. With rare exceptions, all of the seventy-nine children and their families have kept in contact with us throughout the years by telephone calls when problems arose, by periodic follow-up visits and letters, and by treatment of other members of the family. Some came in for periodic follow-up examinations or at critical periods such as college application. For the seven children for whom no 1983 follow-up data were available, their status at their last visit was recorded.

Forty of the seventy-nine were originally seen and treated in 1956–1965, a follow-up of fifteen to twenty-four years. Eighteen of our original group were studied and treated between 1966 and 1970, a follow-up of ten to fourteen years, eleven seen in 1971–1975, a follow-up of five to ten years, and six seen after 1975. At follow-up, thirty-six were twenty-five to thirty-five, twenty-five twenty to twenty-four, thirteen fifteen to nineteen, four ten to fourteen, and one nine. The follow-up period thus ranged from twenty-four years to five years, with the greatest number (fifty-eight, or 73 percent) in the ten to twenty-four year follow-up period; ages at follow-up range from nine years to thirty-four years with the greatest number (sixty-one, or 77 percent) twenty to thirty-five years.

The overall findings in occupational status and academic achievement may be seen in tables 2, 3, and 4. As adults, twenty-one (27 percent) are in professional or technical occupations, including engineers, filmmakers, art historians, attorneys, teacher, journalist, advertising copywriter, accountant, commercial photographer, and medical illustrator. In addition, twenty-three (29 percent) are in managerial, clerical, or sales occupations. Of these, fourteen are in the family business, seven of them taking an active and responsible role in management. Five of the total group are service workers, nineteen still in school or college. Two have been hospitalized, one for an acute psychotic episode in the course of schizophrenia, the other suffering from a progressively degenerating neurological disease (subacute sclerosing panencephalitis). One is unemployed; another, with an attention deficit disorder, drowned in an accident at age sixteen.

As can be seen from the educational data in table 5, thirty-eight sub-

TABLE 2
LEARNING DISABILITIES
PRIVATE PRACTICE FOLLOW-UP STUDY:
OCCUPATIONAL STATUS

Professional and technical	21
Managers, proprieters, clerical, sales	23
Service workers including armed services	5
In school or college	19
Hospitalized	2
Unemployed	1
Deceased	1
No data	7
Total	79

TABLE 3
LEARNING DISABILITIES
PRIVATE PRACTICE FOLLOW-UP STUDY:
PROFESSIONAL AND TECHNICAL

Engineers	8
Journalist	1
Ad copywriter	1
Filmmakers	2
Art historians	2
Medical illustrator	1
Teachers	1
Podiatrist	1
Accountant	1
Lawyer	2
Photographer	1
Total	21

TABLE 4
LEARNING DISABILITIES
PRIVATE PRACTICE FOLLOW-UP STUDY:
MANAGERS, PROPRIETERS, CLERICAL, AND SALES

Family business:	
Management	7
Workers	7
Real estate	2
Security clerk	1
Sales, department store	1
Office workers	3
Lab technicians	1
Manager/rock musician	1
Total	23

TABLE 5
LEARNING DISABILITIES
PRIVATE PRACTICE FOLLOW-UP STUDY:
EDUCATIONAL STATUS

College:	
Completed college	29
Completed graduate school	9
Left before graduation	4
Currently enrolled	9
Vocational training:	
Art school	3
Optics	1
Paraeducation	1
Beauty culture	1
Occupational training	2
Left high school before graduation	6
Below college age	6
Deceased	1
No data	7
Total	79

jects completed college, nine have gone on to graduate school, four left college before graduation, and nine are currently enrolled in college. Eight completed vocational school, six did not complete high school, six are still below college age, one is deceased, and, again, no data were obtained on seven. This group of seventy-nine individuals with learning disability appears to have been relatively successful as adults vocationally and academically. The data, however, were subject to further analysis.

Each subject was evaluated in occupational and academic adjustment on a five-point scale, with ratings as follows: an evaluation of excellent is used when the patient was judged to have (1) attained his full potential in the working world, achieving local or even national recognition for contributions; (2) achieved honors in a competitive college or university. Eight (10 percent) of our original group are in this category, one a nationally recognized art historian, another a journalist with administrative responsibilities in a large New York City daily, another a helicopter pilot, another an engineer responsible for a patentable invention, another a prominent realtor, and the remaining three doing honors work in Ivy League colleges. Good adjustment (4 on the scale), was attained by forty (approximately 50 percent) of our children. An evaluation of "good" means that the individual has attained what could be expected on the basis of his estimated abilities but has not attained outstanding success in his field.

These people are still considered successful. Eight of these good achievers have successfully completed graduate studies in psychology (one), law (two), podiatry (one), optics (one), art history (one), business administration (one), architecture (one); six of the group are engineers, two filmmakers, and seven have managerial positions in the family business.

Average achievement (scored 3) was attained by twenty-one (27 percent) of the total group. By average, we mean: (1) the individual has attained what could be expected of him, but his abilities are not great enough to take him past high school; or (2) he has not attained the potential we had expected, yet, objectively, is managing to support himself and his family. An example of the former is Cindy, whose overall function was in the mildly mentally retarded range. Cindy, at age twenty-one, attends a sheltered workshop. However, she finds her way about the city alone, has a group of friends, and manages an independent existence appropriate to her intellectual level. She is well liked, conscientious, and reliable. An example of the latter is Daniel, the son of a prominent family. His overall cognitive functioning is in the superior range. Yet he never could manage written examinations. Although he was admitted into a law school, the work was too much of a burden and he left at the end of two years. He then went to work in one of the many businesses in which his family was involved and soon took over management of the entire operation. Unfortunately, he never did and still does not care for the work and looks on it as just a job.

A rating of 2, attained by eight (10 percent) of our patients, represents a marginal adjustment. Those people are managing to work but at a level that is not consistent with their potential. Ann is an example. Now twenty-one, she was first seen in 1968 at age eight years nine months. At that time, it was noted that Ann was suffering from two major problems: evidence of perceptual dysfunction and an emotional disturbance characterized by severe anxiety, feelings of inadequacy, and fear of being deserted by her divorced mother and father. Neurological examination showed gross choreoform movements, an abnormal extension test, marked synkinesis, and poor motor coordination. On neuropsychological examination, there was marked angulation difficulty in visual-motor function, severe praxic errors, gross difficulty with right-left discrimination, and auditory sequencing errors. Remedial work went on for thirty months, but it was not until age twelve that she returned for the psychotherapy which had been recommended three years before. Progress was made; she earned her high school equivalency diploma. At age eighteen, she entered a special college program for learning disabled. She was never able to keep up with the work demanded of her and left college two years later to work with her father. Her work is unskilled, and she is really biding time until she marries.

Two children of the seventy-nine had extremely poor outcomes: one was hospitalized intermittently with acute exacerbations of schizophrenia; the other suffers from a progressive neurological disease.

However, the occupational and educational outcomes of the original group were generally favorable, with 10 percent classed as excellent, 50 percent good, 27 percent average, and 13 percent marginal and poor.

There was no significant relationship between occupational and educational outcomes and length of remedial education or age at onset of treatment. However, 26 percent of the children with an organic diagnosis, contrasted with 7 percent of the SLD group, had poor or marginal outcomes, while 14 percent of the SLD, in contrast to 5 percent of the "organic" children, achieved excellent outcomes (fig. 4 and table 6).

An individual, however, is more than his occupational and educational skills. Ivan, for example, age thirty-four at last evaluation, is a successful real estate operator. His income is well into six figures. He has a devoted wife with a doctorate in biology and two children, still of preschool age, who appear to be developing normally. Ivan was first seen in our office

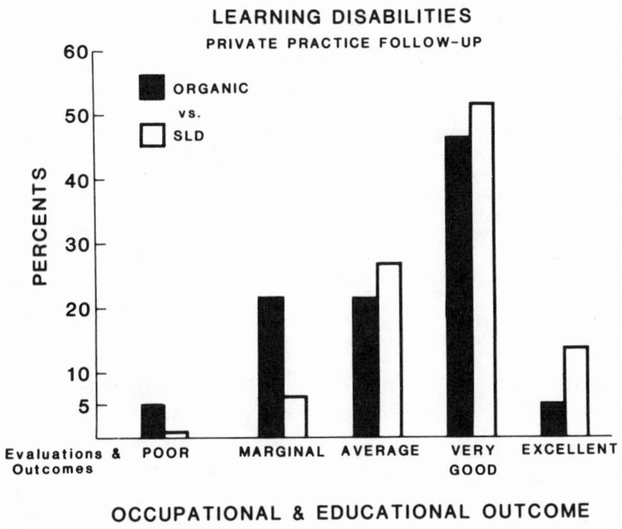

FIG. 4

TABLE 6
LEARNING DISABILITIES
PRIVATE PRACTICE FOLLOW-UP:
OUTCOME AND DIAGNOSIS

	Excellent		Good		Average		Marginal		Poor		
Diagnosis	*N*	%	*N*	%	*N*	%	*N*	%	*N*	%	Total
Organic	1	5	9	47	4	21	4	21	1	5	19
SLD	8	14	29	52	15	27	4	7	0	0	56

in 1953 at about age five years, brought primarily because of unintelligible speech. He was in constant clumsy motion with persistent rhythmic activity, poor fine-motor coordination, increased muscle tone on the left, and choreoform movements on intention. Deep tendon reflexes were increased with ankle clonus and questionable Babinski on the left. Severe perceptual immaturity was found in all perceptual avenues. He was apprehensive, phobic, clinging, and ritualistic. It was felt that this was indeed structural CNS defect, possibly as a result of premature birth weight of two pounds eight ounces, followed by pneumonia and atelectasis in his first month of life. His EEG was moderately abnormal with bitemporal paroxysmal features. He received speech therapy from ages nine to twelve and remedial reading from ages twelve to seventeen. However, he did not have the benefit of specific perceptual training. Psychotherapeutic help was given to Ivan and to his family through those years.

Repeat evaluations at age five, eight, twelve, and eighteen (table 7)

TABLE 7
IVAN: CHANGES IN COGNITIVE FUNCTIONING

	5 Years	8 Years	12 Years	18 Years
IQ	Stanford-Binet, 108	Stanford-Binet, 119	WISC 112 (verbal, 120; performance, 100)	WAIS 116 (verbal, 128; performance, 98)
Reading, oral ..	...	...	3.3 (Jastak)	14.8 (Jastak)
Comprehension	...	...	4.1 (California Primary)	Fifty-seventh percentile DRT
Spelling	...	...	2.6 (Jastak)	5.2 (Jastak) Speed Second percentile

revealed consistently high verbal abilities but persistently average performance abilities. Perceptual errors persisted with consistent problems in spatial orientation including visual-motor, visual figure ground, auditory sequencing, and body image. At age eighteen years, he was still confused in right-left orientation and praxis. His reading had improved to a college level, but his reading speed score was only at the second percentile. He did go to college; he dictated his reports, which were then typed by a secretary, went into a real estate venture with a relative, married a girl who is completely supportive, and bought a house near that of his parents. His conceptualization of real estate deals, however, shows a firm grasp of his business; his holdings are in the millions. Ivan's history illustrates the tenacity with which perceptual deviations remain, particularly in an individual with organic CNS findings. Even under the best of circumstances, evidence of the old learning disability persists. With appropriate treatment and support, however, his abilities were developed and utilized in a successful and productive life.

Conclusions

The prognosis for academic achievement and occupational adjustment in children and adolescents with learning disability who have the benefit of appropriate and sufficient educational intervention and receive optimal and necessary environmental support is favorable. For most, their potential, as suggested by their cognitive abilities, may be reached in adulthood. In children with more limited environmental supports, as seen in the Bellevue study, a majority learned to read, although subgroup differences were apparent when reading adequacy was examined. However, in spite of adequate social and vocational adjustment and neuropsychological maturation in some areas, the problems of spatial and temporal organization persist through adolescence and into adulthood. This was particularly true of those with learning disability who are found on neurological examination to have, in addition, complicating "organic" factors.

One cannot assume that children will outgrow their learning disability spontaneously. Specific intervention and continued support for the children and their families appear to offer the best chances for optimal adult functioning. As we review the occupational status of our private practice group, we are impressed with the patterns of occupational choices in our sample. Two-thirds of our group who attained professional and technical occupations chose work which required strengths in the visual perceptual and quantitative areas. These fields include engineering, filmmaking, art history, medical illustration, accounting, and finance. Only five of our group chose professions requiring language competencies as found in journalism, advertising, and law. This suggests to us the importance of guiding these patients through important transitions in their lives so that they may utilize their strengths and avoid fields in which their weakness would only doom them to disappointment (see cases of Danny and Ivan for unwise and wise decisions). Our experience indicates that, even when the intervention with the learning problem has been successfully completed, adolescents need assistance as they reach such decision points as college planning and occupational choices. Despite the many variables contributing to educational achievement and occupational status of children and adolescents with learning disability, prognosis for the most part is favorable.

REFERENCES

Rawson, M. 1968. *Development Language Disability: Adult Accomplishments of Dyslexic Boys*. Baltimore: Johns Hopkins University Press.

Satz, P.; Taylor, H. G.; Friel, J.; and Fletcher, J. M. 1978. Some developmental and predictive precursors of reading disabilities: a six year follow-up. In A. Benton and D. Pearl, eds. *Dyslexia: An Appraisal of Current Knowledge*. New York: Oxford University Press.

Schonhaut, S., and Satz, P. 1983. Prognosis for children with learning disabilities: a review of follow-up studies. In M. Rutter, ed. *Developmental Neuropsychiatry*. New York: Guilford.

Shaffer, D.; O'Connor, P. A.; Shafer, S. Q.; and Prupis, S. 1983. Neurological "soft signs": their origins and significance for behavior. In M. Rutter, ed. *Developmental Neuropsychiatry*. New York: Guilford.

Silver, A. A., and Hagin, R. A. 1964. Specific reading disability: follow-up studies. *American Journal of Orthopsychiatry* 34:95–102.

Spreen, O. 1978. *Learning-disabled Children Growing Up*. Final report to Health and Welfare Canada, Health Programs Branch. Ottawa: Health and Welfare Canada.

ADDITIONAL REFERENCES

Ackerman, P. T.; Dykman, R. A.; and Peters, J. E. 1977. Learning disabled boys as adolescents: cognitive factors and achievement. *Journal of the American Academy of Child Psychiatry* 16:296–313.

Balow, B., and Blomquist, M. 1965. Young adults ten to fifteen years after severe reading disability. *Elementary School Journal* 66:44–48.

Carter, R. P. A. 1964. *A Descriptive Analysis of the Adult Adjustment of Persons Once Identified as Disabled Readers*. Ph.D. diss. Indiana University.

Dykman, R. A.; Peters, J. E.; and Ackerman, P. T. 1973. Experimental approaches to the study of minimal brain dysfunction: a follow-up study. *Annals of the New York Academy of Science* 205:93–108.

Gottesman, R.; Belmont, I.; and Kaminer, R. 1975. Admission and follow-up status of reading disabled children referred to a medical clinic. *Journal of Learning Disabilities* 8:642–650.

Hardy, M. E. 1968. *Clinical Follow-Up Study of Disabled Readers*. Ph.D. diss. University of Toronto.

Howden, M. E. 1967. *A Nineteen-Year Follow-Up Study of Good, Average and Poor Readers in the Fifth and Sixth Grades*. Ph.D. diss. University of Oregon.

Kline, C., and Kline, C. 1975. Follow-up study of 211 dyslexic children. *Bulletin of the Orton Society* 25:127–144.

Muehl, S., and Forell, E. R. 1973. A follow-up study of disabled readers: variables related to high school reading performance. *Reading Research Quarterly* 9:110–123.

Preston, R. C., and Yarrington, D. J. 1967. Status of fifty retarded readers 8 years after reading clinic diagnosis. *Journal of Reading* 11:122–124.

Robinson, H. M., and Smith, H. D. 1962. Reading clinic: ten years after. *Elementary School Journal* 63:22–27.

Rourke, B. P., and Orr, R. R. 1977. Prediction of the reading and spelling performances of normal and retarded children: a four-year follow-up. *Journal of Abnormal Child Psychology* 5:9–20.

Rutter, M.; Tizard, J.; Yule, W.; Graham, P.; and Whitmore, K. 1976. Research report: Isle of Wight studies, 1964–1974. *Psychological Medicine* 6:313–332.

Trites, R., and Fiedorowicz, C. 1976. Follow-up study of children with specific (or primary) reading disability. In R. Knights and D. J. Bakker, eds. *The Neuropsychology of Learning Disorders: Theoretical Approaches*. Baltimore: University Park Press.

PART III

PSYCHOPATHOLOGICAL ASPECTS OF ADOLESCENCE

EDITORS' INTRODUCTION

It seems reasonably clear that there has been an upsurge in the incidence of the more serious forms of adolescent psychopathology in recent years. Statistics are unequivocal regarding adolescent suicide, which now represents a major public health problem. The numbers are less explicit, but clinical impressions support the observation that such disorders as anorexia nervosa, bulimia, and severe character disturbances are sharply on the rise and are making ever larger demands on the attention and concern of adolescent psychiatrists.

Derek Miller and Barry S. Carlton consider the biopsychosocial etiology and differential diagnosis of a variety of organic and psychological illnesses that result in excessive weight loss. As a final common pathway of attempted solutions to developmental conflict, anorexia nervosa is described as a symptom complex without specific etiology but with a dynamic related to issues of control, helplessness, sexual identity, and generalized identity confusion. There is a notable relationship between the psychological effects of starvation and the underlying dynamic conflicts and problems of treatment. Miller and Carlton state that successful treatment is directed toward relief of starvation, amelioration of pathological personality distortions, and resolution of underlying emotional disorder. They recommend, when clinically indicated, hospital adolescent psychiatric care and discuss the quality of social systems in hospitals, indications for hospital treatment, management of severe anorexia, psychotherapeutic issues, and termination of therapy.

Peter L. Giovacchini considers identity sense in adolescents as being closely related to self-representation and concentrates on its psychopathological distortions as the adolescent encounters difficulties moving into the adult world. Giovacchini relates these difficulties to specific types of infantile traumas that become clinically evident as borderline constellations manifesting a lack of psychic continuity.

Frederick J. Stoddard, Sue S. Cahners, and Kambiz Pahlavan present an integrated study of suicide attempted by self-immolation during adolescence. The authors found that these adolescents came from dysfunctional families and manifested severe psychopathology. In a separate chapter Stoddard and Cahners review the psychotherapeutic efforts made with this group and describe, rather pessimistically, their outcomes.

Perihan Aral Rosenthal and Mairin B. Doherty focus on the intrapsychic conflicts and catastrophic rage exhibited by a group of violent adolescent girls. They found that the rage and violence had psychodynamic origins in their early relationship with their mothers and other significant care givers.

15 THE ETIOLOGY AND TREATMENT OF ANOREXIA NERVOSA

DEREK MILLER AND BARRY S. CARLTON

Excessive weight loss in adolescents is caused by a multiplicity of biopsychosocial factors, and its differential diagnosis includes both organic and psychological illnesses. It may occur in athletic young males who misunderstand the need for adequate food intake as well as in young people who suffer from anorexia nervosa, in which running is the manifestation of a symptom of excessive exercise (Chapman 1983).

Organic causes are tuberculosis, neoplasms, and endocrine dysfunction. The latter, particularly, includes panhypopituitarism, pituitary tumors, and thyrotoxicosis. Plasma growth hormone is below normal in starvation. Psychosomatic causes include the affective disorders and the schizophrenic syndromes, particularly when they involve delusions about food and one's body. Psychological causes include a variety of personality problems, including both histrionic and borderline character disorders, depression due to acute and chronic emotional deprivation, and phobias.

Anorexia nervosa has been thought to occur independently of these syndromes (Bliss 1960), but this is questionable. Although the symptom complex has specific determinants, we hypothesize that the underlying biopsychological etiology is not specific, and ultimately this is the determinant of successful therapy. The syndrome has been called a "dance macabre" in which young people may starve themselves to death in a sea of plenty.

Anorexia nervosa was probably first commented on in the thirteenth century in the description of the personality of Princess Margaret of Hun-

0-226-24058-4/85/0012-0016$01.00

gary, who died at the age of twenty-five (Konradyne 1973). It was described in the medical literature by Morton (1694) and later by Gull (1874). In recent years, along with bulimia, its incidence has become pandemic among relatively affluent groups. It is statistically more frequent among girls (Halmi 1974) and is reported to have a mortality rate of between 3.6 and 6.6 percent.

The Anorexia Nervosa Syndrome

Although the onset of anorexia may appear sudden, often there has been an insidious dietary preoccupation for long periods before the illness becomes evident. Typically the illness occurs in "the best little girl in the world," often a bright, personable child who has never given any particular trouble to her family, friends, or school. Commonly, there is no previous known illness and no history of thought disorder. The characteristic features of the primary syndrome are the pursuit of thinness in the struggle for an independent identity and a striving for perfection. A delusional denial of excessive thinness occurs along with hyperactivity and a preoccupation with food. Body image distortion is often related to the preoccupation of being enslaved and exploited both by one's own body and by others.

All anorectic patients show conflicts over issues of control, but these conflicts are present in many other psychological disturbances. For example, in the initial phase of a bipolar type of mood disorder in adolescents, there is often a rapid, inexplicable type of mood fluctuation. This almost hourly reaction, which is felt as incomprehensible and arouses intense feelings of helplessness, may produce a wide variation of symptoms. Self-starvation is only one method the individual uses in an attempt to gain a feeling of mastery of the self and the environment.

Problems of identity, especially those which manifest themselves with the denial of a wish to be sexual, typically appear in anorexia nervosa. The denial of sexuality may also be present in other syndromes, especially those associated with histrionic personality disorders. Often anorexia nervosa sufferers are particularly competent and cooperative young people whose identity confusion is reinforced because they are unsure whether they are loved for themselves or for their ability.

In all eating disorders the struggle over control is projected onto food. Self-starvation, bulimia, and self-induced vomiting become issues over which the control battle is fought both with the family and the self. In bulimia, the vomiting appears to be an attempt to control a chaotic eating pattern (Johnson and Berndt 1983). Patients often feel that if they allow themselves to eat, all sense of control will be lost. Should this happen, there is then the magical recourse to self-induced vomiting.

The essential dynamic has been discussed many times. Kestemberg (1972) sees the illness as related to oedipal conflicts and the acceptance of one's own sexuality. However, commonly it seems to be an issue of control over a sense of helplessness and it is the patient's projection of this into others who are seen as powerful, particularly the family and therapeutic personnel. The goal is the estalishment of a personal sense of autonomy. These dynamic conflicts do not necessarily have the symptoms of self-starvation.

The choice of anorexia nervosa represents a psychosocially determined final common path that is an attempted solution of many biopsychological conflicts: histrionic characters with conversion symptoms, borderline personalities, neuroendocrinologically based schizophrenia syndromes, and mood disorders. The reason for the appearance of an eating disorder may lie in conflictual social system values which impinge on the individual. Once the syndrome is adopted, the disorder is likely to continue because of the feedback it creates in a vulnerable individual.

Through self-starvation the individual efficiently controls the reactions of others, helplessness is projected, and a false sense of mastery is obtained by controlling the uncontrollable. Bodily induced helplessness produced by pubertal change can also be dealt with. Producing amenorrhea, for females, and decreasing the frequency of erections, for males who abhor masturbation, mean that the body is finally under control. Since starvation in itself increases the sense of omnipotence in these patients, with a dynamic reinforcement they become terrifyingly omnipotent. They have bodies that do not need food; if they die, they will survive. Furthermore, since the individual who feels helpless may feel tormented, there is an additional need to resolve confusion by making this experience real. The symptoms of anorexia are thus reinforced as the experience of persecution may be confirmed.

Many therapeutic modalities—particularly coercive behavioral techniques, such as increasing isolation as a response to weight loss (Maloney and Klykylo 1983)—replay family attitudes of rejection and coercion. Furthermore, the denial of nutritional need, the pleasure in food refusal, and the unusual handling of food (Feighner 1972) all reinforce the negative response of both family and therapeutic personnel to the syndrome.

In addition, when these youngsters induce emesis, use cathartics, and exercise excessively (Lippe 1983), they are likely to produce coercive responses from the environment. Approximately 93 percent of all individuals who suffer from anorexia nervosa deny illness (Rollins and Piazza 1978), which reinforces negative environmental responses. This is a particular issue in those 4 percent of all sufferers who are boys, who are most resistant to treatment (Crisp and Toms 1972).

As with all psychosomatic symptoms, the patient's problems commonly appear to regulate the family system in which they become enmeshed. A marital conflict may be converted into a family conflict over issues of caring for the child. Separating parents may come together over their child's survival. None of this, however, explains why one individual will experience the symptoms of anorexia and another will not. Perfectionistic individuals with identity problems develop other psychosomatic illnesses and have many other psychological syndromes.

Social System Determinants

Two-thirds of the patients in Bruch's (1982) series were only daughters, often with older-than-average parents. The family constellation around anorexia nervosa is typical of that seen in all psychosomatic illness. In particular, the patient has a sense of being enmeshed in the family. There is excessive parental overprotection, rigidity or dishonesty over moral and other issues, and an inability on the part of the family to solve interpersonal conflicts (Minuchin 1978). These are usually controlling rather than impulsive families (Miller 1980).

It is probable that the initial choice of symptom is related to implicit family and societal conflicts over food and weight. It is common for anorexia to appear in families that have been highly preoccupied with issues of diet, health food, and overweight. One of us (D. Miller) saw four boys who suffered from anorexia nervosa; all of them had parents who were involved in the food industry. It is not unusual for anorectic girls to have mothers who have conflicts about cooking. Often these mothers have returned to school or to work, and their homemaking tasks have become more onerous. It is as if their daughters' refusal to eat is partially in obedience to an implicit message from mothers who no longer wish to cook. This may also partially represent a depressed response to perceived lack of parenting. If the situation is compounded by marital stress in association with the new maternal role and fathers who are controlling individuals, precursors for the development of anorectic symptoms exist.

Often the conflicted adolescent appears to develop the symptoms by chance. The typical family situation involves the quiet, good child who is relatively ignored by the family at mealtime. The girl begins to diet, either because of social system pressures, particularly from peers, and/ or internal conflicts over issues of helplessness, control, and sexuality. When the child's poor appetite is noticed, it becomes the focus of the family's attention. Self-starvation is reinforced as the symptom begins to dominate mealtimes and then the whole intrapersonal situation of the family members.

Many adolescent girls who suffer from anorexia nervosa appear to be victims of group contagion. Among girls in a high school setting, there is often an intense preoccupation with weight. These girls often have a group leader who shares the conflicts of the larger group over weight and issues of sexual attractiveness and encourages group dieting. The member of this group who becomes anorectic is likely to be the youngster with preexisting family conflicts over autonomy, with confusion about sexual and personal identity, and with preoccupation with issues of helplessness. Such an individual becomes the group's representative insofar as difficulties over food are concerned. The anorectic adolescent becomes used by the peer group; the starving one is both devalued and protected. The peer group is seemingly tolerant of the increasing starvation, as are the patient's family, until it becomes apparent that the condition is serious. Then peers become highly preoccupied with the feeding of their starving member.

The Effects of Starvation

There is no primary hypothalamic abnormality that causes anorexia nervosa. Rather, the effects on hypothalamic function are secondary to food deprivation. Weight loss that is greater than 20 percent of expected body weight begins to produce psychological and physiological effects. Bradycardia, hypotension, and hypothermia indicate increasing physical danger. An increase in plasma growth hormone with decreases in LH, FSH, and T3 are all clear evidence of interference with hypothalamic function. Weight change not only creates disordered hypothalamic function, it may also produce secondary pituitary dysfunction. Starving patients have a high level of plasma growth hormone and a low level of plasma LH and

FSH; some have an increase in plasma cortisol. Amenorrhea occurs with lanugo hairs. There may be a slowing of the heart rate, and if it falls to less than sixty beats per minute, heart block may occur; thus the result of starvation may be death. Starving individuals lose a sense of appetite and do not know when they are empty and when they are full. There is an absence of appropriate hunger and satiation experiences.

Apart from the physiological symptoms of starvation, its psychological effects influence the development of personality. Starvation produces a psychological regression, a narcissistic preoccupation with the self, and often psychotic-like thoughts. It is associated with hyperacuity and hypersensitivity. These all tend to create a feeling of being super special. The bodily changes of starvation influence the perception of one's body image, but what differentiates the anorexia nervosa picture from other eating disorders is the unawareness that the loss of weight makes the individual look unattractive.

All chronic psychological and physical illness affects personality development. The maturational age of an individual when such an illness occurs is highly significant. If illness occurs prior to puberty, it interferes with the development of adolescence, and secondary separation-individuation may not take place. If the disorder occurs in middle adolescence, the first steps toward the development of autonomy have taken place, but the final consolidaton of identity does not occur.

Successful treatment is directed toward the relief of starvation, the amelioration of pathological personality distortions produced by the syndrome, and the resolution of the underlying biopsychosocial determinants of the syndrome. Thus, adequate diagnosis includes not just a determination of what type of eating disorder is present but also its underlying etiology. For example, the typical primary symptoms of organic depression in adolescence include sleep disturbances in which the youngster falls asleep and is then intermittently wakeful, morning irritability, and an appetite disturbance which does not normally improve until midday. In an appropriate psychosocial field of conflict, this can appear as a profound anorectic syndrome.

Some adolescents with this type of depression/self-starvation syndrome do not see themselves as being more comfortable if they "lose another two or three pounds." They are acutely aware of their own inappropriate appearance and do not normally engage in excessive exercise. Others, however, may show typical symptoms of anorexia nervosa.

Depression may be present in adolescents who are confused about their own identity. It is not unusual to find a mood disorder along with self-starvation and a specific psychological conflict:

> Karen, aged sixteen, had a history of intermittent depressions each year which lasted for about three months. This was first noticed when she was approximately fifteen months old. Her paternal grandmother had been hospitalized for depression, and her mother was clearly depressed. When Karen was eight, a sixteen-year-old male babysitter had sexually assaulted her over a period of about one year. At age thirteen she dated a boy of seventeen who attempted to engage in some "heavy necking." She became very conscious of her breasts. After a rapid weight loss of more than a third of her body weight, she was admitted to an adolescent treatment center. She was excited, grandiose, and elated, but within two weeks she became overtly depressed. She demonstrated marked affective lability. A diagnosis of bipolar affective disorder was made. An appropriate dosage of lithium carbonate ended her mood swings, but she continued to feel that she must be as asexual in appearance as possible. Her weight returned to a safe level at which she remained amenorrheic, and she began to adapt to this. Therapy was still needed for her chronic sexual confusion, her body image distortions, and her pervasive anxiety.

Problems of Treatment

Anorexia becomes difficult to treat when the self-starvation is not controllable on the basis of the interpersonal relationships that an individual may have with the family, significant others, peers, or, when treatment is initiated, with therapeutic personnel. Difficulty also arises when the self-starvation does not respond to any indicated specific psychopharmacological interventions. This especially applies to those individuals who suffer from unipolar or bipolar illness or schizophrenia where anorexia is a secondary symptom.

Almost all difficult cases require hospital treatment which may be in a variety of settings: a pediatric unit, an encapsulated inpatient setting, or a treatment center that provides comprehensive and continuous care from the same treating personnel in a critical care unit, with available partial hospitalization and outpatient facilities.

The quality of the social system of each of these settings needs to be understood if treatment is to be rational. A general medical pediatric ward often is served by multiple attending physicians. Each may have an idiosyncratic policy toward the treatment of anorexia. Some are preoccupied with diet, others with weight; some use minor tranquilizers, sedatives, or antidepressants without a formal diagnosis of depression. Nursing staff are often exposed to multiple house officers, and, in a system in which positive reinforcement is difficult to produce, staff easily become coercive. Those who require tube feeding in such settings may masochistically eroticize the experience.

In general psychiatric units, the quality of medical care is often unsatisfactory, and it is doubtful whether the developmental needs of young people who suffer from emotional disturbances are well met. Adolescent psychiatric wards, in our opinion, offer the best environment to treat anorectic adolescents when hospitalization is indicated, but a great deal depends on the quality of the therapeutic setting.

A hospital experience should provide continuity of therapeutic relationships and, in a highly sophisticated way, meet the specific and nonspecific treatment needs of the patient (Miller and Knesper 1976). A satisfactory treatment center for psychologically and psychosomatically disturbed adolescents should have a clear philosophy of treatment. Tension is alleviated, symptoms are attenuated, and specific therapeutic interventions become more effective if a holding environment (Winnicott 1971) is created into which the patient projects tension and from which she or he receives emotional support. This requires genuine continuity of care. The patient should not be exposed to frequent separations from significant therapeutic and educational caring personnel as he or she becomes able to be more responsible for the self. As the patient matures, the opportunity is given to reject staff, rather than vice versa.

It should be recognized that in some ways the social system of a therapeutic environment for disturbed adolescents can be detrimental for functioning in society at large. Periods of passive television watching and confused idleness are antitherapeutic and hinder personality maturation. The setting should have a school able to provide both remedial and normative education, occupational and recreational therapy, and provision for adequate creative and imaginative stimulation. Individuals who no longer need intensive care should not lose contact with therapeutic personnel when they move to partial hospitalization, to their own families' or a group home, and eventually to outpatient care. Separations from emotionally significant people in a therapeutic setting may be a repetition of destructive early trauma.

A satisfactory holding environment has consistent implicit and explicit messages. All psychologically disturbed individuals have to attempt to alleviate intolerable feelings of helplessness that are worsened when the individual feels in conflict with the internal or external environment. The implicit messages of certain systems, which in themselves are often conflictual and pathological for individuals, tend to be consistent; explicit messages often are inconsistent and contradict implicit communication. Behavioral symptoms commonly are significantly determined by implicit (constant) messages in conflictual systems; it is important that this be recognized if recovery is to occur.

A therapeutic holding environment does not punish, is noncoercive, assists the patient to develop or reinforce the capacity to be ambivalent, is realistic, and offers appropriate controls through skilled interpersonal relationships and understandable consequences to behavior. It allows both intimacy and privacy. It does not create an emotional deficiency disease (Bettelheim and Sylvester 1948) or teach patients to lead a life that is sociologically aberrant (Miller 1957). In particular, it provides a high degree of creative stimulation which helps alleviate the anaclitic state from which all emotionally disturbed young people suffer. Creativity and imagination, cognitive and physical achievement should all be valued. Help should be provided in all these spheres of human functioning.

The treatment center should provide that which is required for normal biopsychosocial development. The therapeutic staff should be able to differentiate between the symptoms of psychological illness and those created by developmental impasse. Serious psychological illness is always an assault on normal psychological development; the failure to recognize this has allowed the pervasive fantasy that brief treatment is appropriate for major psychiatric illness.

Personnel skilled in the psychotherapeutic resolution of specific conficts should be able to provide sophisticated psychopharmacology and appropriate physical care. In self-starvation syndromes, competent specialized medical care is a necessity. Finally, the environment should not produce iatrogenic symptoms. Many settings—psychotherapeutic, intrafamilial, and residential—may implicitly set the stage for the vulnerable patient to develop institutional symptoms which vary from catatonia to self-mutilation and violence.

Indications for Hospital Treatment

The intensity of anorectic symptoms indicates whether hospitalization is necessary. The denial of a need to eat may not be only verbal but may also be present in association with an unrealistic level of exercise, bulimia, vomiting, and food hiding. The effects of starvation are apparent but are denied. The patient may comment that with the loss of a few more pounds, she or he will feel satisfied.

The physiological effects of starvation are likely to be apparent in those who require hospital care. In those who vomit, potassium and sodium levels are lowered. The lower potassium levels produce abnormal EKG changes. Depending on the chronicity of the self-starvation, there may be bone marrow hypoplasia, hypercarotenemia, hypercholesterolemia, and a low sedimentation rate. Electrocardiograph examination, apart from a lowered pulse rate, may also show ST depression, flat T-waves, and a lengthened QT interval.

An indication for urgent intervention is a halving of the pulse rate and/or a shift from a state in which the youngster is hyperactive and convinced that the loss of weight is appropriate to a state of lethargy and general apathy.

The interfamilial and social environments may become psychonoxious for the anorectic patient. Family psychopathology which joins the patient in a denial of the severity of the illness can lead to the patient's death. Some families, perhaps in response to anorexia, begin to behave as though they would like to destroy the child. One family proposed to solve the child's serious loss of weight with a voyage in the Caribbean on a sailboat.

The pathological family interaction which results from anorectic behavior, apart from the place of parental pathology in the etiology of the syndrome, cannot be rapidly resolved despite the optimism of some (Minuchin 1978). Invasive parents who cannot allow their children emotional or physical privacy help create a situation in which total or relative withdrawal from the family becomes necessary for the survival of the child.

The Management of Severe Anorexia

When anorectic adolescents are admitted to the critical care unit of our treatment center, depending on their height and potential optimal weight, they are told that if they gain one-half pound a day, they will be able to take part in all program activities of the treatment center. Most adolescents cannot tolerate more than 3,000 calories daily, so a weight gain of more than one-half pound daily cannot be expected. Stuffing an individual with excessive food produces vulnerability to bulimia. Furthermore, such an approach does not reinforce the concept that staff can be trusted to offer appropriate external controls over gorging and loss of control. The patients are weighed daily but are not told what their weight is because this encourages dietary manipulation.

There should be no implicit or explicit permission for the child to vomit. Since it is well known that self-induced vomiting occurs in anorexia nervosa, to leave the child alone for any period of time may be perceived as giving permission to vomit, to exercise excessively, to not stay in bed, or to cheat when he or she is weighed by drinking excessive amounts of fluid. While the patient is on bedrest and awake, she or he requires constant adult supervision and companionship. The role of the adult is to be companionable, play board games with the patient, and assist with schoolwork. Nevertheless, this is perceived by the child as highly persecutory, because all but the most depressed have an implicit desire for autonomy and privacy.

While the adolescent is on bedrest, contact with peers and parental visits are not restricted. Peers are essential messengers from the environment, thus reinforcing the desirability to the patient of leaving the regressive state of bedrest. With this regimen, plus individual psychotherapy from a therapist who is not concerned with environmental management, patients in our therapeutic system began to gain weight within three to five days. Of thirteen anorectic patients admitted to the treatment center since 1979, only one has ever required intubation. She had been tube fed on a pediatric ward prior to her psychiatric hospitalization and had eroticized this experience.

Weight gain is thus produced by an implicit technique of positive reinforcement. Other than bedrest, no social deprivation is used. Food is an indirect issue. If the patient has become so anxious about excessive food intake that she feels unable to eat enough to gain weight, a food supplement may be offered, but the patient is at liberty to refuse this. We do not believe that isolation can ever be helpful as this may be seen as developmentally assaultive.

The issue of weight should be managed by a physician who is not the patient's psychotherapist; in our setting, this is a pediatrician who is also a child psychiatrist. The criteria for recovery are the restoration of normal weight along with the processes of normal psychological development. Adaptation around a safe, suboptimal weight without the resolution of conflicts about control and sexuality is prognostically unsatisfactory.

Psychotherapy

Issues of projection, helplessness, denial, and control of the environment by dietary manipulation can be dealt with only by a therapist who is not directly involved in therapeutic management. Furthermore, if psychotherapists become preoccupied with management, the patient may create an impasse which becomes an intolerable resistance. None of these dynamic conflicts is specific to anorexia nervosa, but they are among those typical to this syndrome.

Patients are usually seen in expressive-supportive psychotherapy three times weekly. Supportive clarification helps the patients see how they attempt to control their environment and how issues of helplessness begin to be addressed. In addition, problems around the desire for magical solutions and sexual conflict have to be resolved. There are usually clear issues around a failure to resolve oedipal conflicts. Many have little sense of autonomy and appear as borderline personalities. As they recover, they become aware of emotional dependence.

Family therapy in our setting usually begins as the patient shows some sense of autonomy. The therapy is particularly designed to focus on the issue of how the patient is entrapped in the family and how the patient's illness becomes the focus of family conflict. Family therapy may not be possible if parents refuse to share parenting, or if the parental conflict is so great that the parents' narcissistic involvement with each other means that they cannot emotionally involve themselves with their child. Some parents may need a disturbed child as a focus for the projection of their own anxieties. This is particularly likely with parents who themselves suffer from borderline personality syndromes. Some parents unconsciously reinforce the symptoms because of their need to retain a dependent child, and this is a particular issue in those who adapt to a suboptimal weight. This problem is also likely to occur with a younger sibling when others have already left home. Other symptomatically regressive syndromes, such as those connected with drug and alcohol abuse, are also likely to be actively colluded in by some conflicted parents.

The Termination of Therapy

After the patients reach outpatient status, their inclination is often to terminate therapy before the return of the normal menstrual cycle. Although at this point therapy may cease because of overt demands for autonomy, we believe the ultimate prognosis for successful adult adjustment is then impaired. The normal menstrual cycle occurs when 22 percent of body weight is fat, although the cycle is maintained when 17 percent of weight is adipose tissue.

A particular problem is created by those anorectics who adapt to a subnormal weight that does not allow the return of normal menstruation but presents no danger to life. These young people are unable to accept their own sexual identity or normative helplessness. The acceptance of the latter is necessary for the former, but an androgynous solution is not a satisfactory resolution of developmental conflict. Some decide that therapy is no longer needed when their periods return, although they may know, and the therapist certainly does know, that significant issues have not yet been resolved. A number of these youngsters may return at a later date with more conscious motivation to resolve disturbing inner conflicts.

Conclusions

This paper considers the biopsychosocial etiology and differential diagnosis of syndromes which present themselves with a symptomatic picture that is called anorexia nervosa. Although there is a typical dynamic to this, it is not specific; the dynamic is related to issues of control, helplessness, sexual identity, and generalized identity confusion. Projection and denial are prominent defenses. There is no specific biological etiology, but many cases show disorders of mood as well as schizophrenic syndromes. There is a notable relationship between the psychological effects of starvation and the underlying dynamic conflicts and problems of treatment. Proper medical care, relearning to eat appropriately, psychotherapy, and genuine continuity of care are stressed.

REFERENCES

Bettelheim, B., and Sylvester, E. 1948. A therapeutic milieu. *American Journal of Orthopsychiatry* 18:191–206.

Bliss, E. L., and Branch, C. H. H. 1960. *Anorexia Nervosa: Its History,*

Psychology and Biology. New York: Hoeber.

Bruch, H. 1962. Perceptual and conceptual disorders in anorexia nervosa. *Psychiatric Medicine* 24:187–194.

Chapman, J. 1983. Excessive weight loss in the athletic adolescent. *Journal of Adolescent Health Care* 3:247–252.

Crisp, A. H., and Toms, D. A. 1972. Primary anorexia nervosa or weight phobia in the male: report on 13 cases. *British Medical Journal* 1:334–338.

Feighner, M. P. 1972. Diagnostic criteria for use in psychiatric research. *Archives of General Psychiatry* 26:57–63.

Gull, W. 1874. Anorexia nervosa (apepsia hysteria, anorexia hysteria). *Trans-Clinical Society of London* 7:22–28.

Halmi, K. A. 1974. Anorexia nervosa: demographic and clinical features in 94 cases. *Psychosomatic Medicine* 36:18–26.

Johnson, C., and Berndt, D. J. 1983. Preliminary investigation of bulimia and life adjustment. *American Journal of Psychiatry* 140:776–777.

Kestemberg, E. 1972. *Le Faim et le corps*. Paris: Presses Universitaires de France.

Konradyne, G. M. 1973. *Margitsziget*. Budapest: Kossath Nyonida.

Lippe, B. 1983. The physiologic aspects of eating disorders. *Journal of the American Academy of Child Psychiatry* 22:108–113.

Maloney, M., and Klykylo, M. D. 1983. An overview of anorexia nervosa, bulimia and obesity in children and adolescents. *Journal of the American Academy of Child Psychiatry* 22:99–107.

Miller, D. 1957. The treatment of adolescents in an adult hospital. *Bulletin of the Menninger Clinic* 21:189–198.

Miller, D. 1980. Family maladaptation reflected in drug use and delinquency. In M. Sugar, ed. *Responding to Adolescent Needs*. New York: Spectrum.

Miller, D., and Knesper, D. 1976. Treatment plans for mental health care. *American Journal of Psychiatry* 133:65–80.

Minuchin, S. 1978. *Psychosomatic Families*. Cambridge, Mass.: Harvard University Press.

Morton, R. 1694. *Phthisiologia, or a Treatise of Consumptions*. English translation. London: Smith & Walford.

Rollins, N., and Piazza, F. 1978. Diagnosis of anorexia nervosa: a critical reappraisal. *Journal of the American Academy of Child Psychiatry* 17:126–137.

Winnicott, D. W. 1971. *Playing and Reality*. London: Tavistock.

16 THE BORDERLINE ADOLESCENT AS A TRANSITIONAL OBJECT: A COMMON VARIATION

PETER L. GIOVACCHINI

Adolescence is a transitional life phase in which the child undergoes a consolidation of character that will form the adult psyche. Adolescents have to relinquish, to a large extent, adaptive techniques that served them in infancy and childhood, and they have to acquire modalities that are in synchrony with the standards of adult interactions, modalities that are integrated in the ego's executive system. The adolescent in the process of becoming an adult also forms an identity which is in a very significant way determined by newly learned adaptive interactions, by the methods the ego uses to relate to the outer world and cope with external problems and inner needs.

There are other psychic structures and processes beside the ego's executive system that contribute to the structure of the self-representation. In this chapter I consider the identity sense as being closely related to the self-representation. In my mind, it is a sensory manifestation of an ego system, the subjective awareness of the self-representation. I have discussed various aspects of the identity sense in detail elsewhere (Giovacchini [1968] 1975). Here I will concentrate on its psychopathological distortions as the child passing through adolescence encounters difficulties moving into the adult world. These difficulties are related to specific types of infantile traumas that become clinically evident as borderline constellations.

There are, however, specific features to these psychopathological or-

0-226-24058-4/85/0012-0012$01.00

ganizations that have both diagnostic and technical implications. They highlight developmental factors during infancy, childhood, and adolescence. The structural cohesion that is effected during adolescence does not occur in this type of borderline condition, or, rather, there is a particular type of structural defect that contributes to the unique features of this subtype of borderline patient.

There are some parallels to infantile and adolescent development, although I do not believe, as Blos (1962) does, that adolescence represents a second chance and is a second stage of individuation. True, considerable individuation occurs during adolescence, but this refers mainly to expansions and modifications of the self-representation. The first individuation concerns the establishment of ego boundaries and the distinction between the inner and outer world. Object relations are progressively structuralized. During adolescence, these boundaries are fairly firm, and the outer world is perceived as separate. Adolescents do not recapitulate this early infantile phase. Instead, they develop one facet of individuation further; they develop greater sensitivity, depth, and concern for external objects. Nevertheless, in order to achieve synthesis and continuity of various psychic levels, there are transitional processes at work during adolescence that are similar to the transitional phenomenon of infancy. This becomes apparent when there are disturbances in adolescent development that accentuate childhood traumas and illuminate the developmental process in general.

Clinical Perspectives and Transitional Phenomena

The adolescent patients I am about to describe have had traumatic backgrounds, but they were not as severely deprived as many psychotic patients and other patients suffering from severe character disorders. Their parents related to them and, to some extent, were able to respond to their needs. As infants these patients did not suffer from privation as Winnicott (1958b) has described. They knew what it meant to be gratified, but satisfaction of needs was, nevertheless, a traumatic experience. This was partially due to the fact that the parents did not accept their children as being individuals in their own right. They could relate to material necessities but could not give any emotional sustenance.

The most striking structural defect consisted of a poorly structuralized self-representation. This was obvious in treatment as these patients constantly demonstrated the blurred boundaries between the external world and the internal world of the mind. They emphasized their tenuous identity by not knowing who they were, what the purpose of their lives might be, or where they fitted in the general scheme. They had little sense of themselves as distinct and separate, even separate from their surroundings. One adolescent patient saw himself as being merged with both external objects and inanimate objects. If he sank into an armchair, he would feel himself as part of the chair. He did not experience panic as so often happens when patients merge and lose their ego boundaries. On the contrary, he felt comfortable and did not distinguish between animate and inanimate. His tendency was to consider everything around him as animate, and he would talk to the furniture. At night he would say elaborate good nights to the various chairs and tables in his room.

This patient, as well as those in the group I am discussing, was treated as if he were an inanimate object. He was never related to as a human being with a mind of his own and distinct needs. He believed his parents looked after his material needs, but after he was fed and cleaned, they more or less ignored him. If he evinced any curiosity or showed enthusiasm or interest, he had no one who would respond to him. Winnicott (1958a) would have described his dilemma as being due to a lack of ego relatedness; his id needs were met but not those of his ego.

The lack of cohesiveness of the self-representation was the outcome of a specific type of defective mothering. As stated, id needs were usually met. During the earliest developmental stages, what I believe to be presymbiotic (Giovacchini 1979), there is an endopsychic registration of the nurturing experience. Progressing to the next stage, however, is difficult and traumatic. The mother of the patient described above used the child as a narcissistic extension of herself, a not unusual situation when we are dealing with patients suffering from character defects. But with these patients this narcissistic extension is unique.

Ordinarily we think of a mother-infant relationship as involving the mother treating the child as a *selfobject* (see Boyer and Giovacchini 1967, p. 269), usually on the basis of projecting the devalued parts of herself, her bad introjects. In other words, we conceptualize narcissistic attachments as being based on elements of part-object relationships. Children who have experienced such a symbiotic phase usually develop a hateful image of themselves. They revile themselves because of their badness and are, in general, self-destructive.

The self-representations of the patients who are being explored here are somewhat different. Although they may also revile themselves, this is not a consistent response. They are often grandiose, but in this respect they are no different from other patients who have passed through a traumatic symbiotic phase. Grandiosity represents an overcompensatory attempt to overcome their miserable sense of unworthiness. What is striking is how often they feel that they do not exist. This is not a typical existential crisis. They do not panic. As the adolescent mentioned above demonstrated, he did not distinguish animate from inanimate, nor did he separate himself from his surroundings. These patients did not feel real, and all of their feelings were also felt as unreal. They did not exist as live entities; they considered themselves much as pieces of furniture.

During infancy, the parents did not relate to the children's emerging sense of aliveness. When these infants were made comfortable by being fed and changed, they were then ignored. If they showed any interest in the environment or indicated a wish for play, they were simply not responded to. As they reached toward the external world, there was no reciprocity.

One of my adult patients whose manifest problems emerged during adolescence complained that the only games she knew how to play were games that required intellect, such as bridge and chess. She felt very awkward around children and was astounded when a friend, a young mother, in a relaxed manner played pat-a-cake and peekaboo with her seven-month-old son, who was hilariously delighted with these games. She was as confused as if she were witnessing a ritual performed by strangers from an alien planet.

As a rule, inasmuch as these patients were not related to as live objects during childhood, they do not have intimate object relations as adults. Their object relations are marginal. They may have friends, in some instances many friends, but there are no close ties or emotional attachments. The absence of feeling may be so pervasive that we get the impression that they relate to objects in a literal sense, that is, as objects rather than persons.

Their methods of relating to the external world suggest that they might have been dealt with in a similar fashion. If they are incapable of forming relationships on a person-to-person basis, then perhaps they were treated as nonpersons. I have emphasized how they do not distinguish between animate and inanimate. I repeat that in treatment there seems to be an absence of transference, implying that these patients do not project feelings or parts of themselves into the analyst. Furthermore, they have periods in which everything is considered in a concrete, mechanistic fashion devoid of any unconscious connotations. An inanimate object does not have an unconscious. On the basis of these phenomena, it is reasonable to assume that they experience the external world in the same way. I conjecture that their mothers did not project elements of their inner psychic life into their children. Rather, I propose that they treated them as inanimate objects in general and transitional objects in particular.

I recall several female patients who were named after their mother's favorite doll. For these mothers it was important that the doll remain a doll, that she not grow up and become a girl. When he was less than one year old, a high school senior was given the same name as a pendant the mother was given that looked like Pinocchio. The patient would burst into tears if he heard the story of Pinocchio or saw a movie or cartoon about him. His psychic equilibrium would become totally disrupted when he thought of the wooden puppet becoming a boy. He was overcome by a poignant longing that was unbearably painful. Ordinarily he was without feeling, and during the first part of his treatment there was a wooden quality about him.

The transitional object as described by Winnicott (1953) is an object that serves the function of being a tentative entrance into the external world. The child's behavior toward it is ruthless, not because of organized hate or because anything is projected into it. It is part of an in-between space, an inanimate object on which the child's security depends and which emboldens the unformed psyche to structuralize progressively and to form boundaries between the self and nonself. In the in-between space where the transitional object resides, the infant, supposedly within a symbiotic context, exercises omnipotent control, and the transitional object is the target of that control.

Ordinarily, we are not much concerned with the transitional object and the way it is treated. Its fate and reactions are of little interest since traditionally the transitional object is inanimate and inanimate objects have no feelings. The problem with our patients who have represented transitional objects for their mothers is that they were not, in fact, inanimate; they were simply treated as if they were. This has led to specific constellations of psychopathology.

The concept of the transitional object is confusing since there are various formulations about it that are not altogether consistent with each other (Grolnick, Barkin, and Muensterberger 1978). I will outline a developmental sequence which is compatible with Winnicott's. I had the opportunity to discuss what is to follow with him, and he agreed that my views of the transitional object were a reflection and a restatement of his. I emphasize different facets of this developmental phenomenon because my intention is to focus on its relevance to various structural defects and the psychopathology I am discussing.

Winnicott (1953) wrote about the transitional situation and the transitional object, elements which he definitely located in the symbiotic phase. As the child emerges from the symbiotic phase on the path to individuation, he constructs an intermediary space between the inner and outer world that will eventually help in consolidating ego boundaries. This is the transitional area between the me and not-me, and it houses the transitional object. It is also an extension of ego boundaries in which the child believes he or she can exercise omnipotent control, according to Winnicott. Thus, the transitional object is both part of the child and the external world, but it still resides in a space that is completely under the developing ego's control. The mother supports the illusion of omnipotence.

I asked Winnicott if the transitional situation is characterized by an ego that contains a nurturing matrix. By "nurturing matrix" I mean an endopsychic registration of the nurturing situation. Winnicott agreed and added that the transitional situation could be considered characterized by the establishment of this matrix. The child who has had optimal mothering gains the conviction that the source of nurturing resides within the psyche rather than in the external world. Actually the external world is not yet recognized since the child is still in the stage of symbiotic fusion. This is an infantile state of omnipotence, according to Winnicott.

I believe the word omnipotence is an unfortunate term because it connotes megalomaniac, grandiose feelings and a heightened sense of importance and power. These reactions are much too sophisticated for a preverbal infant. What we usually mean by infantile omnipotence is a child who is tranquil and satisfied and experiences the maximum security that inner needs will be met. In a sense, the child has the feeling that he is the source of his own nurture, a situation which can be interpreted as omnipotence since he is in complete control of his destiny in that he needs no one. These formulations are obviously adultomorphic and should not be taken literally. I am referring to tendencies, states of satisfaction, and emotional equilibrium. What the infant actually feels is difficult, if not impossible, to ascertain. Our language is geared mainly to an adult perspective, and perhaps we do not have the proper words to describe these early psychic states and developmental stages.

With this caveat in mind, we can say that the in-between space is the area over which the infant has omnipotent control. Winnicott (1971) conceptualized three spaces: (1) the inner space of the psyche, its periphery being the ego's boundaries; (2) an extension of those boundaries, with their periphery bordering on the external world; and (3) the external world. The second of these spaces is the most important for my purpose of understanding a particular type of borderline psychopathology.

Winnicott called this second space the in-between space, the transitional space which is the area of play and creativity. The nurturing matrix characteristic of the transitional situation is projected into an object in this middle space, and through such a projection it becomes the transitional object, which is then subjected to the infant's omnipotent control.

Again we need to clarify a term because what I have described is not exactly projection. In order to project, which is a primitive mental mechanism but considerably more advanced than what I am describing, the ego boundaries have to be more distinct and structured than the lack of such boundaries found in the symbiotic phase. The external object is discernible and clearly recognized. It requires a certain amount of separation to be able to project. The infant who is emerging from symbiosis by creating transitional phenomena has only blurred ego boundaries, so there is not sufficient psychic structure to project in that it is not possible to transfer psychic content from one distinct ego system into another. Instead, the child's psychic periphery seems to stretch outward much like the pseudopodia of an amoeba engulfing an external object and making it part of itself. This is an incorporation, but the psyche reaches out into the world which it believes is part of the self.

We have become accustomed to conceptualizing this early developmental phase in terms of symbiosis, selfobject (see Boyer and Giovacchini 1967, p. 269), or secondary narcissism. In the individuating process, the child emerges from a state of fusion, the "hatching" phase described by Mahler (1963). Still, what evidence do we have that supports such formulations? From the study of psychopathology we have innumerable examples in which patients during the transference regression have reproduced states of symbiotic merger, sometimes blissful and on other occasions terrifying. Still, the ego states that are being recapitulated are the outcome of distortions caused by infantile trauma. We cannot conclude that there is a direct correspondence in the sense that if we observe a state of pathological symbiosis, then there must also be a developmental sequence in which normal symbiosis plays a prominent role. Symbiosis at such an early stage may not occur.

Nevertheless, with both patients and nonpatients we find examples of symbiotic fusion that are neither idealized nor traumatic. They are sometimes followed by creative accomplishment, a sense of well-being, and heightened self-esteem. They seem to represent optimal adjustments rather than defensive overcompensation. They are characterized, however, by mobility, that is, the ego can move in and out of a fusion state with ease. This would indicate that the boundaries between the inner and outer world are well established, if they are not threatened by temporary dissolution. The corresponding infantile phase of development must have progressed beyond beginning individuation to a stage in which external objects are fairly well perceived as separate and distinct. Thus, a symbiotic fusion ordinarily is a psychic process that characterized already well-established object relationships. When we see manifestations of fusion in a more primitive ego organization, we are undoubtedly dealing with traumatic incursions into the developmental sequence that encompasses progression through the transitional space into the outer world, a progression that involves the relinquishing of control. Children then acknowledge a nurturing source outside the self, and they feel sufficient trust and confidence in their caretakers that they can allow dependency feelings to develop.

Regarding the transitional phenomenon, the adult's and child's viewpoints are different. To the adult, the in-between transitional space belongs to the external world, but the child does not recognize an external world and feels this middle space as being part of his psychic world. According to Winnicott (1953), the good mother does not challenge the infant's viewpoint. With optimal mothering the child's needs are met in such a fashion that he does not recognize that nurture comes from the external world, that world that is outside of the area of his control. The mother supports the illusion that the source of nurture resides within the psyche.

What happens when the mothering interaction is traumatic and the illusion is not supported? What are the psychopathological consequences if the mother does not support the formation of the in-between space and the construction of the transitional object? Some mothers may have such a need themselves for omnipotent manipulation that they cannot let their children feel that they have some control over their immediate surroundings, their transitional object, and the nurturing experience.

The mother's character may have many psychopathological variants. Clinicians commonly encounter women who project hated parts of the self into their children. The mothers of the patients focused on here cannot allow them to individuate. They oppose their separation and individuation (Mahler 1963). However, this is not the same as Masterson (1976) and Rinsley's (1982) formulations, which state that borderline patients exhibit fixations during the stages of separation-individuation. The impact of the traumatic environment is felt from the very beginning of life, and distortions of ego development and defects occur in all phases, but particularly those that involve the transitional phenomenon.

This type of interaction seems to involve states of symbiotic fusion, but what is a symbiotic attachment for one person need not be perceived in the same way for another. The mother's assault on the infant or her using him as a nonhuman object so that she can protect herself from her fears of being destroyed by him can be defensive reactions to her terror of a destructive merger. Thus, she fuses with her child in her own way, in such a fashion that permits her to maintain psychic equilibrium. The effect on the child would not necessarily involve his feeling fused with the mother during infancy. Later, with further emotional development, when object relations are partially constructed, the child or adolescent is terrified of intimacy because, now that fusion can be experienced, he or she fears being destroyed by emotional closeness.

Consequently, when we discuss symbiosis in an individual treatment setting, we must keep in mind that we are listening to one psyche only and cannot make accurate inferences about a corresponding process in the other person. This is not always the case. When we are dealing with marital partners, the patient's mental state is often a reflection of the spouse's (Giovacchini 1958). Between adults, fusion states increasingly approach the biological qualities of symbiosis in that the needs of the partners stem from the same level of psychic development. This is not true of the mother-infant relationship, and the mother's needs are at a much more advanced structural level than those of her child. Furthermore, the infant depends on the mother or caretaker for total survival, whereas the mother has alternatives to insure her survival that permit her to relate to different objects in interactions that encompass a variety of functions.

These mothers in analysis reveal that they are afraid of letting their children grow up because they unconsciously believe that they will be murdered by them if they achieve separation and automony. This is frequently a projection of similar feelings that they had toward their mothers. Consequently, they have to keep their infants at an immature level of psychic development by impeding separation and the construction of distinct boundaries as occurs with the construction of the inner space, the transitional in-between space, and the external world. The mother finds herself somewhere on the periphery of what would be the in-between space if the infant were to structuralize progressively. Then she would feel controlled by her child, which could mean being destroyed by him. The child moving into the external world is also perceived as dangerous.

From the analyses of both mothers and their children, as adults, I have noted some characteristic defensive patterns the mothers have used that produced various reactions in their children that define their borderline psychopathology. As mentioned, these mothers do not allow their children to separate and individuate. They achieve this by treating the child as if he were their transitional object.

Putting the child in their transitional space reverses the threat. They now have control instead of being subjected to what they feel as their children's murderous omnipotent manipulations. By keeping their infants in the sphere of their omnipotent control, they feel protected. They render their children helpless and safe.

Mothers relate to children as transitional objects for many reasons, besides needing a protective defense. Often it represents an attempt to move into the external world as they use their children as an intermediary step, that is, they are trying to recapitulate infantile emotional development that they were unable to achieve during their childhood. They do not succeed in progressing, because obviously as an adult a person cannot develop further emotionally by using techniques and relationships that would have been appropriate in infancy. However, using their children in such a fashion enables these mothers to achieve a sufficient degree of psychic equilibrium that permits them to function relatively well in the external world. But this is at the expense of their children.

Even the in-between aspects of the transitional space that houses the transitional object are reflected in patients' reactions and behavior. They feel their whole life is a transition, and they do not know what their goals are or where they should be going. An adolescent patient told me of a repetitive dream he had since childhood in which he was jumping back and forth between two objects but never reaching the object he was jumping toward. He found himself suspended in air and would, on occasion, become anxious because he was afraid he would fall. Frequently these patients also bring dreams of bridges, but the shores are not discernible. The transitional quality of their lives is even more striking in their relationships with people.

CASE 1

A young man in his early twenties sought treatment because he saw no direction in his life. He had the pervasive feeling that he did not really know who he was, partially because he saw no purpose to his existence, nor could he define himself from the viewpoint of having a function in his milieu.

He could accomplish nothing when alone, but he felt extremely uncomfortable when he was with people. He explained his distress as being the outcome of feelings of intense alienation. His position in the world was of being on the periphery, and this was experienced as not belonging to a group, a cause, or even a family.

At first, I thought of him as having a fairly typical borderline constellation. He never had any overt psychotic episodes, but at times he would withdraw sufficiently so that he might have been diagnosed as schizoid. In contrast, there were periods when he was eminently effective. This happened especially during his sophomore year in college when he distinguished himself athletically and did well both academically and socially. Later in college he continued being successful, but he nevertheless remained unhappy and dissatisfied with himself.

As a child, he was used by his mother to soothe her and as a defense against her sexual relations with her husband. When she felt that her husband was sexually interested, she would go to bed early and bring her infant son into bed with her. Husband and wife slept in separate twin beds. She continued sleeping with her son until he was seven years old. As an adolescent, he was often seduced by older women and had innumerable affairs. However, in spite of his successful sexual experiences and his exceptional attractiveness, he was consumed by painful feelings of inadequacy. He considered himself worthless, ugly (if not in body then in spirit), and incapable of doing anything worthwhile. He did not trust his motives and questioned whether there was one good feeling in his "miserable soul." This is another example of extremes of behavior that indicate some fragmentation of the psyche.

Psychic Discontinuity

Severely disturbed patients demonstrate varying degrees of uneven development reflected in symptoms and maladaptive modes of coping with the external world. As discussed, the identity sense is never spared, indicating that there have been serious disturbances in the earliest developmental stages when separation of the inner and outer world, the self and nonself, has not yet occurred.

We frequently encounter, among these patients, many concretely oriented egos that seem to have little if any capacity to get in touch with the primitive parts of the psyche. There are wide gaps between various levels of the personality; instead of a smooth continuum leading to a hierarchal layering of psychic structure, there is a lack of connecting bridges, which gives the psyche a fragmented quality.

I have seen young adult patients who have taken the stance that they have nothing to say. I assume that this was an adolescent quality, and perhaps it is, inasmuch as adolescence is a developmental phase in which the character is still unconsolidated and has not yet achieved synthesis and cohesion of the self-representation. Not being being able to talk—that is, being incapable of free-associating in the treatment setting—often turned out to be a manifestation of not being able to allow unconscious derivatives into the sphere of awareness. I am referring to an ego defect that has to be distinguished from repression. As I have been discussing, I am postulating a lack of a continuum between consciousness and the unconscious. When these patients state that they have nothing to say, they literally do not; they are not withdrawing, resisting, or repressing.

CASE 2

The following short vignette illustrates these concepts in a clinical therapeutic interaction. The patient, a nineteen-year-old college student, had just resumed his studies after having dropped out during his first year. He had had what was described as an identity diffusion in that he experienced waves of panic. His personal hygiene deteriorated to the point where he was unkempt and unwashed, and he withdrew completely from everyone. He just sat in a corner of his room, mute and motionless.

Initially he was diagnosed as schizophrenic, but once he was hospitalized and his parents came to visit him, he quickly recovered. The psychiatrist and the family mutually decided that he should be given a moratorium, and he returned home with his parents. The next semester he returned to school, but it was felt that it would be prudent that he begin treatment at the same time.

This patient used splitting defenses, and even his movements had an uncoordinated, fragmented quality. He was clumsy and inept with his hands, although he was intellectually superior. He was also likable, and his friends maintained a protective attitude toward him.

His treatment had many difficult moments because he was unable to modulate unconscious derivatives, that is, subject them to secondary process revision so that he could communicate his inner life by his associations. He produced either primary process outbursts or all secondary process expressions, as evidenced by his concrete thinking and the endless, monotonous, obsessive expositions of everyday events unconnected to mental processes.

He complained about his inability to make progress, and even though he blamed himself, I still felt he was covertly reproaching me. In this context, he vociferously lamented that he had nothing to say. It was only when I was able to agree with him that he, indeed, had nothing to say that we could understand the psychic discontinuity that caused him to experience such dilemmas in treatment. He also felt disconnected from me in the same way he was isolated from unconscious processes.

During the final phase of therapy, he viewed his having nothing to say as an inability to energize the deeper parts of his personality. At the same time he was unable to relate to me because, at these times, I did not exist for him. I existed for others but not for him. This was depicted in a dream that was very similar to a fantasy I was having about our relationship and my nonexistence. In the dream he and I were in a dark room, but he did not know whether I was actually there because he could not see me.

Conceptually speaking, I felt the patient was describing a form of psychic discontinuity in which he was relatively unable to cathect his unconscious, that is, the primitive aspects of the self. As a consequence, he was unable to cathect me as well, and therefore I did not exist. He could not form and hold a mental representation of me juxtaposed with the id. In other words, in order to set the process of free association in motion, he had to initiate an energetic current between the deeper recesses of the personality and an external object—both had to be cathected. In the dream, turning on the light in the room would have illuminated both his mind and myself. At that period in treatment he could not achieve this.

Fraiberg's (1969) discussion of the lack of object constancy applies to my patient and many others with similar structural problems. Her description focused on the inability to form and hold a mental representation without the reinforcement of the actual presence of the external object. These patients demonstrate a similar phenomenon but emphasize reciprocity in that the internal world cannot cathect the external object in order to make communication between the mind and the external world possible.

Some Countertransference Problems

This lack of acknowledgment of the therapist and the insistence that they have nothing to say make these patients particularly difficult to treat. They often lament that they are wasting their time coming to appointments, and they frequently miss or cancel them. The therapist feels useless, and the patient seems to strive to reinforce this feeling.

What we often fail to grasp is that, in spite of the cavalier treatment we are subjected to, we nevertheless are valued by the patient. Similarly to the transitional object, we are psychically manhandled and abused but our presence is vital. This was impressed on me by a borderline psychotic adolescent who constantly reviled me as being useless and saw no point in continuing the therapy. He emphasized the latter because he felt strongly that he could not talk to me. During one session, my attention momentarily lagged in that I looked at a digital clock, and the patient had a tantrum. He cried and screamed, paced around the room, and tore his hair. He shouted that here he was trying to open up to me (actually he was, as usual, denigrating me) and I reacted like everyone else by withdrawing and abandoning him. He impressed on me how important it was that I survive his deprecations and that I be there. I became so aware of this that I felt terrible about having failed him, and I profusely apologized for my momentary inattention. He finally realized that I was truly sorry, and, although he was disgruntled when he left, he returned for subsequent sessions.

To maintain a sense of being, adolescents especially have to keep what, for them, is an optimal distance from external objects. They are afraid of emotional entanglements because they threaten their tenuous character organization. This, to some measure, occurs with most adolescents in our culture, but when the fear of inroads on their developing self-representation is pathologically exaggerated, the defensive need for emotional isolation is correspondingly increased. This also has its effects on the treatment relationship and stimulates uncomfortable countertransference reactions. The adolescent patient is often attempting to preserve a sense of inner calm by making the therapist feel disrupted, and this is another example of using him as a transitional object that has to be controlled.

This type of patient uses a variety of adaptive defenses to calm inner agitation. The basic pattern is to have someone else absorb it, and in treatment that role is assigned to the therapist. The therapist does not necessarily retaliate. He nevertheless feels considerable discomfort, and his therapeutic acumen may diminish to the point that he is no longer useful.

My patient acted as if the treatment were an interaction that could be taken for granted and placed in a position of low priority. At least, this was the way he presented himself, but it was a defensive, protective interaction that impelled him to attack or isolate himself from whatever he valued. In any case, I felt excluded, and this must have caused me to feel tense. Other patients are especially adept at creating tension, accompanied by moderate amounts of guilt, in their therapists. This is another situation in which the analyst absorbs the patient's primitive agitation, but it is also a reproduction of a paradoxical soothing interaction (Boyer and Giovacchini 1980).

The eighteen-year-old daughter of one of my patients, an alcoholic dowager, suffered from a chronic state of tension that caused her to be functionally paralyzed. She could calm herself only with drugs or alcohol. Her mother had described to me how she fed her infant daughter. She would literally grab her baby out of the crib and in a jerky, awkward fashion swing her in a wide arc to settle her in her arms. From the clumsy motions she displayed, there seemed to be no neck support. She would then pinch her as she gave her a bottle. True, the mother was somewhat inebriated when she reenacted this early feeding experience, but I surmised that she was drunk most of the time and that must have been her state when taking care of her children, all of whom were alcoholics.

Thus, feeding was accompanied by a background of agitation and intrusive assault. The nurturing process can be divided into two components, a foreground of actual nurture (i.e., the food itself) and a background of soothing. Ordinarily the child is held, supported in a comfortable position so that the ingestion of food is pleasurable and satisfying. These distinctions correspond to Winnicott's (1958a) dividing needs into id and ego needs and his concept of the holding environment. The latter refers to the soothing interaction that makes the satisfaction of id needs a progressive and integrative experience. My patient's daughter had a traumatic holding environment, although she was adequately, and from what I could gather, promptly fed.

The young lady found peace in smoky, crowded discotheques. She found contentment when she was surrounded by chaos. This was accentuated by a recurrent fantasy in which she was in her locked car smoking a cigarette. The car was parked on a layer of ice in the lot adjoining the high school she attended. Since it was illegal for students to park in this lot, two police officers were trying to get to her, but they could not since the doors were securely shut. The policemen became increasingly disturbed as their frustration mounted because they could not break into the automobile and arrest her.

This fantasy was acted out with several therapists she had seen. She would sit in the consultation room calmly smoking and saying nothing. One therapist who saw me for consultation confessed that he found the situation unbearable. He could not stand it and felt a painful urge to get her to talk to him. At times he also felt sexual and murderous feelings that became sufficiently intense that he had to stop seeing her. Other therapists apparently had similar reactions as the patient would sit back, smirking and triumphantly silent. Finally, she was transferred to an older therapist who did not react to her isolation or absorb her inner chaos. He was able to provide her with a soothing environment devoid of assaultive and traumatic elements.

The therapist's survival of the patient's destructiveness and his acceptance of the role of a transitional object for the patient enables the patient to use him as a connecting bridge between unconnected parts of the psyche and as an entry into the external world. This can be a painful experience for the therapist, but he is absorbing the vulnerability and misery the patient had to endure during infancy because of being treated as nonhuman. The treatment process attempts to bring humanity into the relationship even if the therapist has to face the inner disruption of an existential crisis and dehumanization.

Conclusions

In view of the relative lack of consolidation of character structure during adolescence, adolescents as patients frequently reveal psychopathology that has borderline features. In this article, I describe a particular type of ego defect that emphasizes a lack of psychic continuity. The patients presented here could have been considered borderline, although psychic discontinuity can also occur in other types of character defects and schizophrenia.

The backgrounds of these patients indicated that their material needs had been attended to but their caretakers did not encourage or relate to their attempts to individuate into persons in their own right. They were treated as nonhuman objects, as transitional objects used by their mothers for a variety of purposes. They were controlled, manipulated, and not allowed to separate from them.

Being treated as a transitional object leads to characteristic defenses, defenses that are found in many different types of psychopathology but which in combination with other adaptations create specific technical difficulties and countertransference problems. The therapist's existence as a person is sometimes denied as the patient uses him as a transitional object. This occurs as the outcome of the repetition compulsion within the transference context, but, as occurs in the repetition compulsion, the patient converts passive vulnerability to active mastery. There is a reversal of roles as the patient becomes the controlling manipulator and the therapist is the transitional object.

These patients sometimes seem to thrive in chaotic surroundings. Their early backgrounds were devoid of soothing as we ordinarily understand soothing. In treatment they often succeed in getting the therapists to absorb their inner agitation, and the patient is able to maintain calm. Therapists, especially young therapists, may feel sexual urges or murderous impulses toward these adolescents, especially if they are physically attractive. These can become sufficiently intense that they may have to terminate treatment.

In spite of their concrete orientation and treating us in a cavalier fashion, as if we had nothing of value to offer, these adolescents can become covertly dependent on us. We may be the only emotionally significant persons who have acknowledged their emerging sense of aliveness. Surviving their onslaught and withdrawal can help undo the traumatic effects of infantile deprivations and manipulations and set the developmental process in motion once again. The nuances of the therapeutic interaction are intricate and varied and need to be understood further in this conceptual context, that is, in terms of early object relationships and structural defects.

REFERENCES

Blos, P. 1962. *On Adolescence*. New York: Free Press.

Boyer, L. B., and Giovacchini, P. L. 1967. *Psychoanalytic Treatment of Characterological and Schizophrenic Disorders*. New York: Aronson.

Boyer, L. B., and Giovacchini, P. L. 1980. *Psychoanalytic Treatment of Characterological, Borderline and Schizophernic Disorders*. New York: Aronson.

Fraiberg, S. 1969. Libidinal object constancy and object representation. *Psychoanalytic Study of the Child* 19:113–169.

Giovacchini, P. L. 1958. Mutual adaptation in various object relationships. *International Journal of Psycho-Analysis* 38:547–554.

Giovacchini, P. L. (1968) 1975. Psychopathological aspects of the identity sense. In *Psychoanalysis of Character Disorders*. New York: Aronson.

Giovacchini, P. L. 1979. *Treatment of Primitive Mental States*. New York: Aronson.

Grolnick, S.; Barkin, L.; and Muensterberger, W. 1978. *Between Reality and Fantasy: Transitional Objects and Phenomena*. New York: Aronson.

Mahler, M. 1963. Thoughts about development and individuation. *Psychoanalytic Study of the Child* 12:307–324. New York: International Universities Press.

Masterson, J. F. 1976. *Treatment of the Borderline Adult: A Developmental Approach*. New York: Brunner/Mazel.

Rinsley, D. 1982. Object relations theory and psychotherapy, with particular reference to the self-disordered patient. In P. L. Giovacchini and L. B. Boyer, eds. *Treatment of the Severely Disturbed Patient*. New York: Aronson.

Winnicott, D. W. 1953. Transitional objects and transitional phenomena. In *Collected Papers*. New York: Basic.

Winnicott, D. W. 1958a. The capacity to be alone. In *The Maturational Process and the Facilitating Environment*. London: Hogarth.

Winnicott, D. W. 1958b. The mentally ill in your caseload. In *The Maturational Process and the Facilitating Environment*. London: Hogarth.

Winnicott, D. W. 1971. Playing: creative activity and the search for the self. In *Playing and Reality*. London: Tavistock.

17 SUICIDE ATTEMPTED BY SELF-IMMOLATION DURING ADOLESCENCE I. LITERATURE REVIEW, CASE REPORTS, AND PERSONALITY PRECURSORS

FREDERICK J. STODDARD, KAMBIZ PAHLAVAN, AND SUE S. CAHNERS

Burning oneself is a rare, terrifying, and especially tragic form of completed or attempted suicide. When chosen by an adolescent, who feels no longer able to cope with life and whose efforts to find hope for the future seem doomed to failure, self-immolation is a catastrophe—a living nightmare—for the adolescent and his family. Those who survive self-immolation attempts today are often near suicides and might have died without modern advances in care (Burke, Bondoc, and Quinby 1974; Feller, Tholen, and Cornell 1980). Their very survival can evoke ethical questions in family and staff over whether to use modern lifesaving measures or, later, whether they should have been saved.

How should fire come to be used so destructively by a young person? Fire has constructive and destructive, conscious and unconscious meanings in all cultures and languages (Scott 1974). It is used in the Roman Catholic purification ritual of "making a new fire" before Easter and in the Buddhist fire-walking ceremony. In Hebrew and Christian ethics, fire symbolizes not only purification but also sacrifice and punishment, as in the destructive visions of hellfire. For centuries, this has been one of the earliest terrifying images of fire of which children become aware. Today's children learn not only of its symbolic meanings but also of its actual destructive power in war, accidents, political protests, and thermonuclear holocaust (Beardslee and Mack 1982). The vulnerable ado-

0-226-24058-4/85/0012-0020$01.00

lescent bent on self-destruction may carry a seemingly provocative threat into actuality. Fiery language begins to convey the intensity of adolescent sexual or aggressive excitement in phrases such as "Baby, won't you light my fire?" and "Burn, baby, burn." The potential for self-destruction when adolescent excitement is experienced as evil or is cruelly punished is portrayed through the tales of Joan of Arc and Romeo and Juliet. The phenomenon of self-immolation and its occasional association with substance abuse recently became public knowledge as a result of Richard Pryor's burning himself while free-basing cocaine and his acting out the event and his burn treatment in the film *Richard Pryor Live on Sunset Strip*.

Self-immolation generally refers to suicide or parasuicide by self-burning. The term derives from *im* and *mola,* originally referring to the "custom of sprinkling victims with sacrificial meal" but now referring to the "action of offering in sacrifice; sacrificial slaughter of a victim" (*Oxford English Dictionary* 1979). The sacrificial meanings seem to apply to our patients who were influenced in part by fundamentalist religious beliefs. In this chapter we present the epidemiology and what could be learned of the diagnostic and psychological precursors of self-immolation in adolescence in a study of all cases which could be identified at this hospital and two from elsewhere.

Literature Review

For American males between ten and nineteen years of age, suicide rates more than tripled between 1950 and 1977. For American females the same ages and during the same years, suicide rates doubled but were about one-quarter of the male rates. These rates are probably underestimates owing to labeling of suicides as accidents to avoid further grief through public shame (Eisenberg 1980a, 1980b), but Teicher (1979) reported suicide as the second leading cause of death among all adolescents and youth in the United States. The low reporting probably is relevant to burns since most incidents are termed accidents regardless of cause (although this may be changing), when in fact the majority are not strictly accidents but are preventable.

Self-immolation is an unusual method of suicide or attemped suicide. In the Western Hemisphere, there are few reported cases and fewer still involving adolescents. For adults, the mortality rates are high—34 percent and 36 percent in two studies (Andreason and Noyes 1975; Neilsen, Wachtel, and Kolmen 1983). In the Department of Health and Human Services National Burn Program, completed in 1981, only twenty of 1,192 cases of burns in persons under age twenty were reported as self-inflicted, a rate under 2 percent.[1] At this hospital, less than 0.5 percent of patients under age nineteen had the most severe self-inflicted burn injury, self-immolation.

Bernstein (1974) reported one (table 1, case 4) of the only psychiatric cases, one of the four at this hospital. This was a fifteen-year-old Catholic boy from an intact family who suffered 75 percent body surface area (BSA) gasoline burns. His history included childhood fire setting, exhibitionism followed by an unsuccessful psychiatric intervention, and accident proneness. Psychological testing revealed "primitive and bizarre associations," pervasive depression, fears of mutilation from destructive attack, and homosexual fears and impulses.

In contrast, most reports are nonpsychiatric and include few data regarding personality and the psychiatric treatment course of survivors. Crosby, Rhee, and Holland (1977) reported on a sixteen-year-old boy from France who burned himself for political purposes and who was followed by six more cases under age twenty-one, all in 1970. In their series of fourteen cases at the University of Iowa Hospitals, Andreasen and Noyes (1975) refer to a sixteen-year-old boy with an unspecified mental illness. A series of fifty-six cases in France included two adolescents (Brehant and Roger 1973). The fourteen-year-old poured gasoline on his head after stealing a book, but no mental illness was reported. In that series, eight adults attempted suicide by inhaling natural gas which exploded when they lit cigarettes. One of our cases resembles this type.

Self-immolation for political, religious, or consciously sacrificial motives is not unusual, but it is not addressed here since in those situations a different population may be involved (Bostic 1973; Dabbagh 1977; Modan, Nissenkorn, and Lewkowski 1970; Topp 1973). Self-immolation is much more common in cultures outside of the Western Hemisphere and, therefore, is little studied from a psychiatric perspective.

Method

All cases of acute burns admitted to the Shriners' Burns Institute, Boston, from 1968 to 1980 were screened for evidence that they were due to suicide attempts. Burns from playing with matches, accidents without suicidal intent, fire setting, and suicide gestures were excluded. Four patients were identified who had been interviewed and treated both sur-

TABLE 1
DEMOGRAPHIC AND DIAGNOSTIC VARIABLES OF ADOLESCENTS

Case	Age	Sex	Religion	DSM III Diagnosis	Type and Percentage BSA Burned
1	14	F	Muslim	Major depression†	Gasoline, 60%–70%
2	15	F	Fundamentalist Christian	Alcohol and cannabis abuse major depression; borderline personality	Gasoline, 80%
3	16	M	Fundamentalist Christian	Major depression with psychosis; borderline personality	Electrical, 15%
4	16	M	Catholic	Schizophrenia or depression,† exhibitionism	Gasoline, 75%
5	18	F	Catholic	Major depression with hypomania, narcissistic character	Propane, 50%
6	18	F	Jewish	Schizophrenia	Gasoline, 80%

NOTE.—BSA = body surface area.

*The risk-rescue rating is from Weisman and Worden (1972). The combined rating is higher lethality of the attempt. Mean R-R rating for cases 1–6 was 63.1. This compares of 40 (range 17–83). (Weisman and Worden 1972.)

†Insufficient data were available on these patients to make conclusive diagnoses.

gically and psychiatrically with their parents throughout their acute hospitalizations. Consensual DSM III diagnoses were made by a psychiatrist and psychologist. Two cases were added, one from an affiliated hospital and another from one author's (K.P.) medical experience in Iran. Several additional cases have been reported to the authors by colleagues. Because of embarrassment and secrecy surrounding these cases, and the psychiatric treatment within the consultation-liaison context, these reports are less detailed than for patients in long-term intensive psychiatric treatment. In some cases referral was made for long-term treatment following burn treatment.

Results

Subjects were four females and two males (table 1). There were no deaths due to suicide by burning during the period of the study. Although

WHO SURVIVED SUICIDE ATTEMPTS BY SELF-IMMOLATION

Risk-rescue Rating*	Previous Suicide Attempt	Previous Psychiatric Treatment	Family History of Mental Illness	Intact Family
50	?	No	?	Yes
71	Yes	Yes (1 month inpatient treatment, and 3 × per week outpatient psychotherapy with child psychiatrist)	Yes	Yes
63	No (but recent self-caused severe accident)	Yes (weekly with school psychologist and 4 psychiatric visits)	Yes	Yes
56	No	Yes (parents discontinued psychiatric treatment)	?	Yes
71	Yes	Yes (4 evaluation interviews by child psychiatrist; parents refused hospitalization advice)	Yes	Yes
71	Yes	Yes (3 × per week by psychologist)	?	Yes

derived from a risk rating and probability-of-rescue rating. The higher scores signify with a mean for 100 cases of suicide seen at the Massachusetts General Hospital in 1965

diagnoses varied, a significant depressive tendency was present in all patients but major depressive disorder in only three. One was diagnosed as schizophrenic by psychological testing elsewhere. All patients suffered from disturbed thought processes and impaired judgment at the time of their attempts—they were at least briefly psychotic, and one was mildly intoxicated. None had a history or evidence of a specific neurological disorder. Five had histories of previous psychiatric treatment, and three had previous suicide attempts. Rebelliousness at parental rigidity, especially about sexual matters, was frequent. All but case 4, who had a comparable loss, suffered the loss of a major heterosexual relationship where parental opposition to it was overt. All had rigidly religious backgrounds: two Catholic, one Jewish, two fundamentalist Christian, and one Muslim. None burned himself or herself out of social protest. In four of the five U.S. cases the high schools were aware of the suicidal risks but failed in their efforts to intervene owing to strong family opposition. Four cases are presented in more detail.

CASE 1

A fourteen-year-old girl from a devout Muslim family in Iran was beaten and threatened with death by her father after she dated an eighteen-year-old boy. She burned herself out of guilt that was reinforced by her family for committing such an "unethical act" and from fear of her father killing her. Her 60–70 percent BSA second- and third-degree burns were treated for over four months, but no psychotherapeutic treatment was available. A few minutes after discharge she attempted suicide again in front of the hospital by pouring gasoline on herself and lighting a match. She was reacting to her father saying that he would not forgive her for having burned herself and embarrassing him before family and neighbors. It is uncertain to what degree his rejection was due to her disfigurement, but he preferred her to be dead rather than to return home. This time she suffered 30–40 percent BSA second- and third-degree burns. She remained suicidal, pulling all her intravenous lines out in the middle of the first night and cutting her face and hands badly. She was treated with phenothiazines and antidepressants but remained suicidal. Her mental status vacillated from shy, remorseful, tearful, and depressed to very angry and destructive. She felt guilty, blaming herself for what she had done to her family, but at other times condemned them for their cruel and unforgiving attitudes. Her later treatment course and outcome are unknown.

CASE 2

Alice was a fifteen-year-old girl from a fundamentalist Christian family who inflicted 80 percent BSA third-degree gasoline burns on her face, neck, trunk, and extremities. Just after admission, with the cause of the burn unclear, she was asked what had happened to her. She flushed with anger and refused to talk, an unusual response in burn victims. Alice was reported to have been a religious, conscientious, "good girl" when younger, but after age eleven, with menarche, her personality changed. She began to gain weight and manifest insomnia, psychomotor agitation, and feelings of worthlessness. She made two suicide attempts with pills which required brief psychiatric hospitalization and intensive outpatient psychotherapy. It had been felt that through her promiscuous, threatening, and self-destructive behavior she was vicariously acting out the wishes of her parents. Shortly before burning herself, she threatened her peers and became involved with a man who provided her with drugs. There were rumors that she was involved with underworld figures and that her injuries were due to a homicide attempt. While she was receiving surgical care for her burns, Alice's complaints of pain, demands for her mother, and criticism of the treatment alternated with euphoria and delight. After recovering from her acute burns, she reported that she had been very depressed and drinking before burning herself. She was not psychotic but was evasive and affectively labile. During the acute postburn phase she had intermittently wished she had died but was not suicidal. Psychological testing revealed ego constriction and intense preoccupation with her disfigurement. Impulsive escape fantasies were present. Intelligence was high average. Despite loss of all her fingers as a result of her burns, her determination was evident when she would draw or write with a pencil in her mouth. Diagnoses were major depressive disorder and borderline personality disorder.

CASE 3

Bobby was a sixteen-year-old who was admitted with deep fourth-degree electrical burns to his feet and legs caused by climbing a pole and standing on a step-up voltage transformer. He was devoutly religious during his pre- and early teenage years but was beginning to rebel against the religious strictures that he felt set him apart from his peers. Bobby had been treated for suicidal depression by his school psychologist and had been seen a few times by a psychiatrist. He had started taking imipramine three weeks before, and his dosage had been increased to 100 milligrams two days before his burn. In the hospital he was initially confused, regressed, and missed being "treated like a baby" as he had been at the previous hospital. His predominant defensive styles, which emerged in the subsequent weeks, were denial, projection, disavowal, and pseudoautonomy. A month before his burn, while enraged at his father's prohibiting him from seeing his girlfriend, he caused a serious motor vehicle accident but was uninjured. Similarly, before causing his burn, he was angry and confused and with herculean effort shinned up a transformer pole which lacked footholds. He denied suicidal intent, saying only, "I don't know how I could be so stupid." On psychological testing major findings included poorly sublimated incestuous fantasies directed toward his mother and a weak masculine identification. Overwhelming denial did not successfully contain his anxiety and depression. On the WISC his performance score was 159, and his full-scale IQ was 123.

Our focus here is on his confusion to the point of psychotic decompensation at the time of his injury. The sources for this seem to be unresolved conflict between his parents as well as conflict with his father about religion and sexuality. The possibility of self-sacrificial motivation is underscored. It is unlikely that imipramine altered the protective function of any suicidal thoughts he may have had or induced a psychotic decompensation in this borderline boy. Hereditary predisposition to depression or psychosis could not be established.

CASE 5

Secrecy is an essential part of life during adolescence (Teicher 1979). However, secrecy can place the suicidal adolescent at a special disadvantage, especially when the family reinforces it, as in this case in which self-immolation was termed an "accident" even though the adolescent had attempted another form of suicide.

Clara was an eighteen-year-old, devoutly Catholic girl of above-average intelligence who was admitted with 50 percent third-degree burns on her face, neck, arms, and trunk because of an allegedly accidental explosion. At no time during acute care was a suicide attempt considered likely, and it remained a secret for months. Eventually, while still hospitalized, she chose to participate in psychotherapy and began to speak of her depression. She had become depressed prior to her burn and after the loss of her boyfriend following his family's interference. She reported that she was able to hide her severe depression from her family despite increasing isolation, insomnia, and suicidal ideas. Others came to her aid only when she was discovered holding a hunting knife to her throat. She had also made a previous secret suicide attempt with opiates. She was taken to two child psychiatrists who both advised hospitalization, which was refused by the family; in addition, the patient was unable to agree to hospitalize herself, apparently out of fear of her family. After a quarrel with her father, she turned on the gas stove in order to gas herself; she reconsidered her suicide plan but exploded the gas with a spark when she turned on a fan. In psychotherapy after her burn, she was self-centered but without evidence of suicidal ideation. Once she was able to share the facts of her suicide attempt, she made some efforts to use help for herself and her family. Clara's mother had always been close to her and shared antagonistic feeling toward the father. It seemed that a symbiotic mother-daughter relationship had been acted out by ganging up on the father. It was later learned that the father harbored enormous rage, lashing out violently at times. A history of untreated affective disorder with paranoid elements was present in both parents, paternal grandmother, and more distant relatives.

The seriousness with which Clara pursued suicide should be noted and seems even greater than with the other patients in this group. In planning further care, the psychiatric treatment team had to weigh the relative risks of suicide with little or no treatment against the risks if treatment was recommended against the wishes of the family.

Discussion

This group of adolescent survivors of suicide attempts by burning have certain traits in common both before and after their burns. In focusing on the situations preburn, the goal is to understand, if possible, the suicide process and to contribute to prevention. Centering on postburn similarities leads to appreciation of the high suicide risk (table 1) and to the treatment approaches used for this vulnerable, disfigured group of adolescents.

Before the suicide attempts, similar traits included individual mental disorders, family psychopathology, religiosity, psychiatric treatment history, hereditary factors, and the lack of response or failure of response of the caretakers to their cries for help. Sorosky (1981) summarized the situation of the suicidal adolescent in a way that applies to these patients: "Suicidal fantasies and behavior are frequent sequelae of the pain of depression, the emptiness of the borderline syndrome, and the confusion of drug and alcohol abuse. The ultimate act is more likely to occur when cries for help have gone unheeded and the patient's fears, frustrations, and feelings of helplessness have developed into feelings of isolation, panic, and hopelessness. Therefore, therapeutic intervention is necessary as early as possible in the suicidal process, as repeated attempts are typical and of graduated severity."

INDIVIDUAL PSYCHOPATHOLOGY

These patients differed widely, as did the findings in studies of adults who burned themselves (Andreasen and Noyes 1975). Although all had diagnosable mental disorders, they differed in age, sex, intentionality, psychodynamics, degree of severity of psychopathology, substance abuse, and genetic predisposition. For example, although depressive symptoms were present in several patients, one (case 3) made a suicide attempt on sudden impulse, after drinking alcohol, when she found gasoline available; another (case 4) disavowed suicidal intent and was most likely psychotic at the time of the attempt; a third (case 6) was severely depressed and was burned by accident, having decided not to commit suicide by another means.

Although these patients differed diagnostically, there were psychodynamic similarities: narcissistic issues that were intensified during adolescence; rage directed toward the father or another male figure; recent loss of a loved person; and helpless, hopeless, and powerless feelings, particularly in relation to parents and peers (Berkovitz 1981). In accord with the observations of Hendrick (1940) and Maltsberger and Buie (1980) about suicidal patients, these, too, suffered from gross disturbances in the sense of self. Referring to adolescents, Miller (1981) states that "except for those young people who avoid significant drug abuse, who have an intact family, who have significant extrafamilial relationships which are valued, and who participate in a broad educational experience which includes cognitive, creative, and imaginative stimulation, the traditional norms of adolescence hardly exist in some parts of Western society. Many young people have difficulty in developing an autonomous sense of self—becoming instead, 'other directed' adults (Reisman 1954). A feeling of one's self-worth comes to depend almost entirely on the approval of others often perceived as an amorphous 'they,' with autonomy hardly present."

In these adolescent self-immolators, it is likely, although not proved, that biological factors were contributory causes. Biological factors are now implicated in patients with major affective disorders (cases 2, 3, and 5), schizophrenia (case 6), and some types of borderline disorders (cases 2 and 3). Evidence for hereditary factors is suggested by the presence of major mental illness in the families of four of the six patients. Regarding possible biochemical mechanisms which might mediate such violent suicide attempts, recent studies of depressed adults (Asberg, Traskman, and Thoren 1976) and adults with borderline personality disorders with depression (Brown et al. 1982) found that a history of suicide attempt, especially violent suicide, was associated with lower levels of cerebrospinal fluid 5-hydroxyindoleacetic acid (5-HIAA), a serotonin metabolite, than that found in patients with the same diagnoses but no history of suicidal behavior. This was suggested as a possible biochemical suicide predictor.

FAMILY PSYCHOPATHOLOGY

All of our patients came from families that were technically intact, that is, the natural parents of these adolescents were married and living together with their child or children. However, they might more accurately be described as "divorce within marriage" or "parental divorce" (Miller 1981) because of the lack of meaningful communication and the intensity of the largely unverbalized conflicts within the entire family. The children were "expendable children" for their parents, either consciously as with case 1 or unconsciously as with several others. Sabbath (1969, 1970) proposed that term "to account for one of the multiple factors contributing to adolescent suicidal behavior. It presumes a parental wish, conscious or unconscious, spoken or unspoken, that the child interprets as their desire to be rid of him, for him to die." The adolescents we have described had reached developmental impasses and were psychologically entrapped within highly restrictive families, a situation which Berkovitz (1981) has identified as driving the adolescent's autonomous striving and repressed rage toward violent action. Shapiro and Freedman (1983) described a family dynamic in some cases of adolescent suicide which specifically addresses the precursors of pathological family interaction. They state that in adolescence, when the child's body changes and dependency needs increase, there is regressive repetition within the family of derivatives of early experiences of psychological abandonment. These, in interaction with the child's own ego deficits, may evoke the unbearable rage or feelings of abandonment which can lead to suicide.

RELIGIOSITY

A surprisingly consistent trait of these patients and families was their religiosity, in most at the time of the burn injury, but in case 2, several years earlier. The specific denomination seemed less relevant than adherence to a fundamentalist, literal interpretation of scripture, accompanied by severe guilt for real or imagined sins and strict notions of punishment. Some studies have correlated religious beliefs with suicide, for instance, finding that those who commit suicide more frequently express belief in an afterlife than other suicide groups and that a relatively high percentage of those who threaten or attempt suicide are Catholic (Petzel and Riddle 1981).

PSYCHIATRIC TREATMENT HISTORY

Five of these patients were in or had recently had psychotherapeutic outpatient and, in one case, inpatient treatment. Although this is consistent with the finding reported by Roy (1982) in adult studies of past psychiatric patients, the recent report by Carlson and Cantwell (1982) of their study of seventeen adolescent suicide attempters found no statistically significant difference in percentage of chronic psychiatric illness in attempters from nonattempters. Shaffer's (1982) concern for sampling techniques certainly applies to our population, which might represent a sample biased in favor of past psychiatric treatment.

Family therapy was recommended in several cases, without success or with very limited parent cooperation. The schools were aware of the suicidal risk in these cases but were unable to effect psychiatric treatment at the time of the risk or were unable to do so successfully. The past psychiatric treatments were especially difficult because of parental reluctance to accept help, the adolescent's secrecy and/or impulsivity, and the severity of family conflict. There was evidence in three of the patients in psychotherapy at the time of self-immolation that they may have experienced transference psychoses and were unable to talk about their intense rage and sexual feelings with their therapists.

RESPONSE TO THE CRY FOR HELP

In each case, the parents, teachers, and, at times, psychotherapists did not respond to verbalized suicidal threats or did so inappropriately. An effort to make sense of this phenomenon is presented in Mack and Hickler's (1981) discussions of the diary of an adolescent girl who committed suicide by hanging. The therapist of one of our patients allegedly responded to a patient saying he would burn himself with "I know you wouldn't do that," which the patient seemed to take as a challenge. In another case, helpers had difficulty knowing when and how to respond effectively since the patient threatened suicide so often. In several instances parents refused or resisted recommendations for psychiatric hospitalization shortly before the self-immolation occurred.

Conclusions

We report six cases of adolescent self-immolation that, with review of the literature, suggest certain conclusions. These adolescents came from technically intact families with long-standing psychopathology, fundamentalistic religious beliefs, and a family history of mental disorder in a majority of the reported cases. Each adolescent had failed to separate and individuate, but each had made an initial effort in an extrafamiliar love relationship which was lost. These adolescents vacillated psychologically between depression and rage, projection and introjection, alternatively perceiving relationships as all good or all bad, and they resorted to violent, self-destructive actions leading to severe burns when their efforts to cope failed and isolation became unbearable. The self-immolation suicide attempt seemed in some but not all to occur during brief psychotic episodes. The range of DSM III disorders from which these patients suffered was diverse and included affective disorder, substance abuse, borderline personality, and schizophrenia. Whether our findings of high lethality, individual and family psychopathology, religiosity, past psychiatric treatment, and missed cries for help are limited to our population, which might be biased, or are consistent with other populations of adolescents who attempt suicide by self-immolation, remains to be studied.

NOTE

1. J. Locke, New England Regional Burn Demonstration Project, personal communication.

REFERENCES

Andreasen, N. D., and Noyes, R. 1975. Suicide attempted by self immolation. *American Journal of Psychiatry* 135:554–556.

Asberg, M.; Traskman, L.; and Thoren, P. 1976. 5-HIAA in the cerebrospinal fluid: a biochemical suicide predictor. *Archives of General Psychiatry* 33:1193–1197.

Beardslee, W. R., and Mack, J. E. 1982. The impact of nuclear developments on children and adolescents. In American Psychiatric Association, *The Psychosocial Impacts of Nuclear Developments*. Task Force Report 20. Washington, D.C.: American Psychiatric Association.

Berkovitz, I. H. 1981. Feelings of powerlessness and the role of violent actions in adolescents. *Adolescent Psychiatry* 9:477–492.

Bernstein, N. R. 1974. *The Emotional Care of the Facially Burned and Disfigured*. Boston: Little, Brown.

Bostic, R. A. 1973. Self immolation: a surgery of the last decade. *Life Threatening Behavior* 3:66–73.

Brehant, J., and Roger, L. 1973. Les suicides par le feu en France [Suicide by fire in France]. *Nouvelle Presse Médicale* 2:2923–2324.

Brown, G. L.: Ebert, M. H.; Goyer, P. F.; Tomerson, D. C.; Kline, W. J.; Bunney, W. E.; and Goodwin, F. K. 1982. Aggression suicide and serotonin: relationship to CSF amine metabolites. *American Journal of Psychiatry* 139:741–746.

Burke, J. F.; Bondoc, C. C.; and Quinby, W. D. 1974. Primary burn excision and immediate grafting: a method of shortening illness. *Journal of Trauma* 14:389–395.

Carlson, G. A., and Cantwell, D. R. 1982. Suicidal behavior and depression in children and adolescents. *Journal of the American Academy of Child Psychiatry* 21:361–368.

Crosby, K.; Rhee, J.; and Holland, J. 1977. Suicide by fire: a contemporary method of political protest. *International Journal of Social Psychiatry* 23:60–69.

Dabbagh, F. 1977. Family suicide. *British Journal of Psychiatry* 2:130.

Eisenberg, L. 1980a. Adolescent suicide rate. Annual meeting of the American Academy of Pediatrics. *Psychiatric News*.

Eisenberg, L. 1980b. Adolescent suicide: on taking arms against a sea of troubles. *Pediatrics* 315:320.

Feller, I.; Tholen, D.; and Cornell, R. G. 1980. Improvements in burn care, 1965–1979. *Journal of the American Medical Association* 244:2074–2078.

Hendrick, I. 1940. Suicide as a wish fulfillment. *Psychiatric Quarterly* 14:30–42.

Mack, J. E., and Hickler, H. 1981. *Vivienne: The Life and Suicide of an Adolescent Girl*. Boston: Little, Brown.

Maltsberger, J. T., and Buie, D. H. 1980. The devices of suicide, revenge, riddance, and rebirth. *International Review of Psychoanalysis* 7:61–72.

Miller, D. 1981. Adolescent suicide: etiology and treatment. *Adolescent Psychiatry* 9:327–342.

Modan, B.; Nissenkorn, I.; and Lewkowski, S. R. 1970. Comparative epidemiological aspects of suicide and attempted suicide in Israel. *American Journal of Epidemiology* 91:393–399.

Neilsen, J. H; Wachtel, T. L.; and Kolmen, P. B. R. 1983. Suicide and parasuicide by burns. Paper presented at annual meeting of the American Burn Association, March 17.

Oxford English Dictionary. 1979. Compact ed., s.v. “immolation.” 1:1380.

Petzel, S. V., and Riddle, M. 1981. Adolescent suicide: psychological and cognitive aspects. *Adolescent Psychiatry* 9:343–398.

Reisman, D. 1954. *The Lonely Crowd*. Garden City, N.Y.: Doubleday Anchor.

Roy, A. 1982. Risk factors for suicide in psychiatric patients. *Archives of General Psychology* 39:1089–1095.

Sabbath, J. D. 1969. The suicidal adolescent—the expendable child. *Journal of the American Academy of Child Psychiatry* 8:272–289.

Sabbath, J. D. 1971. The role of parents in adolescent suicide behavior. *Acta Paedopsychiatrica* 38:211–220.

Scott, Donald. 1974. *The Psychology of Fire*. New York: Scribners.

Shaffer, D. 1982. Diagnostic considerations in suicidal behavior in children and adolescents. *Journal of the American Academy of Child Psychiatry* 21:414–416.

Shapiro, E. R., and Freedman, J. 1983. Family dynamics of adolescent suicide. Unpublished.

Sorosky, A. D. 1981. Introduction—adolescent suicidology. *Adolescent Psychiatry* 9:323–326.

Teicher, J. 1979. Suicide and suicide attempts. In *Basic Handbook of Child Psychiatry*. Vol. 2. New York: Basic.

Topp, O. D. 1973. Fire as a symbol and a weapon of death. *Medical Science and Law* 13:79–86.

Weisman, A. D., and Worden, J. W. 1972. Risk rescue rating in suicide assessment. *Archives of General Psychiatry* 26:553–560.

18 SUICIDE ATTEMPTED BY SELF-IMMOLATION DURING ADOLESCENCE II. PSYCHIATRIC TREATMENT AND OUTCOME

FREDERICK J. STODDARD AND SUE S. CAHNERS

Psychiatric treatment of patients who have attempted suicide by self-immolation (Stoddard, Pahlavan, and Cahners 1984) has not to our knowledge been described. The principles of treatment we have used and describe here are derived from those used with burn victims from other causes (Bernstein 1982; Stoddard 1982a, 1982b), psychotic patients (Van Buskirk and Semrad 1969), borderline adolescents (Mack 1975; Groves 1978; Shapiro 1978), and patients who were medically hospitalized following suicide attempts (Guggenheim 1978; Yacoubian and Lourie 1973). The degree to which one or another approach is used with a particular patient varies with that patient.

This chapter is based on the treatment of the adolescents and families described in Part I, initiated within the burn unit context. In addition to our contacts with them, we refer to their treatment in other psychiatric settings. Efforts have been made throughout this report to respect the sensitive nature of the experiences of these adolescents and their families.

The outcomes for these patients can be summarized simply: to our knowledge, all but one of the patients are alive and making gradual progress in burn and psychiatric rehabilitation. One patient (case 5) committed suicide by stabbing, two years after her burn injury.

0-226-24058-4/85/0012-0004$01.00

Method

Psychiatric and social service records, as well as the general medical record, were reviewed to identify case examples and patterns in management during acute care, family characteristics and their responses to intervention, psychopharmacological treatment, subsequent psychiatric treatment, and what could be learned of outcome.

Psychiatric Care on the Burn Unit

MANAGEMENT OF ACUTE REACTIONS TO THE BURN

At the time of the initial psychiatric consultation, all of these patients were hospitalized for acute treatment of a severe injury. Usually the family, previous medical personnel, or our medical staff requested psychiatric consultation because of a known suicide attempt or suspicion about it. Despite this, the immediate psychiatric care did not have to do with the suicide attempts directly but, rather, with acute care of the severely burned patients and their families (Ravenscroft 1982; Stoddard 1982a; West and Shuck 1978). The patients as a group were more confused and hostile in the acute postburn phase than other similarly burned patients. They were less tolerant of physical pain and the frustration involved in waiting for staff and family than were other burn victims. They progressed best with simple, clear explanations of the seriousness of the physical condition and with appeals to them to cooperate with care. The acute phase was no time for exploratory psychiatric interviewing which might overwhelm their fragile coping and distract them from energies needed for physical survival. At this time, intensive, supportive psychotherapy with the families secondarily helped the patients through this phase, since the families were in turn more capable of supporting the patient; in addition, very close work with the surgical and nursing staff was essential in managing the patients' confusion and hostility and their parents' grief, anxiety, and guilt.

EFFECT AND MEANINGS OF THE SUICIDE ATTEMPT

Among several meanings of self-immolation which may be present, two were clinically important. The first was to draw attention to feelings of powerlessness, breaking through a barrier to communication with family and others and consequently obtaining help (Noyes, Frye, Slyman, and

Canter 1979). An example of this and the factors contributing to it are shown in treatment of case 2.

CASE 2

Psychiatric interviews began a month after admission and permitted this fifteen-year-old girl to express feelings about the events preceding her burning herself. She told different versions at first but gradually became more consistent. She related, "Two months before I got burned a guy I know got shot and killed—he had 'good drugs.' When I tried to kill myself I thought maybe I'd see him. I probably wouldn't have tried it if he had been around because he had good drugs." She added later that after she broke up with her boyfriend two weeks before the burn, she went out with another boy who also "expected too much sexually." She repeatedly said, "I wasn't that kind of a girl." He was "a little stiff . . . like a wild animal," and "I was afraid he'd rape me." Later therapeutic material indicated that this may have been a hallucinatory projection. "I was angry and I smacked him . . . I'd had no previous sexual contact, except kissing"; "I went to church the next day. I just wanted peace and escape." She said that before burning herself she wrote the following suicide note to a friend: "Things were pretty tough. Is there no end to this insanity that I go through? There must be, and I'll find a way. There has to be an end and I'll find it."

When discussing religion, she said, "I think the devil was really pissed and that's really why he worked harder and harder on me all the time—he really wanted me—my Dad to me is just purely evil and bad, possessed by the devil."

In telling the psychiatrist and other staff about what she had experienced, she gradually oriented herself following her survival, coped more effectively with her physical care, and reestablished relationships with others, including family members. Prior to her burn, she was isolated and unable to seek or use help. Later in her course, despite severe deformities, she resumed previous maladaptive patterns of craving and demanding attention, sexualizing relationships, and eliciting hatred from those endeavoring to provide treatment. Her psychiatric treatment continued at a psychiatric hospital following discharge.

Another meaning of self-immolation was to provide a needed self-experience, different from the example where the goal seemed to be to obtain help and attention, if the patient survived. Case 4 appears to have been such an example of self-therapy (Anthony 1975); the patient's coping improved following the burn, making ongoing psychiatric treatment unnecessary at that time.

MANAGEMENT OF PREEXISTING PSYCHOPATHOLOGY

The burn unit staff looked for help in assisting and managing suicidal risk. "He's your patient—you're in charge" was a frequent interaction in these cases. At times, medical or nursing staff overlooked the patients' saying that they wished to be dead or wished they had not survived, since such statements can occur with other severely burned patients who have not been suicidal. Assessment of suicide risk in such instances was urgent given the ready availability to means of self-harm, such as throwing themselves out of bed, extubation, pulling arterial or venous lines, destroying grafts, or suddenly moving during risky procedures. None of these patients required the sedation, tranquilizing, or muscular paralysis used at times in such situations.

SUICIDE ASSESSMENT AND PRECAUTIONS

Whereas the burn team is experienced more than many with life and death, many staff members may be less comfortable dealing with suicidal risk. They valued clarification of the motivations and the cognitive and affective styles of the suicidal adolescents, and they appreciated clear procedures for management and detailed physician's orders for management when needed. Suicide precautions were needed for only two patients (cases 1 and 2) and in case 2 only briefly when the patient became anxious about discharge. We attribute this to the availability of attentive nurses, minimal frustrations, and the possibility of low recurrence of suicidal risk in psychiatrically treated children who have attempted suicide (Cohen-Sandler, Berman, and King 1982) or who have had near death experiences.

Assessment of suicide risk is ongoing during burn care of these patients and is part of assessing the effects of the stress of intermittent surgery, dressing changes, other painful procedures, isolation, family visits, and especially discharge planning. An assessment of a patient's response to her severe disfigurement, pain, and physical therapy is seen with case 5. At this time she was not judged to be suicidal. In retrospect, she was, like most burned patients, regressed under severe stress, but also more pessimistic and dependent than others at her age. Much later she committed suicide.

CASE 5

She sat gaunt from weight loss, bald from donor sites from her scalp, and wrapped in silver nitrate dressings from head to lower trunk. It was painful for her to be still or to move. She had a hard time talking with the psychiatrist because neck contractures pulled her head back. She asked him to turn her chair so that she could look more directly. He explained that the surgeons and physical therapists had asked that she maintain tension on the contracture on her left neck, in the hope of lessening the likelihood that a surgical release of the contracture would be needed. She was in constant discomfort, moving to new positions such as pushing her leg down and rigidly shifting her trunk. Her severely burned face moved little and was healing actively; there was considerable discoloration and thickening edges to the graft. Her head was badly scarred and partially covered by white bandages so that one could not see that she did not have ears. Several times she asked that the psychiatrist speak louder. He reinforced the burn nursing staff's perceptions of the patient's realistic needs for bodily care rather than attribute her irritability to her psychopathology.

Ego supportive interventions were focused on her rehabilitative efforts; for example, she told the psychiatrist that her mother had reported a message from the surgeons that "you're going to get worse before you get better." She complained that many people were stressing the importance of eating and of her cooperating with physical therapy. The psychiatrist disagreed with what her mother had said and explained that was not what the surgeons had said; rather, they had emphasized that she was progressing very well and that improved nutrition certainly would facilitate healing. She was responding negatively to being in a more directive rehabilitative program than previously and tried to collude with the psychiatrist in opposition to the surgical and physical therapy plan. While such collusion might have helped build the relationship with her, it ultimately would have been a repetition of earlier maladaptive relationships and would have undermined her overall care.

It appeared that she was responding to her care with regression and resistance, leading staff to treat her as a stubborn, younger child. One nurse recognized the pattern of infantilization and said firmly, "You're not five," and responded willingly to her requests for water and other things, rather than regarding her as seeking inappropriate attention. Such regression and struggles with parents and staff are common with burn patients but are accentuated in those with severe preexisting psychopathology.

OPENNESS OF THE ADOLESCENT AND FAMILY TO HELP

Interventions, as mentioned, with distraught, grief-stricken patients and their families may make acute burn care a time when there is a good opportunity to initiate a psychotherapeutic relationship. However, in these cases the parents usually did not welcome the opportunity. Most families meet with a social worker soon after admission and welcome the opportunity to sit in privacy, share their grief, and receive support from an empathic, nonthreatening professional. In these cases, however, the parents avoided the opportunity to communicate in other than superficial ways and resisted sharing the depth of their feelings and various pertinent facts. In each case parents were pleasant and polite, essentially insisting that "everything is just fine in our family" or resisting with "we are handling the problem in our own way, thank you." This is a red flag warning to pursue further information about the accident and prior history.

CRISIS INTERVENTION WITH PARENTS AND SIBLINGS

These interventions were even more difficult and requiring of psychotherapeutic expertise than treatment of families of burn victims without such severe preexisting psychopathology. At the core of feelings that were addressed was parental guilt. Parents frequently find reason to blame themselves when a child is injured, and this must be eased in order to prepare the family for a productive future. When a child has chronically demonstrated self-destructive behavior, the guilt of the parents has been concealed and has festered. Their ego strengths must be identified and carefully encouraged to eventually establish trust.

The parents of these adolescents felt overwhelmed with guilt, angry at the patients for having burned themselves, and reticent to share feelings, particularly the fathers. For instance, one father did not appear in the hospital for several months despite efforts to bring him into the treatment process. In most of these cases, the parents did not take seriously the fact of their child's suicide attempt and the probability that ongoing psychiatric care would be needed. They attributed the entire problem to the burn injury and denied or avoided the reality of the suicide attempt and their feelings about it, in some instances to avoid their own homicidal wishes toward their child (Sabbath 1971). Their reactions could be attributable in part to ego constriction, an emergency adaptive mechanism first described by Hamburg, Hamburg, and deGoza (1953) in burn victims but which we have observed in families also. Siblings tended to be excluded from the psychotherapeutic treatment process because of parental distress over the acute burn and the fact that most siblings were younger than the patient and lived far away. After the acute phase, some siblings were more involved, but the parents were unwilling to discuss openly the suicide attempt with them. It was unusual for the social worker to have a secure therapeutic alliance with these parents. In addition to the factors mentioned, the lack of a secure alliance was due to severe marital conflicts that interfered with their grieving the loss of their child as he or she was before the burn and responding helpfully to their child after the burn.

SPECIAL PSYCHOTHERAPEUTIC ISSUES

The central psychotherapeutic issues, as with any burned patient, were the grief and painful suffering which the patient and family endured as a result of these devastating injuries (Bowden, Feller, Tholen, Davidson, and Hames 1980; Stoddard 1982b). The embarrassment about the nature of the injuries and the responses of others to them may make the emotional working through even more difficult. Each stage of work raised questions of secrecy and confidentiality which lessened as the patient became more trusting of the psychotherapist. Confidentiality issues occurred in relation to family, previous medical personnel, staff on the burn unit, and particularly the previous treating psychiatrist or other psychotherapist. For example, in three instances, the patients resisted providing information and giving permission to the staff to contact previous psychiatrists.

PSYCHOPHARMACOLOGICAL TREATMENT

Many psychopharmacological agents are used on burn units but with scant scientific basis for dosage, effects or side effects, toxicity, or pharmacokinetics. Treatment is empirical as a result, with even less scientific basis in children than in burned adults. Commonly used pain medications were opiates, particularly morphine and Demerol during acute phase (Perry, Heidrick, and Ramos 1981). Antidepressants are rarely used (Forrest,

Brown, Brown, Defalque, Gold, Gordon, James, Katz, Mahler, Schroff, and Teutch 1977; Webb, Smith, Evans, and Webb 1978). Major depression, although present in the histories of these patients, was not seen during acute burn care, except for case 1, but it is probable that a larger sample of self-immolators would reveal some who suffer from weight loss, severe sleep disorders, withdrawal, and persistent depressive mood during the acute burn period, since we have seen this in a few other burn patients. Many burn patients have one or more of the above symptoms but fail to qualify for a DSM III diagnosis of major depression, if symptoms are assessed regardless of acuteness of the trauma, metabolic state, drugs, and so forth. Some burned adolescents not in this group required antidepressants and appeared to respond well. An alternative to tricyclic antidepressants is stimulants which have a shorter duration of action. Psychotic symptoms as part of delirium were seen in two patients during their acute course. These patients responded to fifty to 100 milligrams of chlorpromazine or thioridazine, although one patient with severe breast scarring had the side effect of lactation in response to thioridazine; this was very embarrassing to her. Haloperidol (one to ten milligrams per day) has been effective for delirium in other cases but was not used here (Lerner, Ewow, Levitin, and Belmaker 1979). Diazepam is currently being favored in tranquilizing of acute patients where respiratory depression is not a concern, but a recent adult study suggests risk of drug accumulation due to impaired hepatic metabolism, possibly due to co-administration of other drugs such as cimetidine (Maartyn, Greenblatt, and Quinby 1983).

PLANNING PSYCHIATRIC AND SURGICAL AFTERCARE

This planning was begun within the psychotherapeutic work with patients and families on admission, and this preparatory process provided them with education and some control over their futures during the acute, middle, and rehabilitative phases of burn recovery. This was true from the acute phase, where life and death issues were primary, to the middle phase, where body image change predominated, to the rehabilitative phase, where adaptation to physical limitation and return home supervened. In all cases they were reluctant to accept the presence of a mental disorder despite the suicide attempt and past treatment, and they were likewise resistant to recommendations for further psychiatric care, particularly inpatient evaluation or treatment. We understood that their resistance resulted from ambivalence about past psychiatric care, from their suffering from the stigma of being scarred, and from reluctance to have the added stigma of more intensive care in a psychiatric unit. Nevertheless, in the parents' resistances to psychiatric care there was a sense of their not caring for their adolescent or their adolescent's survival.

In case 1, as summarized in Part I, the father consciously encouraged his daughter's suicidal actions. In case 2, the father-daughter relationship was similar to that in case 1, but establishment of a trusting therapeutic relationship with the mother resulted in her becoming able to sever her marriage and assume responsibility for herself and her child. In case 3, psychiatric referral was accomplished only with the aid of local school personnel who shared our concerns and appreciated our support of their plan. In case 5, the most that was possible was parental acceptance of treatment in the home community, which provided them with the privacy they required.

In addition to planning follow-up with the families, there was need to educate the psychiatric staffs receiving the referrals since they were inexperienced with burns. As in school or industrial consultation, we worked with the psychiatric staffs to learn of their medical and psychiatric resources and explain the long course of burn rehabilitation. Psychiatric hospital staffs provided needed expertise in management of suicide risk and depression, but they were overwhelmed at seeing severely scarred patients and apprehensive about arranging for physical therapy and ongoing surgical care.

Long-Term Psychiatric Care

It is a dilemma for psychiatrists treating adolescents who have burned themselves to determine the severity of the ongoing suicide risk. It was our experience that the acute risk postburn was low, but the long-term risk was in some cases high. The risk required careful, regular reassessment, if possible, and psychiatric treatment planning distinct from, but coordinated with, reconstructive surgical treatment. It was not possible to predict the stress on these patients caused by return to family, school, or work and the prospect of years of surgical reconstruction. For five of these patients (table 1), prognosis for survival is guarded and uncertain. A factor contributing to survival for several patients was their families' and hospital staffs' rallying to the patients' cry for help and providing much needed emotional sustenance during and after burn care. Some of the patients responded to loss of the protective surgical hospital environ-

TABLE 1

TREATMENT AND OUTCOME VARIABLES OF ADOLESCENTS WHO SURVIVED SUICIDE ATTEMPTS BY SELF-IMMOLATION

Case	Surgical Hospitalization	Psychiatric Hospitalization	Treatment Method(s)	Psychotropic Medications	Ongoing Suicide Risk	Outcome
1	Several months	?	Medication	Tricyclic antidepressant; chlorpromazine	Yes	?
2	7 months and many readmissions	3 months	Individual and group psychotherapy; medication	Various phenothiazines	Occasional	Continued in psychotherapy; completed high school
3	3 months and 1 readmission	2 months	Individual and group psychotherapy	None	No	Dropped treatment and high school, is working
4	3 months	No	None	No	None known	Alive and well after several years
5	4 months and 5 readmissions	6 weeks	Individual and group psychotherapy; medication	Trilafon	Yes	Suicide
6	Several months	No	Individual psychotherapy Medication monitoring	MAC inhibitor	None known	Continued treatment, finished high school, and alive before lost to follow-up

ment with severe depression, particularly on return to a hostile environment (cases 1 and 5). All caretakers involved with case 5 were aware of the severe suicide risk, which was why she was psychiatrically hospitalized and followed intensively after psychiatric discharge. Prior to her suicide, it was clear that she was not succeeding in key areas of both her burn rehabilitation and psychiatric rehabilitation. Specifically, her physical therapy did not progress well and she did not return to school or work, and thus she was left alone with much unstructured time. In addition, psychiatric hospitalization was shorter than recommended, and the alliance with the family was weak.

SELECTION OF PSYCHIATRIC TREATMENT

Some patients (cases 4 and 6) did not require inpatient psychiatric treatment following their burn care (Frances and Clarkin 1981). They may have achieved a form of "self-therapy" as a result of the burn injury and elicited enough emotional support so that the degree of suicide risk was low. However, in cases 1, 2, 3, and 5 inpatient care was the more judicious course following acute burn treatment. All modalities of treatment (individual, family, group, psychopharmacological) were used during psychiatric hospitalization.

The phase of transition into the psychiatric treatment setting was fraught with various types of regression and resistance and with the patients' rejecting psychiatric patienthood and wishing instead to be treated like "normal" burn patients. None of the patients transferred to psychiatric hospitals was suicidal at the time of transfer, and none required civil commitment. In contrast with their attitudes toward psychiatric hospitalization, these patients and their families more readily accepted outpatient treatment, but in cases 3 and 4 they did not pursue it for long. Outpatient individual psychotherapy was usually only once a week, and families participated actively *only* in case 2, despite this being recommended in all cases. A variety of antidepressant and antipsychotic medications was prescribed, as shown in table 1.

PHYSICAL AND SOCIAL REHABILITATION

Planning surgical reconstruction required as much preparation as possible for patient, family, school, employer, and mental health personnel. All patients needed preparation for their return for ten to thirty plastic surgical procedures over several years, and during such readmissions patient regression is common, occasionally including depressive and transient suicidal episodes (Bernstein 1982; Stoddard 1982b). Patient and family participation in choice and timing of surgical procedures was even more essential than usual and may decrease regression (Belfer, Harrison, Pillemer, and Murray 1982; Goin and Goin 1981). The psychological meaning to the patient of readmission for reconstruction should be understood prior to surgery, and postoperative changes in mood or personality should be monitored and reported to the psychiatrist treating the patient.

EFFECT OF THE SELF-IMMOLATOR ON STAFF AND PATIENTS

The reaction when a self-immolator was admitted to the burn unit was increased staff anxiety and disbelief that a teenager could do such a thing. One physician at another facility stated that surgical care of such a patient was a waste of valuable resources. Since the patients tended to be hostile, complaining, and demanding as well as critically ill, early staff anxiety was often replaced by anger at the patients for causing such terrible injuries which consumed so much medical care, as well as hatred at the patient's manipulation of family and staff. It was usual to experience these adolescents as taking so much attention when others nearby, whose burns were caused in other ways, seemed more in need of attention. Other patients occasionally learned that these patients had made suicide attempts, and they became jealous and regressed competitively because of the extra attention these patients tended to attract. Still others tended to regard the patients primarily as burn victims rather than emotional outcasts, but they were at times naive and mercilessly victimized by these impulsive patients. However, it was more usual for the self-immolators to isolate themselves to avoid what they feared would be peer stigmatization. For example, several avoided participation in the adolescent group, which met twice weekly.

The burn team is trained to deal with critically ill patients but not those with severe mental disorders. A potentially suicidal patient is a significant disruption to the unit and requires time for the staff to learn techniques of management and to adapt to this added, unwelcome burden; the possibilities for staff splitting are similar to those seen with similar patients in psychiatric hospitals (Burnham 1966; Stanton and Schwartz 1954). The team turns to the psychiatrist for clear direction.

When direction was provided, the burn team proved capable of assisting in assessment of suicide risk on an hour-by-hour basis and of managing suicide precautions while those patients required burn care. Specifying roles helped, with the psychiatrist directing management of behavioral care and the surgeon focusing on physical care. This decreased patient success in dividing staff but required careful coordination.

A fear was present in all staff caring for these patients who had attempted suicide that they would repeat the act. Staff and patients were very attached to the patient who later killed herself, and our grieving was more difficult because the patient was away from the burn unit for several months before her suicide. Meetings among staff were helpful in sharing grief and in reviewing aspects of her care.

Conclusions

This chapter describes selected aspects of treatment of six adolescents who attempted suicide by self-immolation, and their outcomes. Epidemiology, case reports, and precursors are presented in Part I. Psychiatric care on the burn unit required closely coordinated surgical, nursing, psychiatric, and social service interventions with patient and family. Psychiatric diagnosis and recognition of the suicidal causes of the burns were hindered by secrecy, shame, and in some cases parental anger. These affects were clues that the supposed "accidents" were, in reality, suicide attempts. Guilt and denial were pervasive and were only partially modified in most patients and families. Although suicidal risk did not recur on the acute burn unit, further psychiatric care, both psychotherapy and medication, was indicated for most but was accepted with great reluctance. Coordination of psychiatric and plastic surgical rehabilitation (ten to thirty operations) efforts were crucial but complicated. One patient committed suicide despite extensive rehabilitative efforts. The feelings in staff elicited by various of these patients included fear, anxiety, disgust, anger, vulnerability, devotion, and grief.

REFERENCES

Anthony, J. 1974. Self-therapy in adolescence. *Adolescent Psychiatry* 3:6–24.

Belfer, M.; Harrison, A. M.; Pillemer, F. C.; and Murray, J. E. 1982. Appearance and the influence of reconstructive surgery on body image. *Clinics in Plastic Surgery* 9:307–315.

Bernstein, N. 1982. Psychosocial results of burns: the damaged self-esteem. *Clinics in Plastic Surgery* 9:337–346.

Bowden, M. L.; Feller, I.; Tholen, D.; Davidson, T. N.; and Hames, M. H. 1982. Self-esteem in severely burned patients. *Archives of Physical Medical Rehabilitation* 61:449–452.

Burnham, D. L. 1966. The special problem patient: victim or agent of splitting? *Psychiatry* 29:105–122.

Cohen-Sandler, R.; Berman, A. L.; and King, R. A. 1982. A follow-up study of hospitalized suicidal children. *Journal of the American Academy of Child Psychiatry* 21:398–404.

Forrest, W. H.; Brown, B. S.; Brown, W. R.; Defalque, R.; Gold, M.; Gordon, H. E.; James, K. E.; Katz, J.; Mahler, D. L.; Schroff, P.; and Teutch, G. 1977. Dextroamphetamine with morphine for the treatment of postoperative pain. *New England Journal of Medicine* 296:712–715.

Frances, A., and Clarkin, J. F. 1981. No treatment as the prescription of choice. 1981. *Archives of General Psychology* 38:542–546.

Goin, J. M., and Goin, M. K. 1981. *Changing the Body: Psychological Effects of Plastic Surgery*. Baltimore: Williams & Wilkins.

Groves, J. 1978. Taking care of the hateful patient. *New England Journal of Medicine* 298:883–887.

Guggenheim, F. C. 1978. Suicide. In T. P. Hackett and E. H. Cassem, eds. *Massachusetts General Hospital Handbook of General Hospital Psychiatry*. St. Louis: Mosby.

Hamburg, D. A.; Hamburg, B.; and deGoza, S. 1953. Adaptive problems and mechanisms in severely burned patients. *Psychiatry* 16:1–20.

Lerner, Y.; Ewow, E.; Levitin, A.; and Belmaker, R. H. 1979. Acute high-dose parenteral haloperidol treatment of psychosis. *American Journal of Psychiatry* 136:1061–1064.

Maartyn, J. A.; Greenblatt, D. U.; and Quinby, W. D. 1983. Diazepam kinetics in patients with severe burns. *Anesthesia Analgesia* 62:203–297.

Mack, J., ed. 1975. *Borderline States in Psychiatry*. New York: Grune & Stratton.

Noyes, R.; Frye, S. J.; Slyman, D. J.; and Canter, A. 1979. Stressful life events in burn injuries. *Trauma* 19:141–144.

Perry, S.; Heidrick, D.; and Ramos, E. 1981. Assessment of pain by burned patients. *Burn Care and Rehabilitation* 322:326.

Ravenscroft, K. 1982. Psychiatric consultation of the child with acute physical trauma. *American Journal of Orthopsychiatry* 52:298–307.

Sabbath, J. C. 1971. The role of the parents in adolescent suicidal behavior. *Acta PaedoPsychiatrica* 38:211–220.

Shapiro, E. R. 1978. The psychodynamics and developmental psychology of the borderline patient: a review of the literature. *American Journal of Psychiatry* 135:1305–1315.

Stanton, A. H., and Schwartz, M. D. 1954. *The Mental Hospital*. New York: Basic.

Stoddard, F. J. 1982a. Coping with pain: a developmental approach to treatment of burned children. *American Journal of Psychiatry* 139:736–740.

Stoddard, F. J. 1982b. Body image development in the burned child. *Journal of the American Academy of Child Psychiatry* 21:502–507.

Stoddard, F. J.; Pahlavan, K.; and Cahners, S. S. 1984. Suicide attempted by self-immolation during adolescence. I. Literature review, case reports, and personality precursors. In this volume.

Van Buskirk, D., and Semrad, E. 1969. *Teaching Psychotherapy of Psychotic Patients*. New York: Grune & Stratton.

Webb, S. S.; Smith, G.; Evans, W. O.; and Webb, N. C. 1978. Toward the development of a potent, nonsedating oral analgesic. *Psychopharmacology* 60:25–28.

West, D. A., and Shuck, J. M. 1978. Emotional problems of the severely burned patient. *Surgical Clinics of North America* 58:1189–1204.

Yacoubian, J. H., and Lourie, R. S. 1973. Suicide and attempted suicide in children and adolescents. In S. Copel, ed. *Behavior Pathology of Childhood and Adolescence*. New York: Basic.

19 PSYCHODYNAMICS OF DELINQUENT GIRLS' RAGE AND VIOLENCE DIRECTED TOWARD MOTHER

PERIHAN ARAL ROSENTHAL AND MAIRIN B. DOHERTY

This chapter will focus on the intrapsychic conflicts and catastrophic rage exhibited by a group of violent adolescent girls that had psychodynamic origins in their relationship with their mothers and other significant care givers. The literature on aggression and violence has stressed multiple causes such as organic brain damage or injury (Lewis, Shanok, Pincus, and Glaser 1979; Monroe 1970) and family sociocultural influences (Glueck and Glueck 1950; Shaw and McKay 1931). Psychodynamic theory emphasizes the quality of personal relationships, especially of the earliest interactions between mother and child. Many authors believe (Bender 1953; Eron, Walder, Toigo, and Lefkowtj 1963; Woodmansey 1971) that the aggressiveness of delinquents is the result of cruel experiences at the hands of hostile parents or parent substitutes.

Observers have pointed out that aggression is an inherent human tendency which must be socialized within the matrix of loving and nurturing human relationships if it is to be channeled into benevolent behavior (Freud 1949; Freud and Dann 1951). In psychoanalytic terms, Freud (1970) has noted that aggressive outbursts may be the mark of insufficient fusion between libido and aggression. The cause does not relate to the aggressive drive alone but resides in a developmental failure within the libidinal process. A child's disappointment in the love object, imagined or real rejection, or possible object loss leads to insufficient available libidinal energy to neutralize or bind the aggressive impulses.

0-226-24058-4/85/0012-0023$01.00

Case studies of severely aggressive individuals usually contain much evidence of severe frustration during early formative years and clear models of violence in the home (Capote 1966). Some researchers describe mothers of delinquents as more likely to be careless or inadequate in child supervision. Delinquent girls, especially recidivists, more frequently acknowledge intense murderous impulses to their mothers with reports that their mothers did not care for them (Conger 1973). A child who has been neglected or abused has little opportunity to have inner feelings states validated by cues and clues from his or her environment. This failure of empathic response between the child and caretaker leads to self-doubt and poor self-esteem. That, in turn, interferes with the child's mastery of identity and the development of internalized controls over the discharge of violent and aggressive impulses. Anger and rage may be directed toward significant others with the same lack of empathic consideration as had been previously experienced within the relationship.

Wertham (1941) commented that the shift from a fantasy of murdering mother to actual commission of the act may be due to an overwhelming emotional response which produces an immediate need to act out and may spring from an unconscious hatred of the mother superimposed on desire for her. A variety of ego defense mechanisms may normally serve to ward off both the impulse and its appearance in consciousness. When there is a failure of these defenses, the impulse emerges into consciousness and may result in commission of the act unless the impulse can be discharged in another manner. Linder (1948) discussed four pathways to discharge these murderous impulses toward the mother other than the act itself and included: (1) displacement onto another person; (2) suicide involving the death of the introjected mother image; (3) antisocial acting out; and (4) dreams (Scherl and Mack 1966).

Data

The clinical sample consisted of twenty girls between the ages of thirteen and seventeen with a median age of fifteen years. Thirty percent of this population was black, and 60 percent of the families were divorced. The overall socioeconomic status of the patients' families could best be described as middle and lower middle class on the basis of the mean income and years of education of the parents. These girls had been involved with many mental health agencies since their early years because of acting out. The cases had in common a history of early maternal deprivation, rejection, provocation to anger, harshness, and exposure to continuous abuse of a sexual and physical nature. Fifty percent of the girls had been the victims of an incestuous relationship with their father or father figure, and in more than half of the families there was generational incest as 50 percent of mothers had also experienced incest with their own fathers. The mothers had been unavailable, rejecting, or had failed to protect their daughters from the external abuses and dangers. Some of the parents, for pathological reasons of their own, seemed to need an ill, disturbed, or infantile child. These parents assigned to the child a role in their own pathology, and many mothers acted out through their daughters' symptoms. For these mothers, their attachment to the child depended on the child's representing for them a valued or devalued aspect of themselves or a significant figure from their past. To retain parental love under these conditions, the child allowed her personality to be molded into a pattern which neglected her innate potentialities and led to the development of a pseudoself with intrapsychic conflicts.

The fathers in many cases were extremely passive, failing to protect their daughter from the abusive or neglectful mother. Fathers were for the most part viewed as weak or indifferent, but more than half became involved in forceful sexual abuse of their daughters. There were serious alcoholism, marital problems, and promiscuity in both mothers and fathers.

The delinquent girls had low self-esteem, long-standing depression, and problems with sexual identity. The majority of the sample experienced their mothers as a constant source of deprivation and neglect and had serious identity problems because of the absence of a positive role model. These adolescent girls devalued their mother's role as a mother and female and had difficulty with tenderness and closeness. They sexualized these attributes in other females and frequently became panicked by homosexual anxiety. When overwhelmed by erotic and sexualized feelings, associated with the regressive pull toward mother and females as images of warmth and security, some girls had an immediate need to act out and discharge the anxiety through violent and aggressive acts that reestablished distance and modulated the anxiety. In addition, some of the girls in the group turned toward frantic heterosexual activity during early adolescence to combat this anxiety. These girls were more interested in scandalizing their mothers than in developing an emotional relationship with boys they seduced. They frequently enjoyed shocking people by seducing innocent, moral, naive boys and were often more masculine than feminine in their aggressive conquest of males, showing virtually no tenderness toward the boys and frequently preferring to have many boyfriends. Their attitudes were spiteful toward both their mother and their sexual partners.

Case Study

Mary, an extremely attractive fourteen-year-old girl, was referred for mental health services by her mother following an altercation between them which resulted in the mother's having a black eye and being terrified by her daughter's emerging rage.

Mary was the eldest of three siblings and the only girl in her family. The pregnancy had predated her mother's marriage at the age of sixteen, and Mary's early care was often left to her maternal grandmother, father, or others as her mother found child care and housework boring and difficult. In addition, mother invested Mary with a wisdom and maturity beyond her years. For most of her life, Mary found herself in the mothering role with her siblings. When her parents separated when she was seven, Mary was expected to take on many responsibilities in the family while the mother worked. At that time they moved into a one-bedroom apartment in which mother shared her bed with Mary. At age eleven, Mary began running away, disappearing for several days at a time. She became promiscuous with boys whom she invited to her mother's room to have sex while her mother was working. Around this time, Mary was hospitalized following a fainting episode. She fell to the ground and appeared to be struggling with an unseen force. She cried out several times "he is choking me." She later described this experience as being an encounter with a male force which sometimes appeared as a cloud and at other times as a seven-foot man. She said she had felt the influence of this force for two years, and that it prevented her from going to sleep on certain nights, sometimes made her talk to strangers, and forced her to drink alcohol and smoke pot. There was no evidence of drug ingestion, and laboratory tests were negative.

Mary's therapy lasted one year and terminated when she moved out of the region. Early alliance formation was difficult, but finally Mary began to report many traumatic life experiences. At the age of three, she had been sexually abused by a paternal uncle. She remembered wishing her mother would intervene but recalled not being able to tell her because she feared her mother would become angry and abusive (mother had used corporal punishment for any small behavioral problem). Following her parents' separation, her maternal grandfather moved in with the family, and Mary was again sexually abused. Her grandfather had forceful intercourse with her that caused intense pain, and she remembered her fear that he would kill her if she told anyone. She recalled holding her mother and begging her not to leave her alone with him and the mother's becoming angry and at times physically restraining her. Her grandfather would subsequently goad her by saying, "See, your mother doesn't care about you, she never believes you anyway." Mary remembered hiding in the closet, falling asleep there, and her grandfather dragging her out saying, "You cannot ever get away from me." Following intercourse she felt her body was dirty and she would bathe for several hours to clean herself, a behavior which further infuriated her mother. In spite of Mary's begging her mother to stay, her mother spent most evenings away from home.

When Mary reached puberty, she had difficulty controlling emerging sexual feelings which were associated with a regressive pull toward mother as a need-satisfying object. She pleaded for a room change so they would no longer need to share a bed. Mary's ambivalence about these regressive and sexualized feelings created panic about being homosexual, and she could state that at times she felt like killing her mother to stop her anxiety about the sleeping arrangement. She equated those feelings about her mother with the anxiety, arousal, coercion, and humiliation that she had previously experienced with her uncle and grandfathers, and she frequently showed retaliatory abuse toward her mother. It was around this time that Mary became promiscuous and sought to shock her mother by telling her of her escapades. When her mother showed anger and made disparaging remarks to Mary about being a whore, Mary experienced relief that the threatening homosexual closeness had been avoided and her heterosexual orientation confirmed.

During therapy, Mary was raped by her paternal uncle while intoxicated. In spite of family support from both parents about pressing charges, she refused to testify against him in court. The incident, however, did mobilize mother to report generational incest which she herself had experienced in her family with her stepfather and uncle and which grandmother had also experienced. When the mother openly acknowledged that Mary had been sexually abused and that she had played a role in the process, she became somewhat more supportive of Mary and her problems. However, Mary could not deal with this new closeness. She attempted to force a precipitous separation by becoming pregnant by a boy whom she had just started to date. Her rage attacks then shifted between her mother and boyfriend. Mary finally expressed her frustration, "They can do no more for my needs; I feel so hurt that I have to hit or break things to make them see how much I am hurting."

Discussion

According to Blos (1968), adolescence is an important developmental phase in which the child seeks to establish a sense of continuity with his own previous feeling states, remembered experiences, and the history of his own family. This allows for the resolution of earlier traumas, solidification of a sexual identity, and loosening of parental ties. When a child has been traumatized in that child's family of origin, the remembered experiences and feeling states create conflict and anxiety around the completion of these developmental tasks. During adolescence, the resurgence of sexual and aggressive impulses further influences the defense mechanisms at the ego's command, and the symptom formation may represent either internalization or externalization of the conflict. Blos (1962) described the deprived child's precocious development in situations of extreme stress and deprivation and how the egos of such children remain impoverished in terms of internalized objects and identification. The children are forced to take over self-protective functions before they can establish object constancy and internalization of the maternal function.

During their early development, girls in this sample were not nurtured or protected. They had their dependency needs frustrated by their mothers or other caretakers. They thus retained the ambivalent object relationship of the preoedipal period and were filled with primitive sadistic rage characterized by ego attitudes of clinging, torturing, dominating, and controlling the love object (Freud 1949). Their incomplete separation-individuation from the early love object was combined with a fear of merging and being engulfed by the mother (Mahler 1965). The girls were drawn toward mother in the hope of experiencing the fantasied caring and nurturing figure, but, because of the need to avoid reexperiencing their early frustration and deprivation, it was necessary to remain distant (Rosenthal 1979).

Aggressive and violent behavior served to protect these girls from the regressive pull to the preoedipal mother and the attendant depression when needs were not fulfilled. The onset of puberty and the arousal of instinctual sexual impulses complicated these adolescent girls' attempts to recapitulate the infantile sexual period. Ambivalent feelings related to pregenital object relations, erotic arousal in the relationship to mother, and fears of attack on their body integrity created catastrophic anxiety about closeness. These girls protected themselves by the early defense mechanisms of sensorimotor discharge of aggression and rage against mother.

Research indicates that delinquent females tend to have more self-punishing or escapist symptoms than boys, who are more likely to act out their aggression on things or other people (Caplan 1981). However, in our sample, girls competed freely with men, identified with them, or followed male modes of action with a more archaic form of aggression and violence. This was felt to be partially due to cultural factors, rapid changes in social mores, and new images of womanhood. It appeared that these adolescent girls might be more comfortable in the aggressive and violent mode of action than earlier generations.

Conclusions

Serious problems in early object relations, that is, instability, rejection, deprivation, or abuse during formative years (Freud 1965) create a disturbance in the balanced fusion between libido and aggression, with uncontrollable aggression and destructiveness toward the object. If, during a child's formative years, painful stimuli over which the child has no control are inflicted on the psyche or body, these experiences will be internalized, and the conflict may be expressed by identifying with the aggressor, inflicting pain on others, or inviting an attack on oneself. If a daughter's first love object, the mother, is experienced as a destructive force, the move toward the second separation-individuation phase during adolescence causes the earlier destructive images of mothers to resurface. The painful ambivalence intensifies when the adolescent girl is confronted with closeness, and the resultant panic at the thought of feeling homosexual toward mother may result in catastrophic rage and violent primitive aggression.

REFERENCES

Bender, L. 1953. *Aggression, Hostility and Anxiety in Children*. Springfield, Ill.: Thomas.

Blos, P. 1962. *On Adolescence*. New York: Free Press.

Blos, P. 1968. Character formation in adolescence. *Psychoanalytic Study of the Child* 23:245–263.

Blos, P. 1979. *The Adolescent Passage: Developmental Issues*. New York: International Universities Press.

Caplan, J. 1981. *Barriers between Women*. New York: Spectrum.

Capote, T. 1966. *In Cold Blood*. New York: Random.

Conger, J. J. 1973. *Adolescent and Youth: Psychological Development in a Changing World*. New York: Harper & Row.

Eron, L. D.; Walder, L. O.; Toigo, R.; and Lefkowtj, M. M. 1963. Social class parental punishment for aggression, and child aggression. *Child Development* 34:849–867.

Freud, A. 1949. Aggression in relation to emotional development: normal and pathological. *Psychoanalytic Study of the Child* 3:37–42.

Freud, A. 1965. *Normality and Pathology in Childhood*. New York: International Universities Press.

Freud, A. 1970. The symptomatology of childhood: a preliminary attempt at classification. *Psychoanalytic Study of the Child* 25:19–45.

Freud, A., and Dann, S. 1951. An experiment in group upbringing. *Psychoanalytic Study of the Child* 6:127–168.

Glueck, S., and Glueck, E. T. 1950. *Unraveling Juvenile Delinquency*. Cambridge, Mass.: Harvard University Press.

Lewis, D. O.; Shanok, S. S.; Pincus, J. H.; and Glaser, G. H. 1979. Violent juvenile delinquents: psychiatric neurological, psychological and abuse factors. *Journal of the American Academy of Child Psychiatry* 21:190–197.

Linder, R. M. 1948. Equivalents of matricide. *Psychoanalytic Quarterly* 17:453–470.

Mahler, M. S. 1965. On the significance of the normal separation-individuation phase: with reference to research in symbiotic child psychosis. In M. Schur, ed. *Drives, Affects, Behavior*. Vol. 2. New York: International Universities Press.

Mahler, M. S.; Pine, F.; and Bergman, A. 1975. *The Psychological Birth of the Human Infant*. New York: Basic.

Monroe, R. 1970. *Episodic Behavior Disorders: A Psychodynamic and Neurophysiologic Analysis*. Cambridge, Mass: Harvard University Press.

Rosenthal, P. 1979. Delinquency in adolescent girls: developmental aspects. *Adolescent Psychiatry* 7:503–515.

Shaw, C. R., and McKay, H. D. 1931. *Social Factors in Juvenile De-*

linquency. Washington, D.C.: National Commission of Law Observance and Enforcement.

Scherl, D. J., and Mack, J. E. 1966. A study of adolescent matricide. *Journal of the American Academy of Child Psychiatry* 4:569–594.

Wertham, F. 1941. *Dark Legend: A Study in Murder*. New York: Duell, Sloan & Pearce.

Woodmansey, A. C. 1971. Understanding delinquency. *British Journal of Criminology* 11:155–166.

PART IV

CLINICAL INSTITUTE: PERSPECTIVES IN THE TREATMENT OF ADOLESCENTS AND YOUTH

CLINICAL INSTITUTE: PERSPECTIVES IN THE TREATMENT OF ADOLESCENTS AND YOUTH

ROBERT M. GALATZER-LEVY

Jack Schimel, then President-Elect of the American Society for Adolescent Psychiatry, scanned the audience of three hundred psychiatric professionals. The occasion was the Third ASAP Institute, Clinical Practice: A Broad Perspective in the Treatment of Adolescents and College Youth. He said he had carefully studied the program in search of a unifying theme and had discovered one—coffee. Indeed, the single most frequent program entry was "coffee," but Schimel's remark was correct in a more important way. Although the group who planned the meeting—Jack Buffington, Miepje deVryer, Charles Jaffe, and I—would have phrased it differently, Schimel's observation caught an essential element of our intentions. We hoped, in a context of mutual interest and respect, that colleagues in adolescent psychiatry would meet, learn about, and discuss each other's thoughts and ideas. The informal but serious discussions people have over coffee are what we were trying to achieve, and that spirit pervaded the meeting.

It is increasingly difficult to practice adolescent psychiatry with a limited outlook. American Society for Adolescent Psychiatry Institutes are designed to review the latest developments in the field, refine clinical understanding from long and widely accepted viewpoints, consider new ideas, and present a state-of-the-art overview of clinical work with adolescents. Topics in the February 1983 Institute included adolescent language, countertransference, postdivorce families, adolescent mourning, educational evaluation, interpersonal psychiatry, psychopharmacology, and psychotherapy. A variety of special patient populations were examined—the eleven- to thirteen-year-old, adolescents with eating disorders or drug abuse, and college youth. The following chapters represent a sample of the diverse topics discussed at the conference.

Ideas from linguistics play an increasing role in psychiatry. Theodore Shapiro shows how a psychoanalyst, informed by linguistic concepts, understands the role of adolescent language. He notes that every adolescent lives in at least two subcultures, his group and his family, and there is transference significance in the language he uses with the therapist and the language used to speak of emotion. Shapiro concludes that the appreciation of the uniqueness of tongue is as much a challenge as our understanding of the adolescent's striving for independence. In her discussion of Dr. Shapiro's paper, Bonnie E. Litowitz explores the wide area of mutual interest between psychiatry and psycholinguistics by discussing the use of language in the establishment of identity, object relations, and reassuring communication in adolescents.

A common dilemma in today's world of adolescent psychiatry is the internal conflict of the dynamically oriented therapist practicing brief treatment based on psychoanalytic understanding. Rita L. Love and Helen A. Widen explore the confusion arising from the inadequately worked through idealization of psychoanalysis and show how it can interfere with the application of analytic concepts to brief therapies. The authors demonstrate the usefulness of brief interventions and how the therapist's ambivalence about his work can result in inappropriate technique and less than optimal work.

On the other end of the spectrum, it is rare that adolescents are offered the opportunity for full analytic treatment. In my own contribution, I demonstrate through a case report how well some adolescents can use the analytic situation. I address many of the problems which have been discussed about adolescent analysis such as the nature of the transference, modification of technique, the parents' role, and the timing and nature of termination. I believe there are many adolescents for whom psychoanalysis is the treatment of choice.

Among the greatest challenges of adolescent psychiatry is the treatment of the severely disturbed adolescent. Jacquelyn Sanders describes how the staff in a residential treatment center works with disturbed children and adolescents by virtue of constant attention to their own internal lives and their responses to their patients. Through dealing in an open manner with the various conflicts aroused in the staff, the author finds that it is possible to sort out the most chaotic emotional barrage and achieve empathic understanding and rewarding mastery.

Adolescent psychiatry would be greatly advanced if meaningful preventative intervention were possible. A prerequisite to such prevention is an understanding of the effects of potentially pathogenic crises such as parent loss and divorce. Benjamin Garber uses empirical studies to demonstrate the several patterns of mourning observed in adolescents. Adolescent mourning does not follow one set pattern but may manifest itself in many types of experiences that reflect the fluid state of the psychic structure during this phase of life.

Thus we have tried to provide a sample of the work presented at the Third ASAP Institute. We hope that some of the institute's atmosphere has also been communicated and that the reader will feel tempted to join us as we continue our discussions. Coffee is always available.

20 ADOLESCENT LANGUAGE: ITS USE FOR DIAGNOSIS, GROUP IDENTITY, VALUES, AND TREATMENT

THEODORE SHAPIRO

A colleague told me that, when his son was about to go off to college, he wished to impress on him the importance of using more varied language and a broader vocabulary than he had employed during his high school years. There was no issue or topic that his son had not evaluated as either "awesome" or "gross." Finding the apt moment, the father addressed his son, saying, "I want to say something to you, Johnny, that I hope you will take in the right spirit. Before you go off to college, I wish that you would consider not using two words; they are awesome and gross." The young man looked at his father patiently, waited, and responded, "Go on, what are the words?"

I begin this presentation in this way to illustrate that adolescence is not only a segregated period by virtue of a child's entry into puberty and the formation of separate groups with their own lore and customs, but because there is a wide linguistic gulf that develops rapidly. That gulf is designed to signify the separateness of the adolescent culture from the adult culture and the independence of the adolescent from his home, and at the same time it represents an abiding group cohesion which distinguishes adolescent from child and grown-up.

To be sure, the initial example cited has its ambiguity too, because the grammatical form (though adult and appropriate) is such that it is difficult to know whether "awesome" and "gross" are appositive to "the two words" or were in some ways adjectival evaluations of "the two words" that were

0-226-24058-4/85/0012-0015$01.00

yet to be stricken from the young man's vocabulary. Nevertheless, the young man believed that his father was describing the two words that he found so offensive. They had become so natural to him that he did not bat an eyelash when his father used them as though they were a part of father's vocabulary. The kind of confusion that emerged makes for humor. However, there were other times when an adolescent never would have imagined that his parents would use such words, because the wish implied in creating a new language (strictly speaking, a new sociolect) is to dissociate parents from the new group. "You don't belong to my language group, and I don't belong to yours!" is the message.

Another, now archaic, example from the past approaches separateness, but in the other direction. It comes from a young man from the 1940s who spontaneously responded to a shocking statement by his mother: "No shit!" His mother turned around and said, "What did you say?" Of course the latter example was from the 1940s and not the 1980s, highlighting a central problem in practical linguistics. Both language and social practice change rapidly over short time spans. These diachronic shifts make for difficulties in understanding among people.

These events are important in daily life, in common family situations, and in therapeutic situations. Those of us who do psychotherapy or psychoanalysis with adolescents understand that it is a mutual enterprise between therapist and patient, both of whom are engaged in a quest for meaning (Shapiro 1979). It is not a simple matter to discover what someone is thinking about by what he says if we are not acquainted with the referential system he is using and the particular vantage point from which his words emerge. Thus, we ought to know something as therapists about how meaning organization comes about in adolescence and what the rules of transformation are so that we can make appropriate and significant interpretations of what is being said. Only later will we be able to plumb the significance of what is said in regard to wishing and defensive operations directed toward not exposing. Thus subtleties of new sociolects would allow that an utterance used can obscure as well as reveal.

Let me address the matter of the meaning of adolescent language initially in terms of its most general psychological function: if we accept the vantage point of the dynamic psychotherapist or even a sociologist, we would have to say that entry into adulthood, adult responsibilities, and responsibilities for raising a family have been time segregated from physical maturity and biological preparedness for procreation. That gap between biological readiness and social acceptance into the adult world is called adolescence. In modern times, the time gap is augmented by prolonged periods of education and training before one enters adulthood. In intrapsychic terms, the struggle to remove one's thoughts from oedipal themes, or, in ego psychology terms, the revival of separation-individuation struggles in adolescence, becomes a central problem. Using a number of strategies, adolescents endeavor to take on psychologically new and significant roles in the community and in their own minds that lead to increased self-esteem and peer esteem. One can make a simple parallel from a transindividual vantage point of adolescence to that which has been described for ethnic cohesion.

Following the First World War, the artificial creation of new national boundaries that created countries such as Yugoslavia also created internal problems among Montenegrins, Croats, and Serbs. They all had to band together for their new national interest, but they also announced their separateness by maintaining their own sense of uniqueness as a people and pride in their own dialects. The latter continues to be a marker of their ethnic, rather than national, cohesion. Similarly, Eastern European Jews clung not only to their ways within the Diaspora but to the Yiddish language. That language marked them as separate, though they were diffusely disseminated among a variety of nations marked by political boundaries. It always guaranteed recognition among them as kin, no matter where one found another. Adolescent language or sociolect has a similar function with regard to the wish to maintain psychological and social separateness as a means of group identification within a sea of other individuals who belong to varying categories or groups—whether professions, work groups, unions, or even family circles. Coping with the problems of this period of life is done much better by the normalizing influence of being able to share with others in a similar situation. The shared problems of this developmental stage are better transmitted in a language that signifies and carries meaning in a manner that is not available to others. There is also a creative joy in messing with words that others do not understand—a sense of belonging to a unique social body with group separateness. I would not like to venture that this strategy is new or that it is consciously purposeful rather than that it grows naturally in accord with the normalizing function of adolescents having common goals, common problems, and common needs. Distinctive social group dress as well as ethnic dress also provide group cohesion and separate identity, as individuals migrate hither and yon.

Certainly the notion of the melting pot in the United States seems idealized and mythic from our vantage in the 1980s. It is erroneous to think that only in the Bronx or Brooklyn or on the south side of Chicago is ethnic cohesiveness maintained. In the northern towns of Minnesota or in the hills of Kentucky original languages and dialects hold on, as well as original practices; sometimes even ethnically distinct dress continues. People maintain their languages and cultural heritage not because they are sequestered from larger communities but because they wish to be separated and individual. The adolescent is similarly disposed. He is not welcome in all adult places, and he is also suspect in terms of the usual adult sense of what is good clean fun. In addition to these larger social issues, psychotherapists must be alerted to idiosyncratic languages because sometimes a new language may not be a group phenomenon shared by a peer group. It may be an individual phenomenon and signify pathological separateness and even loneliness. The prepsychotic youngster, for example, who makes up neologisms, or the borderline who lives by and uses a personal code, does not want others, peers or adults, to understand what is going on in his inner thoughts and feelings. Without digressing too far, I may say that poetry may be another special way of coding the emotions—thus, poetic idiom often becomes an adolescent indulgence too. Such romantic visions sometimes encourage the adolescent to cast his thoughts and feelings in a potentially creative idiolect that may in rare instances become popular. More often than not it remains personal and opaque.

From the vantage point of traditional linguistics, there is some question of what that science may have to say about the developmental event called adolescence. Yet there may be some contribution that psychologically sophisticated linguists can make to these considerations. Prior to exploring the matter directly, I would like to run through some of the traditional vantage points of linguistics in order to indicate the modes of language study that have been employed. Clinicians will have to see if they can be useful as an application of a method that permits better understanding of patients.

Traditionally the linguist looks at grammar as the relation of words to words and form or structure. Semantics usually refers to the elaboration of meaning and more specifically to reference. Pragmatics is a shorthand notion of the dialogic aspects of getting things done, viewing language as a useful tool with special regard to affecting other people. Grammar or syntax takes as its study the invariance in form of groups of words in sentences. It considers how that invariance interlocks with semantic aspects of language, but only in regard to how well formed a sentence seems to our grammatical intuition. Well-formed grammatic sentences are easily understood and express relationships, but similar invariances may be found in dialogic rules between and among people and also may be studied in terms of the formal aspects of how one sentence relates to another and how one person's remarks elicit another's utterance. In adolescent argot we can sometimes find new grammaticisms, but by and large I think the study of form in terms of individual sentences is not very much different from the study of form in average sentences spoken by nonadolescents. Thus, in a strictly linguistic sense, they do not create or use new languages but variant sociolects. What does happen sometimes, however, is that adolescent argot employs a unique use of words which might not find their way into sentences in the grammatical slots available in usual good usage.

Chomsky (1957) provided us with an interesting commentary on the latter theme in the phrase, "colorless green ideas sleep furiously." His argument was based on the fact that every one of the words in that sentence is well suited to its position if we consider grammatical requirements, but the words are ill placed considering their function as signifiers and carriers of meaning. Thus, we could have good grammar but poor reference or semanticity. Poetry does it sometimes too—"Spring is like a perhaps hand," wrote e. e. cummings (1926). The latter jars us just as "colorless green ideas" does because "a perhaps hand" seems poorly placed in the sentence. Grammarians use a concept of feature analysis of words to signify that the mathematical formalism of grammar requires that only certain insertions are appropriate within the strict parameters of the grammatical form. For example, what is disruptive in "colorless green ideas" is that, although colorless and green are adjectival, they are nonetheless semantically antithetical. Moreover, ideas are not colored or colorless except metaphorically, nor do they sleep, and therefore the verb form is not appropriate as an action describer for the particular noun. An idea is inanimate and incapable of somnolence.

Let us contrast the latter with another sentence which was popular in the 1960s. "I dig my head." It carries some of the same problems as in "ideas sleeping." It is not that the sentence is incomplete; it has a pronoun, a verb, a possessive pronoun, and an object. However, how does one "dig" a "head"? The feature analysis again has been disrupted, and the sentence is jarring unless one has accepted a broadened usage for "dig," a new polysemy for a single homophone.

A similar problem arises in the language of adolescents of the 1980s. I cite an example from Valley talk (Val Speak), where there are ellipses and omissions as well as new usages. For example, the young ladies of the Valley might say, "like no biggies," which translates to "I'm telling you that it is not a big problem for me"; or "you gross me out"—that is a use of what now has become a commonplace expression that has drifted into the larger community. However syntactically disrupted it is, it indicates that "you make me puke." "Fer suure, gag me with a spoon!" qualifies as an exclamation of surprise. We will return to Valley talk and also to street talk of the 1960s and other adolescent linguistic forms later, but now I would like turn to another aspect of feature analysis as it comes into play in therapy, employing a semantic vantage point.

The instance to be cited is the use of the opposite for the word signified. Freud's (1910) paper on antithetic meaning of primal words addressed similar issues in his historic analysis of a common mechanism of dream work in the light of the linguistic theory of his day. He would have had a heyday studying modern adolescent productions for they tell each other that they are "bad" when they mean that they are "good." Or say that something is "bitchen," strictly speaking a neologism, when they mean it's "the best." Or when they suggest that they are interested in a young man—they describe him as "wicked," meaning "real good," or "tubular," the origin of which is "out of sight."

Bateson (1956), in one of his more whimsical moments, provided an interesting example of the problems of class inclusion of words and how the principles can be utilized in the service of play and cultural differences in carrying messages. He asked a group of scholars to imagine the universe of nameables and to make classes out of them. For example, he offered the word *chairs* and then asked the group to name a number of "not chairs," namely, to sequester a separate class. The volunteers in the group retorted, "tables," "dogs," "people," "autos." Bateson then placidly introduced "tomorrow" and arrested their attention by noting the discomfort in saying "tomorrow is not a chair." He then introduced the notion that there are two senses of not—a proper sense and an improper sense—so that there are two classes of objects which are not chairs: "proper not chairs" (tables, dogs, people) and "improper not chairs" (tomorrows). He then judged that similar reclassifications are at play with regard to normalization processes within communities with respect to rituals and how outsiders may not immediately understand such forms in use.

Aborigines who do not eat kangaroos may not have a confusion between kangaroos and fathers who are not to be eaten, but they may utilize signifiers in categorization to designate nonedibles in a different formal system of negative classes. They nonetheless recognize fathers as cognitively nonkangaroos. Similarly, adolescents, by using words the way they do, may come up with associational pathways that wholly disrupt our formal sense of order. Now, how is the task of the therapist changed if he has to decipher whether an adolescent is ill or just a part of a new and different linguistic group? More important, how can therapy proceed on a common ground of understanding if separateness and group cohesion may be confused with madness or perversity?

The final area concerns the social or pragmatic aspect of language, language as a tool to get things done, that is, language as an area of study that helps to understand the effect of words on people. It should be clear that to do this type of analysis and understand what is said fully we need additional information to supplement grammatical and semantic information. Let me provide an example by making a statement. "Ronald Reagan is the greatest liberal president we ever have had in these United States." To understand that sentence based only on semantic and syntactic grounds—one would have insufficient information. We must add social knowledge, one must know my politics, my state of mind, and even to whom I am addressing my remarks, to know that I am speaking ironically. Similarly, in the case of antithetic meanings, the social, pragmatic, message-carrying aspects of the words become important. A philosopher, Austin (1962), introduced the notion that there is a class of phrases and words that perform acts: "I do" is one, "I promise" is another. Perhaps every sequence of words to someone is a performative, say some. There is a significant body of knowledge to indicate that how and in what sense something becomes a performative is dependent on social convention. The irony intended in my initial sentence about Reagan might not be as apparent in 2084 as it is in 1984. Diachronic shifts make small differences trivial. I am sure scholars who read Aristophanes struggle with his humor insofar as it refers to local and temporally bound politics. Similarly, the humor of Swift's *Gulliver's Travels* may be apparent in 1984, but the political references to English-Irish politics are lost to most.

The social conventions and practices of the adolescent constitute an area laden with problems because adolescents may be accustomed to a set of usages in groups that are not easily transferred to therapy, and their social customs change rapidly. Knowledge of those social and pragmatic rules of dialogue is very important in treating adolescents—even if language were not an issue. In order to provide a runthrough of the formal aspects mentioned, let me contrast the pragmatics of two recent forms of adolescent argot that have made some dent on adult consciousness. The white community adaptation of black adolescent slang and the modern import from California, now prevalent on Long Island also, called Val Speak, provide apt examples.

A historical note is warranted: Before we had the argot of the black ghetto adolescent we had the special lingo of another outside group, that is, the jazz musician, and then the more popular adolescent mode, the bobby-soxer of the 1940s, and finally, in the 1950s and 1960s, the adaptation of a particular subset of dialect that borrowed from black adolescents' language was transferred into the dialect of the white city adolescent. Much of the content of this era had to do with the drug culture but also with mutual insult, raw frank sexuality, and irreverence to parents. The ease with which it penetrated and exposed that which was traditionally hidden in polite society is an interesting example of how a sociologically distinctive group, adolescents, became the exhibitionists of our unconscious and preconscious preoccupations, making everything that had been unsaid conscious, raw, and honest, showing the hypocrisy of the repressed polite adult world while embarrassing it.

The controlled formalized exchanges between black youngsters called *sounding* or *trading dozens* is a prime example that has been studied by linguists such as Labov (1975). Trading dozens or soundings have a characteristic pattern and a set of invariant rules, he says. Insults have never been so elegantly and carefully delivered since Oscar Wilde—but in a unique language form. Not only are they insults but there are audiences for the insults, and there are rules of not jostling or hitting as the exchanges bruise sufficiently while also testing wit. Cleverness and finally the acceptance by the group involve a careful understanding of the rules for exchanges to take place. What is permissible and what is clever are central. Labov notes, for example, that it is important to distinguish what is said from what is done. He notices that from a grammatical viewpoint there are only a small number of sentence types, which are simple in form but reveal an imaginativeness with respect to the ease of their expression—they sometimes even employ rhymed couplets. On the other hand, there is a paucity of variety in the actual words used. And there is a telling preoccupation with the central and basic themes of human dependency and sexuality. Most of the remarks center around insulting via offensiveness about one's mother. The raw aggression in relation to ritualized exchanges reveals a fusion of aggression and sexuality in a way that is unprecedented except perhaps in the recorded curses of the Arab cultures and their extensions into Spain by Moorish invasion. An example of a ghetto couplet:

> I don't play the dozens the dozens ain't my game
> But, the way I fucked your momma is a Goddamn shame.

Or,

> I hate to talk about your mother—she's a good old soul
> She got a ten-ton pussy and a rubber ass hole.

Labov (1975) analyzes these as consisting of disclaiming or retiring first lines; the second lines are contradictions. The format then is not dissimilar to other poetic forms. On the other hand, some of them are not as imaginative. They use common similes and begin with lines such as "Your mother is like," or "Your mother looks like," or "Your mother is." The dialogic rules of the exchanges between people are also well documented, and the returns and refrains do not allow for too lengthy a filibuster. For example:

J1: Hey [whistle]—that's your mother over there [in response to a lady passing].
J2: I know that lady.
J1: That's your mother.
J3: Hell look at the way that lady walks.
J4: She's sick in the head.
J3: Walks like she's got a lizard neck.

This dialogue indicates not only the raw preoccupations of adolescents in regard to what others avoid but also the counterphobic exposure of aggression and sexuality in relation to the adolescents' mothers. It has been institutionalized in a way that is shocking to grown-ups but pleasing and amusing to the teenagers. These are the expressions of poverty-ridden ghetto youngsters who hang together in groups in order to find some support outside of their homes, which are often incest ridden and violent. They expose to their peers the things that may be commonplace at home. So why not express them openly—why not seek group counsel, if you will, and group support, without having to bash heads between groups or even seek out an alien therapist—and bring what was personal and frightening to a peer forum in order to make the associated anxieties less potent? It has been determined that, although there is much intragroup cohesion by virtue of these sociolects, there is also cross-group adolescent migration or linguistic drift of such practices. Take, for example, the fact of transmission of some of these dialect examples into the white community.

The white upper- and middle-class adolescent community during the 1950s and 1960s adopted many of the forms and phrases of groups their parents would not permit to live next door. There is no doubt that some of the language came from blacks and the poor, just as the transmission of jazz had come that route before. However, it was not only in the talk of the adolescent of this period that we recognize the identification with the poor and the black but also in their dress. Indeed, our modern adolescents still dress in blue jeans and denim, originally the cloth of workers and laborers. Such trends in style provide an apt example of how identification with the poor became a symbolic counterattack on affluent parents of adolescents. It was the adolescents' way of saying we are not yours—we want something else in life—we don't want your money—we will shame you by an avowal of your own shameful lost past.

Individuals like this who belong to good cohesive groups do not frequently enter therapy. Linguistic drift in this group paralleled the dress until there was a drift to inarticulate vagaries that were also common in the 1950s and 1960s. Phrases like "I feel," "like," "I am uptight," "like, man," and "you know"—all disguised a mass of inarticulateness and nonexpressibles of adolescents of the white community that was not found in a more glib usage of the black community. This occurred despite opportunity, middle-class education, and encouragement to good speech. It paralleled a negation of the adult community and perhaps even had its parallel negation in the movement toward varying cults that also disavowed the affluence of the larger parent groups. With this in mind, we can understand better phrases such as "After all the shit went down I had to cover my ass, because I was sure he was going to lay it on me." That phrase seems almost understandable and commonplace in the 1980s to adolescents' therapists who have had time to adapt. But imagine having just learned standard English and having to decipher it. As though a testimony to the rapid changes of adolescence and the tendency for linguistic drift, too, we now have yet another new sociolect to consider that represents new identifications and yet another sign of new adolescent values different from those which were espoused earlier.

This new talk is beset with a further negation of that which adolescents affirmed in their admiration of the poor blacks. The following are a few phrases from the newer language:

1. Lets greg on the white zone—I hear there are a bunch of Debbies there who are complete Martians.

Yet one more:

2. *Bite* the ice Melvin—like, I am so sure! That grody tale about that bitchen dude barfed me out. So bag pipe it—I'm gonna buzz the nab and mac out.

The first one represents the surfer indicating that he would like to get together where the waves are good, because he understands that there are a number of sexually stimulating, naive girls there who are from other parts, like the Midwest. The second one translates, "Get lost you weird person—There is no way that I will believe that awful story about the best guy we know. You make me puke. Forget it—I'm gonna leave and get some pizza."

Let's try another one:

3. Fag your face, airhead—you're blitzed and crispy—I'm gonna look for a wicked dude with a cruisemobile. [Get lost, stupid, you're drunk and a drug burnout. I'm gonna look for a real good fellow who has a terrific car.]

I do not think it is just California that created the Valley girls—although it certainly was the waves that created the surfers. However, recent evidence suggests that, with mass media, the drift of the new argot to teenagers in the East is complete. With this behind us—How does the analysis of the language of the adolescent help the psychotherapist? Essentially, it helps because we must understand that the devotion to a particular language form does not preclude bidialectism or bilingualism. Just as a two-year-old who is brought up bilingually seems to know rather quickly to whom he should speak in which language, the adolescent takes a clear stance in relation to the therapist when he or she chooses to use adolescent separatist tongue. If he insists on his adolescent argot, he is challenging the therapist to commitment regarding which will be the language of therapy. If there is a shift in linguistic form during a session, one may be able to look toward the defensive use of either the argot or the therapist's language when the shift comes about. The question for most therapists is whether to intrude or empathize with the presentation by showing we understand the adolescent language nuances and by encouraging use of the language that is closest to his feelings. We are between a rock and a hard place. If we intrude on the talk by suggesting that we do not understand, or if we confront by suggesting that they do not want us to understand, we are offering a challenge. Yet the establishment of a therapeutic contract demands that both parties obey the pragmatic rule of sincerity that an exchange is about to take place. But how is it that we can establish the bargain and the empathy for the problems of the adolescent and indicate that understanding takes more than linguistic jousting?

The adolescent use of new languages is by design a signifier of the difference between the therapist and the adolescent that is similar to the distance that the adolescent has established between himself and his parental group. It may be a designation and statement about his separateness that are ego-syntonic and not to be penetrated. On the other hand, we could interpret the form of the language in terms not only of the sexual obviousness in the themes that recur but of the fact that the adolescent group concerns that are expressed in a separate code sometimes sexualize more than is necessary. This may parallel the tendency described by Blos (1962) to look for a solution to anxiety in masturbation. The soundings of the 1950s, 1960s, and 1970s made an adjectival form out of the word for intercourse (fuck). They also made *mother* half a curse word. They constantly bring the individual to the emotional peak of protection or flying in the face of that protection of his family bonds by insulting family. The need to be cool in both the 1960s and the 1980s has taken on the form of new identifications, first with poverty, and then with a kind of resounding immersion in decadence, laughing at the parental straight and narrow. Yet sexual activity still seems to be the common object of the conflict that it always has been. While dudes are on girls' minds, Joanies are put down, and dresses are shorter than ever and more flouncy and feminine—there is also an ample amount of latency-age play around anality in disgust, grodiness, and that which is awesome by virtue of its smuttiness.

Grown-up attention to being attractive takes on a caricature form—just as the bobby-soxer in the 1940s disguised sexuality by wearing long baggy shirts and in the 1960s by wearing work clothes, the Valley adolescent has invented a chic that is pure kitsch and even little-girl pristine. And yet the evolution has come about and the forms change. The advertising industry also has resexualized denims in the ads for designer labels. While the therapist's stance takes cognizance of the group identifications and their function in the psychological life of the adolescent, serving to keep the adolescent separate from the adult, the therapist also recognizes that the language helps the adolescent to belong and provides a normalizing experience in sharing concerns with peers. Thus, as a therapist, I would not recommend an assault on this identity which, because of its ego syntonicity, seems natural to the adolescent—nor should the therapist treat adolescent lingo as a cute curiosity, because narcissistic injury and anger are sure to be aroused. Thus, our temptation to interpret what we understand as a subcultural phenomenon may have to be kept in abeyance until the symptom is ripe for lancing.

The adolescent may see early interpretation as inappropriate and an uninvited transgression. But to not understand is to be too removed. Thus, therapy must proceed within a balance between being able to listen and infer and being able to accept differences and say, "please explain."

As one gets to know the particular adolescent, one will be able to interpret when the language is used defensively and when a wish has become preconscious. Do not be fooled by the constant reference to sexual and aggressive themes as if the surface language automatically signified deeper latent content, because too rapid an interpretation at a depth level may be the last thing needed. Just as there are no primitive tribes according to anthropologists, because current practices in other cultures have gone through a long evolutionary change just as those in more cultured groups have, the unconscious is not more easily available just because the language seems more primitively referential. The layers have to be peeled in a different direction. The Valley speaker, the jive speaker, the hip speaker are no less conflicted about oedipal and other themes than the polite speaker of standard English, and the ritual language may be less explicit than we imagine. The words may not carry the impact and emotional valence to the natural speaker that they do to the alien auditor. For example, the therapist may be provoked by a short dress or tight jeans, but the interpretation of provocation as an intention must first be dosed and built up by carefully worded preliminary interventions. Mutual regard and therapeutic alliance may permit confrontation in that group practice may coincide with individual wish only once the preliminary work has been done.

What about the individual who comes with a more unique kind of vocabulary? A young man, for example, told me that he wrote poetry and translated it into a secret code because he does not like others to read his poems. This represents a less social form of language, an idiolect. Another patient said he felt "scarable." That was clearly neologistic and, indeed, idiosyncratic. There is no group behind such secret and individual references. They are private, and there is no evidence that the individual authors are about to normalize their creations by easy sharing with peers. It may be the call for something personal, unique, and special, and, while group languages must start with individual creativity, they must similarly become popular. There is no such community for these individual users of their own language. These are the more schizoid—sometimes even preschizophrenic—alone and isolated, seeking restricted understanding, sometimes from a therapist with whom such secrets may be safe. Frequently such practices lead to further isolation and are reflective of the fear they feel for larger communities. Indeed, the normalizing process of sharing both a language and inner secrets during adolescence seems to me to be an extension of a need for community and the potential sign of health that Sullivan (1953) saw in the more limited chumship. When this cannot come about because one's inner secrets and thoughts are so private or considered to be so noncommunicative, then we may be dealing with more serious pathology.

In general, care must be taken in regard to what we know about adolescent language and language use, and special attention should be paid to the task to be done. We must turn always to the pragmatic function of our exchange. If the pragmatics is to hide from the group or isolate the adolescent, it is a more serious defense than that of using a special dialect. If the pragmatics is to share with a community which is narrower than the larger community, then language takes on a highly specialized function which is part and parcel of being an adolescent in the first place but not the only requisite.

Conclusions

The therapist must be aware of a number of facts about language to proceed with this ethnically distinct developmental period. Language usage changes over short time spans, but even as it changes it provides a unique possibility for understanding the ideas and values of each new wave of adolescents. The group expression, however, is not immediately connected to the unconscious wishes, no matter how raw or primitive the utterances seem. Therefore, the therapist should be alert to the new argot as a defensive intrusion as well as a potential royal road to understanding. That fact should make us alert to the bidialectism of every adolescent who lives in at least two subcultures, his group and his family. We may be able to follow our transferential significance by virtue of how we are addressed and which language is accompanied by emotion-laden themes. Tolerance of uniqueness of tongue is as much an adolescent challenge to our tolerance for his individual status as a part of a separatist movement. However, the therapeutic contract ultimately requires signs that trust and information are to be exchanged in the service of potential change. That change is, after all, the aim of the therapeutic talk in the first instance. In the last instance we may have to agree that the exchanges even build toward yet a third language—the language of therapy where, we hope, each party has a new two-person code enabling growth.

NOTE

Presented to the American Society for Adolescent Psychiatry, Saturday, February 18, 1984, Evanston, Illinois.

REFERENCES

Austin, J. L. 1962. *How to Do Things with Words*. New York: Oxford University Press.

Bateson, G. 1956. *In Group Processes: Transactions of the Second Josiah Macy, Jr., Foundation Conference*. Madison, N.J.: Josiah Macy Foundation.

Blos, P. 1962. *On Adolescence*. New York: Free Press.

Chomsky, N. 1957. *Syntactic Structures*. The Hague: Mouton.

cummings, e. e. 1926. *Collected Poems*. New York: Harcourt Brace.

Freud, S. 1910. Antithetic meaning of primal words. *Standard Edition* 11:153–161. London: Hogarth, 1957.

Labov, W. 1975. *Language in the Inner City: Studies in the Black English Vernacular*. Philadelphia: University of Pennsylvania Press.

Pond, M. 1982. *The Valley Girls' Guide to Life*. New York: Dell.

Shapiro, T. 1979. *Clinical Psycholinguistics*. New York: Plenum.

Sullivan, H. S. 1953. *The Interpersonal Theory of Psychiatry*. New York: Norton.

21 THE SPEAKING SUBJECT IN ADOLESCENCE: RESPONSE TO THEODORE SHAPIRO'S ESSAY

BONNIE E. LITOWITZ

Dr. Shapiro has addressed himself exclusively to talking with adolescents in a therapeutic setting. I am not able to comment on the nature of this special kind of communication. However, whatever additional characteristics it may possess, it must share with all communication the multiple uses of language to present oneself to another and be confirmed, to establish a social contract, and—especially—to mutually negotiate meanings. For such communication to progress, one must respect the stage of language development of one's adolescent partner.

Adolescence is a period of increasing awareness of language (we call this metalinguistic awareness). This increasing awareness gives rise to a paradox. On the one hand, adolescents display great verbal art. Shapiro has mentioned "playing the dozens," a verbal insult routine of black ghetto adolescents which, along with "rappin'" and "stylin' out," "sounding," "signifying," and "marking," has been well documented (Kochman 1972; Labov 1973; Mitchell-Kernan 1972). Similar routines are common among adolescents of other cultures. Dundes, Leach, and Özkök (1972) have described the ritualized, rhymed insults on a single theme of anal penetration by eight- to fourteen-year-old Turkish boys. And the apotheosis of antithetical speech must surely be in Walbiri, a backward language used by adolescent Australian aboriginal boys as part of their initiation (Hale 1971).

On the other hand, along with the verbal artistry, adolescents are just as often less sure than we about the uses of language and less confident in their mastery, distrustful about language's ability to express intense

0-226-24058-4/85/0012-0031$01.00

affects and unsure how much can be verbally or nonverbally expressed, and uncertain how to use communication to maintain multiple identities or to indicate closeness of relationships.

I would like to comment on adolescent language from the perspective of a psycholinguist. In the process I shall expand some of the important points Shapiro has made and shall also raise others. At the end, I shall remark on what I find missing in psychoanalytic approaches to adolescents' talk.

I am familiar with Shapiro's work, and the breadth of his reading in linguistics is truly impressive. Equally impressive is his ability to apply insights from often abstruse linguistic theory toward a better understanding of patient speech.

Let me say at the outset that, as a psycholinguist, I make a distinction between language and speech that Shapiro has not made. Language is that abstract, ruled system that we possess when we say we speak English and that allows us to make and decipher examples of English we have never exactly heard before. Speech is actual use of language in real-life situations, in contexts.

Shapiro describes adolescents as bilingual. The assumption that adolescents are bilingual implies that they know two languages. I disagree: they know one language only imperfectly—that is, they are still learning it—and they have several speech styles ("dialects," "sociolects," *façons de parler*). They never speak "*the* language"; they abstract a language from speaking in particular styles in various dialogic contexts. For adolescents in therapy, therapeutic discourse becomes yet another context of learning. Unlike ethnic cohesion, adolescence is a time-limited context. Yesterday's teen talkers are in new contexts today talking about "the downside," "hackers," and "transference."

Linguists, even psycholinguists, are so preoccupied with the structure of language in the limited sense of rules that they can add little to our knowledge of adolescents and how they use language. The rules of phonology and grammar are mastered by five-year-olds. By five years of age most children know the sounds of their language, what sentence patterns string words in acceptable ways, and the relationships among words, objects, and other words. A few linguists have tried to draw the attention of others to the tasks of later years, but even they stop at ten or eleven (Chomsky 1969; Karmiloff-Smith 1979). In general, these authors tell us that between five and preadolescence children are mastering the fine points and subtleties of their language system.

Because language is complex, one usually separates out its subsystems for focus: phonology, or the sounds and intonation patterns; morphology and semantics, or how words are put together and their meanings; syntax, or what constitutes well-formed sentences and how sentences are related; and pragmatics, or how to do things with language.

In each subsystem, subtle changes are occurring in adolescence—conclusive evidence that adolescents are still learning their language (see Appendix). The major accomplishment at this time, however, is the adolescent's awareness of the complex subsystems of language and the attempt to use language more adroitly because of this new awareness. Just as psychoanalytic theorists talk of a revisiting or reworking of the Oedipus complex in adolescence at a different level, there is a circling back to subsystems of language to gain control over them in a new way in adolescence which is termed meta, that is, at a higher level. All developmental theories note this phenomenon during this period, as in the spiral development of Werner and Kaplan (1962), reflective abstraction and formal operations in Inhelder and Piaget (1955), or the raising of higher consciousness in Marxist psychology (Vygotsky 1962). Both what remains of language to master and becoming language's master serve ends which are specific to adolescence: the establishment of an identity, meeting greater adaptive demands of society, and increased independence and control in relation to expanding environments.

What knowledge of the subsystems does not tell us, however, is how language is used, under what circumstances, to accomplish what ends. Linguists, sociolinguists, and philosophers of language study these questions under various guises as language functions, pragmatics, sociolinguistics, and speech act theory. Unfortunately, they have not given us a picture of equal clarity about functions to what we know about language structures. All we do know for certain is that children are increasingly able to "do things with words" (Austin 1962; Bruner 1978) for which they previously had used other systems such as vision, crying, action, and gestures and that they manipulate the complexities of the language system itself.

Some authors are fond of grandly claiming that language has but one basic function—to communicate (see Feldman 1977). Other authors see two functions—to refer and to express (Bloom 1973; McNeill 1970; Nelson 1975). Still others distinguish as many as seven functions (Halliday 1973; Jakobson 1960; Leech 1974; Tough 1977). I mention only three functions which are particularly pertinent for adolescence: (1) the use of language to establish identity, including gender identity; (2) the use of language to establish closeness of relationships; and (3) the use of language for phatic communication—the socially ritualized and reassuring use of language as in "Hi, how are you. Have a nice day."

As Shapiro has shown through many examples, adolescent speech is an endless variation of the theme of establishing group identity. One example is the ingroup-outgroup, boundary-marking function of words and phrases that change for each new generation of teens, such that to be "hep" is not to be "hip," but to be "bad" is to be "good"—and that's "fer sure"! Some expressions are taken from groups (e.g., blacks, musicians) or role models: "Get your ya-ya's out" from the Rolling Stones; "agro" from British Punkers; and most recently from *Fast Times at Ridgemont High,* "Hey dude, what's your problem?" Others, such as Valley Speak, sweep across the country from California. (Note that California also gave us adults psychobabble from Marin County.) The use of language to cement groups is not unique to teens but is represented in all groups by geographical/regional dialects and professional jargons. This phenomenon has its roots in every person's experiences learning language in a family: special words and phrases for bathroom activities, for foods and kin, etc. Adolescence is the first experience, however, in establishing and manipulating this use of language on one's own, outside, and often as opposed to the family.

One of the most interesting phenomena of language acquisition is that both sexes learn language in most cases from hearing female speech (the mother/female caretakers), but little boys must switch to speech patterns like their fathers' or other men's. This they do before and during adolescence. Physiological changes force differences in pitch and loudness; the larynx in men is enlarged, and vocal cords become longer and thicker. But physiology alone is not the reason why men and women speak differently. A ten-month-old boy and a thirteen-month-old girl were observed to alter their vocalizations for fathers and mothers, lowering their voices to fathers (Lieberman 1967). In addition, studies of prepubescent children's voices, where anatomical similarities were controlled, show that listeners could distinguish the sex of speakers. Therefore, there are many stylistic variables besides pitch that distinguish typical male and female speech (Sach 1975; Sach, Lieberman, and Erickson 1973). Some of these stylistic elements of feminine speech patterns include qualifiers ("sort of," "rather," "quite"), intensifiers ("so," "very," "really") and the heightened intonational elements (stress, pitch, loudness) that accompany their use, and greater use of questions (Thorne and Henley 1975).

Learning to speak like other women or other men is part of the complex processes lumped under identification and identity. We know very little about the interplay between these processes and the beginnings of language. Consequently, we do not know how linguistic issues of identification resurface and are worked out in adolescence. Concerning gender-differentiated speech, we do know that in their teens boys give up the great variety of intonation patterns and intensified, qualified speech that becomes negatively connoted as feminine and disempowered in our culture. Many cultures have more elaborately distinguished gender dialects, and these are mastered by adolescence, if not earlier.

While the sounds of language are completely acquired by adolescence, speech accent is usually set at this time but is alterable later in life under specific circumstances. These include conscious decisions to get rid of a Southern or New York accent that may be perceived as a social or professional handicap or identification with a new group (e.g., coming to America from another country). Accents are shaped by positioning of articulators in the oral (and to a lesser degree, nasal) cavities. Variations in these resonating chambers through which the air flows from the tensed vocal chords produce differing vowel sounds that account for the major differences in accent. In this extremely concrete form of identification, the speaker unconsciously shapes his or her mouth to produce sounds that conform to other speakers' sounds.

Another function of language (besides identity formation) is to establish different degrees of closeness in relationships. Joos (1962) has described five styles for five degrees of relative closeness or distance: intimate, casual, consultative, formal, and frozen. Each style differs from the others in (1) how much information is shared and how much needs to be made explicit, (2) how much participation is expected from one's partner, (3) the physical closeness of the communicating partners, and (4) the explicitness and completeness of syntactic construction. For example, intimate speech, used for physically close and maximally participating partners, presupposes much and requires no explicitness of reference. The intimate style uses extraction (an extreme form of ellipsis—leaving out words) and jargon specific to the two partners; it precludes frame markers such as "yeah," "I know," "uh-huh," or "well" to indicate participant or topic changes. In contrast, frozen speech is maximally distant and fully explicit, as exemplified in writing. One of the rules of speech styles is that one cannot move more than one style in either direction at a time—

for example, go from formal to intimate all at once.

Adolescents' speech is colloquial, using casual and consultative styles. They struggle to master other styles and to use them both to signal and to establish varying kinds of relationships with others. They often err: they use the slang and ellipsis of casual style in any situation; they become overly familiar too soon; and they are unclear how to express the intimacy they seek. Therefore, it is important for a therapist working with adolescents to understand that an adult model of closeness or distance as clued by their speech may not be appropriate. In other words, they may not be able to express closeness or may seem overly familiar, disrespectful, and provocative because they are in the process of mastering these aspects of language use. They learn these uses not through maturation but through dialogues with adults.

Another example of a language function developing in adolescents is the establishment and manipulation of language as phatic communication—the socially ritualized, soothing, and reassuring, seemingly semantically empty use of language as in: "Hi, how are ya?" "Yeah," "uh-huh," "Isn't it the truth," "really," "cool." Morris (1967) has equated phatic communication with grooming in monkeys, and others have said it is the later verbal manifestation of stroking and holding in infancy. Phatic communication establishes a turn in conversation (e.g., "well") without saying anything besides "I'm here, I'm listening, I'm socially involved with you." It is a verbal nod of the head or smile, recognizing and acknowledging the presence of the other, and is often accompanied by these gestures. Current adolescent variations include: "like, yeah," "really" (spoken without a questioning intonation), "cool," "fer sure," "hey man, how's it going/what's happenin'?" These expressions are accompanied by their own gestures: handslapping ("give me five"), highly ritualized (often lengthy) handshakes, salutes, and body posturing.

While phatic communication establishes verbal joint attention, it can also serve to frame the messages that follow (Bateson 1972; Goffman 1974). Adolescents are not adept at the use of language to establish frames, especially of new situations such as making dates or becoming more intimate. Very useful in this regard is the "go-between" who serves to translate A's intentions to B: "He really likes you. No, really. He told me so. He wants to take you out." If A asks B, "Are you going to homecoming?" it often falls to the go-between to translate for B whether A is simply making chitchat, is asking for information, or is inviting A to go to homecoming. Adolescents often do not know what their intentions are, and even when they know, the intentions may be hard to accept; but it is always difficult to learn how to set up situations so that intentions are evident.

Adolescents are very vulnerable, and an important function of the go-between is to test the waters: no point in asking B to homecoming if B would refuse. Phatic communication markers enable speakers to maintain a level of confidence that the listener is still in contact, still sharing the negotiated communicational contract (Rommetveit 1974), and still approving. Adolescents need more reassurance than many adults and thus pepper their conversations with "ya know?"s. Every "ya know?" is an opening to let the listener jump in and prevent the speaker from making a fool of himself. Another way to prevent looking foolish in one's listener's eyes is to hedge the certainty and finality of one's statements. Ubiquitous to teen talk, therefore, is the use of "like" to preface all communication. "Like" hedges the certainty of what follows (Litowitz 1981): "*Like,* he's so sure of himself"; "He's *like* so sure of himself"; "He's so *like* sure . . ." "Like" is particularly useful since it can be moved around to qualify the whole proposition or only part of it, but other qualifiers are also used: "kind of," "sort of (sorta)." Therefore, seemingly empty or vague use of language should not be considered necessarily evasive or obstructionistic. All the difficulties adolescents have in mastering the phatic function of language will be evident in therapy as well.

Adolescence is a period both linguistically and psychologically of a circling back in the spiral of development to reexperience issues faced earlier, but now at a higher level. Above all, adolescents are struggling to control the new possibilities in language and in relationships to others by means of language, of which they have become aware. In their struggles with language they are often frustrated and distrustful, and they often misuse or misinterpret it. The struggle to become the master of the language system—to bring it under voluntary control—mirrors other conflicts in their lives at this time in which control is an issue. Issues of control can most clearly be seen in the adolescent's new awareness of speech acts and in the power of coining new word meanings.

For the first part of their lives, adolescents have been the recipients of verbal control by adults who are adept at getting things done with words. Even young children understand that "Isn't it past your bedtime?" is not the kind of speech act called a "request" (for information) even though its form is a question. Rather, it is a "directive" or "command": "Get to bed!" Through speech acts, one can assert, describe, command, request, promise, and so forth (Austin 1962; Searle 1969, 1975). Many sentences convey their speech acts directly: "Stop that!" is a command. Others, such as the example above, are indirect; and indirect speech acts take on great import in adolescence.

Adolescents realize that every utterance embodies through its speech act two different forces: what one is trying to do with language (illocutionary force) and what one is trying to get others to do (perlocutionary force). Aware now of these differences, adolescents often misinterpret all adult statements or questions as directives (to cite but one kind of speech act misunderstanding). A recent example may serve as an illustration:

> Toward the end of a pleasant conversation on girls, dating, and social life at the high school, a father asked his seventeen-year-old son: "Do you think that you should see other girls besides Betty?" Immediately, the son became irate: "Why are you telling me what to do, who to see? You're trying to control my life. Don't you think I'm old enough?" Defensively the father said, "I only asked," and repeated his question. The son replied: "No, you said, 'Don't you think that you should see other girls?' and that means you're telling me to see other girls!"

In contrast, the mutual understanding of adolescent-adolescent, peer communication, seems a haven. This is especially true when that communication is largely ritualized and reassuring but is less so when one is trying to do something with words other than confirming and mirroring: asking for a date, seeking intimacy, or establishing control.

A second example of seizing control of language can be seen in semantics, as adolescents exercise their power to create new word meanings. Very young children take over the verbal labels already present in their world. Their task then in communicational exchanges with adults is to learn what a given label refers to (i.e., the extension of a term) and how that label is related to other labels (i.e., the intension of a term). In the beginning, there are many mismatches between children's terms and adults'. There is overextension when all women are called "mommy" and underextension when only daddy's shoes are "shoes" and all sorts of other incongruities. Gradually, though, children shape their categories and labels to match adults'.

Adolescents, however, turn this process on its head. They become the arbiters of a word's meaning (extension and intension). Only they know what things can be labeled "grody" or what is truly "awesome." They take over words and redefine them or create new words altogether. They invest an adjective such as "gross" with new meaning and then make it into a verb: "he grossed me out." These examples of new word use are validated by consensus of the adolescent peer group.

Other examples may arise in more personal dialogues. For example: A fourteen-year-old boy smarting under yet another refusal by his mother to bend the rules for him said: "God! There sure has been a lot of *stubbornization* around here lately!" Like Shapiro's example of the adolescent who described himself as "scarable," this example arises from an overgeneralization of the rules of productive derivational morphology that are not used by a group—or at least not yet. Unlike true neologisms, however, such examples are not fixed in their usage or truly idiosyncratic; rather, they are legitimate attempts in a dialogue with another to use the rules of language (of which adolescents are now aware) to express a feeling or idea.

There is a period of creativity in early language development when children make up words and delight in silly rhymes and games such as pig latin (Chukovsky 1968; Clark 1982). This brief early period of pleasure in the control over language becomes dormant only to reerupt in adolescence. Extending proper names to become class designators ("Joanies," "Debbies"), for example, is not common during that earlier period but will prove useful in adult communication: "He's a regular Benedict Arnold"; "Put your John Hancock right here"; and "Watergate" for any scandal.

With awareness of language as instrument and object comes an inarticulateness not found before. As in previous periods of increased awareness, confusion and seemingly poorer functioning are often the first response. For example: It is well known that young children who have mastered the individual past forms of verbs such as "he went" and "he talked" will regress to "he goed" in learning the general rules of past tense formation. The seeming regression is actually a hypothesis of a rule being worked out that will, once learned, be more efficient than mere memorization of individual forms. In the same way, a new awareness in adolescence can make teens less at ease with their language than before.

Adolescents may seem suddenly tongue-tied and inarticulate for other reasons. The strength of their emotions at this time cannot seem to find appropriate expression in their speech. They use many intensifiers as if words alone and unmodified could not possibly express the felt affect: "She's really mean"; "no, really"; "he's sooooo cute"; "to the max."

Sometimes words fail altogether. One adolescent told me: "I wish sometimes I could open my mouth and rock music could come out." Music seems to express emotions directly, harkening back to our earliest beginnings in language when in our first weeks of life it was the intonation patterns to which we attended. Intonation patterns carry the affect in language very directly and are therefore the first aspects of language used by infants in making attachments. Full use of all the functions of intonation (attitudinal, semantic, syntactic, pragmatic, social, and psychological) is not mastered until adulthood (Crystal 1979), but with plurifunction perhaps is lost some power of intonation to express its original function, affect.

The importance of music in the lives of adolescents can perhaps be tied to the importance of early intonation in the expression of affect states. Music also permits an instant group identity, much as accent and speech patterns do: "Are you into rock 'n' roll, country 'n' western, R and B, soul, jazz, punk, new wave, classical?" Professor Higgins noted that as soon as we open our mouths we let every one know who we are. By wearing a t-shirt emblazoned with a rock band insignia, one does not even have to open one's mouth.

Shapiro has given many intriguing examples of adolescent dress. As Roland Barthes (1967) has written, dress has its own codes, and if we were to do full justice to adolescent dress we would need to expand our discussion to the "semiotics" (i.e., all the sign systems) of adolescence: dress, language, and body language (kinesics, paralinguistics, proxemics). Surely romance of working-class garments and habits precedes the 1960s and has something to do with the rise of a leisure class. Recall that Marie Antoinette used the Petit Trianon to play dairymaid in special outfits. Work clothes or other outfits are not work clothes when they include a boundary or frame marker: an alligator insignia, designer label, artfully displayed holes on knees, or rump patches. The creation and manipulation of boundary or frame markers in adolescence are interesting in both the nonverbal and the verbal spheres. Clearly, a discussion of the total semiotics of adolescent culture would be a good topic.

Conclusions

When Shapiro describes "a mutual enterprise between therapist and patient, both of whom are engaged in a quest for meaning," he is defining discourse or dialogue. But when he speaks of "translations" or "transformations," we are misled. The psychoanalyst himself does not use a pure language into which the transformed adolescent language must be translated. Like any two participants in a dialogue, the analyst and the adolescent speak partially overlapping dialects, neither of which is ideologically free. The patient must also, to paraphrase Shapiro, decipher the values implied in the analyst's speech. The task in any dialogue is not to translate my jargon into yours or yours into mine but to create a new shared discourse between us that will be new to both of us and change us both.

If there are limitations to Shapiro's approach, they are the limitations of the linguistic theory he has used. American linguists since Chomsky are preoccupied with abstract, formal structures that represent the underlying competence of a lone, ideal speaker-hearer. The limitations of a psycholinguistics that relies on this kind of linguistics are profound: an ideal speaker-hearer has neither cultural nor individual history, no family, no unconscious or inner reality.

Jargon, derivational morphology, verbal games, and language functions can be very interesting and important, but what can they tell us about the speaking subject? Can they tell us with whom he identifies, whether he has individuated/separated? Lest you jump to the conclusion that they can, let me ask, Do we know the role that language plays in identification or in individuation-separation? Psychoanalysts use language (sometimes when they mean "speech") as a footprint that reveals or expresses the real, underlying subject. But what analysts should be focused on is that speech is constructive of the subject; it is through speech that the subject exists. As Shapiro is aware, Victor Rosen (1961/Shapiro 1979) liked to quote: *le style, c'est l'homme même*—"Style, it is the very man."

The speaking subject evolves in dialogues; French analysts and Soviet psychologists like to say, "language speaks the subject." If you did not believe this, why would you want to engage adolescents in a therapeutic dialogue? You must believe that it is through dialogue that they have become what they are and therefore through dialogue with you that they will change. So, as a psycholinguist I look not to my colleagues in American linguistics but to you psychiatrists and psychotherapists to teach me more about the speaking subject in adolescence.

Appendix

Following are examples of changes in language structure of children after the age of five, as reported by linguists, developmental psycholinguists, and psychologists.

1. On a syntactic level, complex verb patterns ("ask"/"tell"/"persuade") take considerable time to work out, as do sentence patterns where the psychological subject and the grammatical subject may differ (e.g., active vs. passive). Sentences that have been rearranged to highlight or focus some information and leave other information presupposed will also be more difficult for young children (e.g., front-shifted clauses and multiple embeddings).

2. After five, children continue to expand their vocabulary and learn how to use productive derivational rules to accomplish this (e.g., "erase" + "er" → "eraser"; "dirt" + "y" → "dirty"; "slow" + "ly" → "slowly"; "bird" + "house" → "birdhouse"). Up until five, these words are learned separately (Derwing and Baker 1979). In the same way, so-called double-function words are learned separately (e.g. "a bright light"/"a bright girl"; "give me a ring"). During later years, children learn that the physical senses, learned first, and the psychological senses are related (Asch and Nerlove 1960).

3. Full understanding of language that depends on underlying cognitive development that occurs in concrete or formal operational stages (eleven to fifteen years) will be mastered only during that period or later. Full understanding of relational terms may require an underlying ability to conserve (e.g., "it's shorter but wider"); and competent use of complex adverbial expressions such as "although," "because," "if . . . then," "nevertheless," "while," and "since" may involve mastery of underlying logical relationships between propositions. According to Piaget (1924), full use of these terms may depend on mastery of concepts such as causality having previously been worked out in actions on concrete materials (see Piaget and Inhelder 1969, pp. 130–155).

4. Children over eight years of age show increased metalinguistic awareness of language as an object itself. Younger children refer to the environment and extralinguistic factors to reduce ambiguities, for example, while older children increasingly look to intralinguistic cues. Older children understand that aspects of language can be plurifunctional, and they struggle to cope with all the complexities of the language system with which they have just become aware. Karmiloff-Smith (1979, p. 323) notes the changes in five- and eight-year-olds in what she calls "metaprocedural behaviour":

> In my view, the gradual passage from juxtaposed, unifunctional homonyms, to plurifunctional systems of relevant options for modulating meaning [see 2 above], may be a general feature of development of noun and verb phrase

after five years [see 1 above]. Related aspects of later language development were shown to include the tagging of general principles with rules for exceptions, the progressive passage from co-ordination to subordination [see 3 above], the gradual capacity to be economical in utterances, to avoid redundant marking, to gauge the communicative burden a morpheme can carry, to understand the presuppositional constraints conveyed by the use of various linguistic means such as intonation. A further characteristic of language development after five appears to be the gradual passage from extralinguistic to intralinguistic reference, both in spontaneous utterances and, later, in metalinguistic awareness. Five years does indeed seem to be a frontier age, representing the beginning of a new phase in language development. Another new phase appears to begin around the age of eight.

REFERENCES

Asch, S. E., and Nerlove, H. 1960. The development of double-function terms in children: an exploratory investigation. In B. Kaplan and S. Wapner, eds. *Perspectives in Psychological Theory: Essays in Honor of Heinz Werner*. New York: International Universities Press.

Austin, J. L. 1962. *How to Do Things with Words*. New York: Oxford University Press.

Barthes, R. 1967. *Systèmes de la mode: The Fashion System*. New York: Hill & Wang, 1983.

Bateson, G. 1972. *Steps to an Ecology of Mind*. New York: Ballantine.

Bloom, L. 1973. *One Word at a Time: The Use of Single-Word Utterances before Syntax*. The Hague: Mouton.

Bruner, J. 1978. Learning how to do things with words. In J. S. Bruner and A. Garton, eds. *Human Growth and Development*. Oxford: Clarendon.

Chomsky, C. 1969. *The Acquisition of Syntax in Children from 5 to 10*. Cambridge, Mass.: MIT Press.

Chukovsky, K. 1968. *From Two to Five*. Berkeley: University of California Press.

Clark, E. V. 1982. The young word maker: a case study of innovation in the child's lexicon. In E. Wanner and L. Gleitman, eds. *Language Acquisition: The State of the Art*. New York: Cambridge University Press.

Crystal, D. 1979. Prosodic development. In P. Fletcher and M. Garman, eds. *Language Acquisition*. New York: Cambridge University Press.

Derwing, B. L., and Baker, W. J. 1979. Recent research on the acquisition of English morphology. In P. Fletcher and M. Garman, eds.

Language Acquisition. New York: Cambridge University Press.

Dundes, A.; Leach, J. W.; and Özkök, B. 1972. The strategy of Turkish boys verbal dueling rhymes. In J. Gumperz and D. Hymes, eds. *Directions in Sociolinguistics: The Ethnography of Communication*. New York: Holt, Rinehart & Winston.

Feldman, C. F. 1977. Two functions of language. *Harvard Educational Review* 47(3):282–293.

Goffman, E. 1974. *Frame Analysis: A Framework for the Study of Language and Communication*. New York: Wiley.

Hale, K. 1971. A note on a Walbiri tradition of antonymy. In D. D. Steinberg and L. A. Jakobovits, eds. *Semantics: An Interdisciplinary Reader in Philosophy, Linguistics, and Psychology*. London: Cambridge University Press.

Halliday, M. 1973. *Explorations in the Functions of Language*. London: Edward Arnold.

Inhelder, B., and Piaget, J. 1955. *The Growth of Logical Thinking: From Childhood to Adolescence*. New York: Basic, 1958.

Jakobson, R. 1960. Linguistics and poetics. In T. A. Sebeok, ed. *Style in Language*. Cambridge, Mass.: MIT Press.

Joos, M. 1962. *The Five Clocks*. Bloomington: Indiana University Research Center in Anthropology, Folklore and Linguistics.

Karmiloff-Smith, A. 1979. Language development after five. In P. Fletcher and M. Garman, eds. *Language Acquisition*. New York: Cambridge University Press.

Kochman, T. (ed.) 1972. *Rappin' and Stylin' Out: Communication in Urban Black America*. Champaign: University of Illinois Press.

Labov, W. 1973. *Language in the Inner City: Studies in the Black English Vernacular*. Philadelphia: University of Pennsylvania Press.

Leech, G. 1974. *Semantics*. Harmondsworth: Penguin.

Lieberman, P. 1967. *Intonation, Perception and Language*. Cambridge, Mass.: MIT Press.

Litowitz, B. 1981. Hypothetical speech. *Journal of Psycholinguistic Research* 10(3):289–312.

McNeill, D. 1970. *The Acquisiton of Language*. New York: Harper & Row.

Mitchell-Kernan, C. 1972. Signifying and marking: two Afro-American speech acts. In J. Gumperz and D. Hymes, eds. *Directions in Sociolinguistics: The Ethnography of Communication*. New York: Holt, Rinehart & Winston.

Morris, D. 1967. *The Naked Ape*. London: Cape.

Nelson, K. 1975. Individual differences in early semantic and syntactic development. In D. Aaronson and R. W. Rieber, eds. *Developmental Psycholinguistics and Communicative Disorders. Annals of the New York Academy of Sciences,* vol. 263. New York: New York Academy of Sciences.

Piaget, J. 1924. *Judgement and Reasoning in the Child.* Totowa, N.J.: Littlefield & Adams. 1959.

Piaget, J., and Inhelder, B., 1969. *The Psychology of the Child.* New York: Basic.

Rommetveit, R. 1974. *On Message Structure: A Framework for the Study of Language and Communication.* New York: Wiley.

Rosen, V. H. 1961. The relevance of "style" to certain aspects of defense and the synthetic function of the ego. *International Journal of Psycho-Analysis* 42:447–457.

Sach, J. 1975. Cues to the identification of sex in children's speech. In B. Thorne and N. Henley, eds. *Language and Sex: Difference and Dominance.* Rowley, Mass.: Newbury House.

Sach, J.; Lieberman, P.; and Erickson, D. 1973. Anatomical and cultural determinants of male and female speech. In R. W. Shuy and R. W. Fasold, eds. *Language Attitudes: Current Trends and Prospects.* Washington, D.C.: Georgetown University Press.

Searle, J. R. 1969. *Speech Acts: An Essay in the Philosophy of Language.* London: Cambridge University Press.

Searle, J. R. 1975. A taxonomy of illocutionary acts. In K. Gunderson, ed. *Language, Mind and Knowledge.* Minneapolis: University of Minnesota Press.

Shapiro, T. 1979. *Clinical Psycholinguistics.* New York: Plenum.

Thorne, B., and Henley, N., eds. 1975. *Language and Sex: Difference and Dominance.* Rowley, Mass.: Newbury House.

Tough, J. 1977. *The Development of Meaning: A Study of Children's Use of Language.* New York: Wiley.

Vygotsky, L. S. 1962. *Thought and Language.* Cambridge, Mass.: MIT Press.

Werner, H., and Kaplan, B. 1962. *Symbol Formation.* New York: Wiley.

22 SHORT-TERM DYNAMIC PSYCHOTHERAPY: ANOTHER KIND OF LEARNING ON CAMPUS

RITA L. LOVE AND HELEN A. WIDEN

In 1954, Fenichel wrote, "Brief psychotherapy is the child of bitter practical necessity." Until recently, most professionals involved in dynamic psychotherapy basically agreed. They believed that the depth, intensity, and effectiveness of therapy were irrevocably tied to a long-term commitment. For the last five years, however, the heart and soul of the Mental Health Service at Northwestern University have been the practice of short-term psychoanalytically oriented psychotherapy. Our theoretical bases incorporate classical ego psychology, object relations theory, and self psychology and are, to that extent, eclectic. Our techniques actively employ an appreciation of the importance of unconscious material, the past determinants of present behavior, and the inevitability that characteristic behaviors will be repeated or transferred into the therapeutic relationship.

We define what we offer rather flexibly as "a quarter or two" of treatment. Along with many college mental health workers, we find that this approach is well suited to the demand for service and the nature of the problems of an essentially young, bright, and capable population and to the exigencies of the academic calendar. Because we had all been traditionally trained to do long-term, intensive work, we tended to view our campus practice from that perspective and brought to it a doubtful and questioning attitude, including some resistance to the time limitations. These were openly shared and scrutinized during our weekly case conference. What has emerged during the last seven years is a rather remarkable growth in confidence in our effectiveness because we have been repeatedly surprised and gratified by our results. These results make us

0-226-24058-4/85/0012-0041$01.00

ask ourselves and each other, "What in the world are we doing, anyway?"

We find that there are certain aspects of the therapist's activity that become emphasized when it is necessary to deal with the fact that time limitations put pressure on both the patient and the therapist. Short-term practice is an intense and active experience. There are ways both to facilitate the process and also to mitigate the potentially negative or disruptive consequences of fast-moving treatment. What we rely on more heavily, we think, are statements that make explicit the fact that therapy is a learning experience and that it is characterized by a learning partnership and by the acquisition of new ways of looking at and learning about oneself and others. Many authors talk about the cognitive process which occurs in insight-oriented treatment (Alexander 1965; Basch 1980, 1981; Bellak and Small 1965; Marmor 1979). We would like to share some ideas about this emphasis with you, along with case examples.

Developmental Aspects of Learning

Learning theory is a useful vantage point from which to survey the therapeutic process, and it is particularly relevant in an educational setting. In addition to the normal transference of expectation and affect that takes place throughout life, whenever anyone finds himself in a position of dependence on another person, certain transferred aspects are highlighted whenever a student comes to us. College students declare a moratorium on assuming a consolidated character structure and independence in favor of greater scope and complexity in their development. Essentially, they contract for a prolonged adolescence and for periodic regression in which old certainties can be loosened to permit new learning. The entire college community is designed to support students during these—we call them "regressions in the service of the ego." They come ready to see us functioning as instructors, teachers, and the idealized mentors on whom all adolescents need to depend. Furthermore, they are a group which values and finds satisfaction and growth in using words and ideas for thinking, communicating, and self-awareness. The capacity for observation that is encouraged in scholarly research is compatible with an early therapeutic alliance based on developing the capacity for self-observation. Other general factors are that all students structure their learning in time-limited segments or courses which have a beginning, a middle, and an end, and that the college years are marked by transience. Our effectiveness is perhaps based in part on these preexisting factors.

The aim of both short- and long-term psychoanalytic therapy is to clarify through verbal interpretation the nature of the defense, the anxiety, and the affect or impulse in each of three sets of relationships (Malan 1976). These are, first, current relationships with significant others; second, figures from the past, usually parents and siblings; and third, the transference relationship. Most important, the aim is to connect or link these areas, thus building a "triangle of insight" (Menninger and Holzman 1973) and thereby exposing a predominant pattern in the patient's life. This aim, of course, is preceded by empathic work to establish a therapeutic alliance in which self-observation is actively encouraged. Simple phrases such as "Can we look at that?" or "Let's look at this so that we can learn something" can appeal to a person to proceed in spite of the pain which may be involved (Winokur, Messer, and Schacht 1981). Following are some other ways to encourage neutral self-observation in the opening phase, as illustrated by case vignettes.

Case Examples

It can be helpful to offer explanation of therapeutic techniques that actively contradict the patient's view of the therapist if that view could be disruptive. For example, a female medical student who early indicated that the therapist's silence at the beginning of the hour was experienced as rejecting was told that he waited in order to better be able to understand what is on the patient's mind. The feelings of rejection were dealt with later as transference.

One might explain the function of symptoms which are causing intense anxiety at the outset: a twenty-one-year-old young woman from abroad presented with the symptom of depersonalization of about three months' duration. By the time she consulted, she was terrified of losing control and was locked into an obsessive preoccupation with her symptom. At the end of the first session, she asked the therapist directly for education of sorts. The therapist spoke about her impression that the obsession was a symptom, that there were underlying conflicts, and that some difficult feelings were being warded off. They explored again the presenting themes of guilt and separation and her thoughts about staying here and going home. In response to her question about what to do when the terror struck again, it was suggested that she think about telling the therapist about it the next time they meet. She asked what else to do, and the therapist said that everyone has ways to help himself or herself feel better, and she should think about what hers have been in the past. She was seen for a total of nineteen sessions while they focused on the division within her and the disavowed rage at her mother that came through at about session twelve. She spent five days in the infirmary, and by the time she left therapy she was beginning to feel more healed and whole.

Self-observation can also be encouraged by commenting aloud on how the patient seems to be needing the therapist to function. An example: A graduate student presented because she could not write the paper to qualify for candidacy. She filled the sessions with witty and pungent social commentary. In the interest of the time limit the therapist had to cut short these luxurious digressions and to explicitly label as one of her functions and that of the therapy to help the patient maintain a focus.

In the opening phase, the authors further act to anticipate with patients that the same flight, avoidance, or acting out of which they complain in their lives will be brought into the treatment. This can help to circumvent disruptive and time-consuming maneuvers.

Another element in establishing an early alliance is that of engaging a student in active self-observation using the "triangle of insight." An early interpretation can further serve to decrease the passive feelings of helplessness which are so threatening to the emerging capacity for independence in this age-group.

A freshman woman (with a psychotherapist mother) presented with a sophisticated cognitive "summary"; she had been unloved as a child and was therefore unable to feel close to anyone, including a current male friend. She wanted to know about the therapist's qualifications and experience, to be sure that she was used to "serious" problems, rather than to "silly" students only, all the while speaking in a clowning manner; similarly, she spoke dramatically of "momentous" life events, while her affect minimized the words and she seemed to be laughing at herself. Relevant history included a parental divorce when she was eleven; she lived with a "phony" and cold mother until fifteen, left after a fight and moved in with father, who was charming but unreliable. Because of her sophistication, it was possible to make an early interpretation using the "triangle of insight"; the therapist pointed out that while she voiced a wish to be taken seriously, she skillfully tried to provoke laughter; it was reminiscent of her telling of a mother who trivialized her concerns and a father who disappointed her—both of which she was setting up in the therapy session. Perhaps this happened also with her boyfriend. She was quickly able to acknowledge and use this insight and apply it to other life situations with less acting out.

In the middle phase, because so much intense dysphoric affect is experienced and expressed in such a short time, the therapist needs to provide empathy and active support. One can do this with genuine and immediate impact by verbalizing what is ordinarily the assumed or "silent" part of the positive therapeutic process. For example, to an inhibited young man who was experiencing intense despair about his loneliness, it was pointed out that his dreams had been full of relationships between and among people. A comment was also made on the capacity he demonstrated to maintain the therapeutic relationship in spite of intense anxiety they had talked about. To an overwhelmed, depressed, and anxious foreign graduate student, the hope for mastery was pointed out in a dream where she conquered her fear of flying and took an airplane trip with her beloved sister. (The therapist chose to do this rather than to make a point of the transference link.)

Before making a transference confrontation or interpretation, the authors make a preface designed to deal with potential narcissistic injury. The preface may go something like this: Something very interesting is happening in here that indicates that your therapy is working just as it should. Up to now we have been talking about the problems in your life out there. Now, we can see that the very dilemma which we have been talking about is right here in the room where we can look at it and work on it together.

The following example from the middle of a case in supervision shows how articulating the here-and-now relationship in the therapy helps a chronically depressed and borderline female graduate student to risk some closeness in the session. Fearing annihilation, she uses anger and despair to distance herself from any human interaction, including the treatment relationship, and insists that "nothing can ever change for me." In the previous session she announced that she wanted to quit school, saying she could not handle it, and asked for help in planning her future. Instead, the therapist explored current difficulties and toward the end of the session suggested that quitting school was perhaps an avoidance of something else. She blurted out that she did not see what good therapy would do, that it would take too long, and that she would have to stop in June only to start all over with someone else. The therapist suggested that her wish to quit school was closely related to her fear of continuing in a treatment relationship. Her response of agreement confirmed the interpretation.

In the following session the patient began with the repetition of her hopelessness and insistence that things would not ever change for her. The therapist asked if she had reactions to the previous session. The patient stated she would never open up to the therapist because such efforts in the past only led to more hurt. She repeated her insistence that no one would ever care for her or protect her, although she desperately wants protection. The therapist shared her increasing urge to argue with the patient about the hopelessness, saying that this would only increase her despairing convictions. The patient responded by stating that the therapist could never understand the despair, softened, and then acknowledged having "opened up a little." The patient then stated that if she allowed the therapist to get any closer she would intrude on what little space the patient had left. After a pause, the following dialogue occurred:

P: What do you think?

T: We do have a relationship, you have been coming consistently, seem very concerned about it ending, and so here we are talking about termination. You express some fear that no one will protect you, and perhaps we can explore how you can use this relationship constructively in the time we have left. You might begin to consider how you can protect yourself in here, and your controlling the distance with me is a good example.

P: It's only one relationship. [Pause] If I did move closer, what would happen? What can I expect? No one has ever told me that.

T: From therapy?

P: Yes, what surprises?

T: You can expect that I will be here consistently for the time we have agreed upon, that there won't be any surprises in what I do, that I won't be much different than what you have already experienced.

P: I'm afraid you'll try and lead me somewhere.

T: I don't see my role as leading you anywhere.

P: I wouldn't go.

T: I know that. Rather, I see my role as attempting to stay with you as you explore your own experiences, to reflect on your struggles and help you gain some understanding that I hope will aid you to risk change.

P: Do you think I'm being melodramatic? Or is there something, some traumatic thing that happened to me?

T: I don't have in mind a single event, no, but I see your fear and pain as very real.

The patient left the session with an expression of appreciation and one month later began a session by stating, "In my last quarter here, I want to spend the three months we have left talking about our relationship."

In short-term therapy, termination is an issue from the start, and it is often a focal issue in the latter half. As such, it is particularly effective in dealing with bereavement and loss. Students very often present with issues of separation and loss—developmentally appropriate as they strive for change and independence. Earlier unresolved conflicts having to do with autonomy are frequently stirred up and worked out through the transference relationship, particularly around termination. In time-limited therapy, these issues become much more quickly joined and dealt with (Mann 1973; Podolnick, Pass, and Bybee 1979).

An attractive sophomore woman with bland affect came in late in spring quarter. The youngest and least successful of three children, her role was to be the "brilliant but lazy one." She acquiesced in her parents' decision that journalism was to be her career, but she was vaguely unhappy and performing indifferently. She was dreading being home for the summer and wondered how to deal with things in the therapist's absence; it was quickly pointed out that she had chosen to come in so late and that she was the one leaving. The therapist suggested that the issue was, in fact, her ambivalence about autonomy versus dependency, and that they could work together on that in the fall.

She returned in the fall and engaged in an examination of that issue, although she continually pressed for advice or opinions from the therapist while actually being able to move away from parental influence despite strong criticism and pressure. The therapist remained neutral as she changed careers, supporting her wish for autonomy and empathizing with her pain at relinquishing hopes for parental admiration of such independence. She was able to associate to earlier bizarre idealization of parents' excessive overprotection and identify with the therapist's confidence in her capacity for growth and change. She was able then to internalize that self-concept and mourn the loss of idealized parental images. She made some attempts to prolong the therapy, and this was interpreted, worked through, and used to facilitate the concept of mourning as being an appropriate and necessary reaction to loss.

In helping students overcome defenses against the sense of loss and disappointment at termination and with the limitations of the treatment, we first provide the most important support of all, which is the empathic acknowledgment of the patient's immediate distress. In addition to this, we often support hope by explanations that therapy may continue to be effective after the sessions come to an end. We may talk about the process of therapy as related to the process of growth or about the inevitability of experiences of loss and mourning. We sometimes articulate the possibility that what has been learned can be generalized to other situations, and that what happened during therapy can serve as a benchmark when the patient is faced with future problems.

Sometimes therapy ends with the expressed need to seek long-term treatment for the problems which have now become clarified. We point out that, through the insights gained and the feelings experienced, both pleasurable and painful, the patient has indeed changed; just as he has applied past experiences to learn to deal with his current life, so he will apply the therapeutic gains to his future life, including the pain of termination. He will find that this has now become part of him and is his to keep, making him able to become his own therapist in a sense. Just as we helped him to see himself as a continuous person in terms of his past, so we hope he adds the future dimension to his sense of continuity. In this way, the "triangle of insight" can be expanded into a "quadrangle of insight."

Conclusions

We have offered case examples from the opening phase, the middle phase, and the termination phase of short-term dynamic psychotherapy. These were chosen to demonstrate the kind of therapeutic intervention which occurs more often than in long-term treatment because both patient and therapist are pressured by time limitations. The therapist functions, in part, as an instructor by commenting on the observing and learning aspects of the process and by being ready, when necessary, to educate the patient about his emotional life and about therapy itself. These interventions seem to facilitate the formation of an alliance in the opening phase, to mitigate the potentially negative or disruptive effects of intense affect in the middle phase, and to help overcome defenses against the grief and disappointment that are often present in the termination phase. If these cognitive interventions are used too often, therapy can become a dry and sterile intellectual exercise, but it is a mistake to eschew them altogether. The judicious use of the instructive function is an important part of the art of short-term treatment.

REFERENCES

Alexander, F. 1965. Psychoanalytic contributions to short-term psychotherapy. In L. Wolberg, ed. *Short-Term Psychotherapy*. New York: Grune & Stratton.

Basch, M. F. 1980. *Doing Psychotherapy*. New York: Basic.

Basch, M. F. 1981. Psychoanalytic interpretation and cognitive transformation. *International Journal of Psycho-Analysis* 62:151–175.

Bellak, L., and Small, L. 1965. *Emergency Therapy and Brief Psychotherapy*. New York: Grune & Stratton.

Fenichel, D. 1954. *The Collected Papers of Otto Fenichel*. New York: Norton.

Malan, D. H. 1976. *The Frontier of Brief Psychotherapy*. New York: Plenum.

Mann, J. 1973. *Time-limited Psychotherapy*. Cambridge, Mass.: Harvard University Press.

Marmor, J. 1979. Short-term dynamic psychotherapy. *American Journal of Psychiatry* 136:149–155.

Menninger, K. A., and Holzman, P. S. 1973. *Theory of Psychoanalytic Technique*. New York: Basic.

Podolnick, E.; Pass, H.; and Bybee, D. 1979. A psychodynamic approach to brief therapy. *Journal of the American College Health Association* 28:109–113.

Winokur, M.; Messer, S. B.; and Schacht, T. 1981. Contributions to the theory and practice of short-term dynamic psychotherapy. *Bulletin of the Menninger Clinic* 45:125–142.

23 THE ANALYSIS OF AN ADOLESCENT BOY

ROBERT M. GALATZER-LEVY

The analytic case study is a tale with a moral. The moral of my tale is twofold: there are many analyzable adolescents, and the analyzable adolescent benefits greatly from analysis. The tale is worth telling because very few adolescents are offered the opportunity to have an analytic experience. I hope to persuade you to consider analysis seriously for adolescent patients.

Much psychoanalytic literature discourages analysis during adolescence. That literature contends that analytic work is incompatible with expectable adolescent development. On the basis of this view, otherwise analyzable patients are offered less intense treatment (Blos 1983; Harley 1974a; Kaplan 1982). Furthermore, even when analyses are undertaken, the prophecy that the adolescent's analysis will not develop along standard analytic lines tends to fulfill itself because the analyst introduces technical variations (Eissler 1953; Sandler, Kennedy, and Tyson 1975; Sklansky 1972). Much literature on adolescent analysis gives the impression that it is a horrendous undertaking: either a task of heroic proportions or one doomed to failure or limitation by external "reality" (e.g., Harley 1974b; Laufer 1981; Pearson 1968). The very first analysis reported, Freud's treatment of Dora, is an example of a failed analysis of an adolescent. Many later reports of adolescent analyses also involve incomplete and not entirely successful experiences. I think these case reports reflect a skewed population. They do not represent adolescents as a group but as a special, doubtful, or difficult to analyze population.

In this chapter I describe what might be called an "ordinary" analysis of an adolescent boy, that is, a case involving the successful treatment of a neurotic youngster by the standard methods of psychoanalysis. I il-

0-226-24058-4/85/0012-0007$01.00

lustrate why I recommended analysis; how the analytic process developed; how his principal modes of avoiding knowing about himself were identified and analyzed, leading to the emergence of his central difficulties within the analytic relationship; how these difficulties were worked through; and, finally, how we separated. Obviously, in the available space I can give only highlights of a complex process which lasted for three and a half years. However, I hope to demonstrate that such undertakings are worthwhile and valuable.

The Case of John

John was referred for a reactive depression precipitated by the parents' divorce. However, John, an attractive, not yet pubescent boy of fourteen, told me that, although the divorce distressed him, other things worried him more. For example, the divorce surprised him even though his parents had got along badly for years. What was wrong with him that he hadn't seen the obvious? Despite reassurance that puberty came late in his family, he was greatly concerned that his penis would always be too short for him to be a good lover. He also realized that for three years he had lost much of his enthusiasm and had lived in a state of dulled experience. The only area where he felt himself to be vigorous was baseball, in which he starred.

His depression had started at age eleven when he asked a girl out for the first time. He liked her, but she quickly lost interest. He tried with another girl, his sister's best friend, but his sister said her friend thought he was "too immature." That ended his attempts at dating. At the same time he lost enthusiasm for everything else. From a stellar pupil he became mediocre and unenthused in school. He gave up clay working, which he had enjoyed as a child. He ceased reading for pleasure. In sum, the boy described a pervasive neurotic inhibition which he had been unable to work on by himself for the past three years. The neurotic difficulties precluded his moving ahead in the developmental tasks of early adolescence. He was bright, articulate, curious about himself, and able to tolerate intense experience. I recommended analysis to him. (For a discussion of the developmental view of the indications for analysis, see A. Freud [1965].)

At first, John was ambivalent. He worried that the analysis might interfere with his athletics. Remarkably, by the time of our next meeting he was entirely agreeable to beginning. His mother wholeheartedly supported the idea, and he was certain the father would do likewise.

His certainty was misplaced. His father doubted that John needed intensive treatment. The father met with me in several increasingly acrimonious sessions, putting forward his very rational objections to the boy's analysis. John complained of passivity in his sessions. He felt unable to influence things as his father and I decided his fate. I wondered if John had unconsciously stimulated his father's resistance, if, rather than experience an internal struggle over the analysis, he had arranged for his father and me to represent the various sides of his conflict. To explore this idea, I asked John what he had done to ensure that his father would support the analysis. On reflection, he realized that he had never told his father of his distress. He allowed the father to believe that the mother's reports of his depression were merely the continuation of her almost hypochondriacal preoccupation with the children's mental health. John resolved to talk to his father that evening, but when he met with father he was unable to tell him how he felt and returned home in tears.

We were able to partially understand the sources of the inhibition in the defensive avoidance of the experience of internal conflict. John was able to talk with his father, who promptly and with consistency thereafter supported the analysis. More important, John and I had succeeded in understanding a convincing example of a major defense, externalization, which he was to employ and which we were to come to understand in great depth in the course of the analysis. By "externalization" I mean the experience that one's internal conflicts are not difficulties within oneself but, rather, are the result of a conflict with or between other people. Such a position is often supported by subtly arranging for the others to enact the role assigned to them, that is, to take up one side of the internal conflict.[1]

John began analysis at four times a week. Let me give you an idea of the opening phase of the analysis by describing some hours from that period of the analysis. While many themes, including fears of passivity and castration anxiety, are evident in this material, the major anxiety concerns the experience of regression as John became engaged in the analysis.

During the fourth analytic hour John said[2] he was much concerned with scheduling problems and that there seemed to be all sorts of difficulties in meshing his school and analytic hours. I said that beginning the analysis was hard. He described his pleasure in playing baseball, how athletic and muscular he feels, how he enjoys working up a sweat and batting the ball very hard even though he lacks control. It's one thing he's really good at. He glanced repeatedly at the couch.

ANALYST: You needn't hesitate to interrupt yourself if something comes to mind.

JOHN: I'm thinking about the couch. I'd be uncomfortable on it. I'd feel terribly exposed. I like to sleep on my stomach or my side. The back is a kind of protection. There is little chance of being seriously injured if you are hit on the back and it doesn't hurt that much besides. If you're hit on the abdomen there are all kinds of vulnerable organs which might be damaged.

ANALYST: Sounds like you're anticipating some sort of assault on the couch.

JOHN: No, don't be silly. It's just what came to mind was about being hit and how I guess when I am in bed alone the thought must come up about being hit in some ways. But you know these things are all quite realistic.

The next day John was thirty minutes late.

JOHN: There was an accident on the train. I was sitting in the train which was stopped past the accident and that's why I'm late. I hated the conductor. He was so indifferent. He didn't seem to care what was happening. I sort of watched all the people and I observed who responded by getting impatient with the delay and got angrier and angrier at how poorly designed the station was and that the crowding on the station must have caused many people to be injured. It must have been some old men who didn't clear the track properly who were responsible for the accident. It's typical of the sort of indifferent, don't care attitude. I hate riding the train. I feel so passive when I do it. There's nothing I can do to alter things. I just have to sit there. If I were an adult I would be able to do things better. I wouldn't have to put up with whatever happened to me.

ANALYST: It sounds again like you're talking about some kind of danger.

JOHN: Yes, the most frightening thing would be to be in some kind of danger and not be able to do anything about it.

On the next day he began talking about how his grandmother bugs him as she rattles on and on.

JOHN: I'm sick of her guilt-tripping me and everybody else. My mother and sister both say they'll try to do something about it, and my father says he'll talk to her directly, but he's done that many times without any effect. My sister says that we should just leave the old lady alone and wait, but that kind of passivity just makes me furious. After all, the old bitch is going to live for a long time.

ANALYST: I think it's worth noticing your urgency about doing something direct and, in particular, how awful it is for you to be passive in this situation here—which may be why your grandmother bugs you so much at this moment.

JOHN: Yeah, I wonder why. She's been the same dreadful person for sixty-five years and I've known her for fourteen of them, but today I felt just like I absolutely had to do something about her. I can't stand to let it ride right now for some reason.

The next day he continued about grandmother for some time.

JOHN: My mother doesn't support an active approach with grandmother, but I think it absolutely essential to do that.

ANALYST: I wonder if it isn't difficult to be direct in the analysis.

He thought of a band director who banished him from the band for a day for fooling around and how he was "grossed out" by the band director's sweating.

ANALYST: You're evaluating your performance and mine and trying to decide if you're misbehaving.

JOHN: I am concerned about my performance. How well I'm doing. It comes to mind as images of buildings. Perhaps what I really feel badly about is that I haven't started using the couch yet. You know, I decided before I came in here that I would start using the couch today, and I was going to walk in and simply lie down, but when I started to move toward the couch I felt afraid, I thought about how I would look lying there, what would happen if I was lying there and I got an erection. You must think that this is pretty silly after a while. Do you mind if I actually try using the couch?

ANALYST: No, not at all. But I think we should notice that it may be less frightening to actually go ahead and use the couch than to talk about what you fear happening if you do.

> JOHN: Well, in any case, I'll try it. After all, I can talk about it after I'm there. [He lay down on the couch and was silent for a few minutes.] Your head sort of sinks down into the pillow. It feels almost like it would be hard to get up again. Are most people as worried as I am about using the couch? You know, it felt like a real act of bravery to walk over here and lie down, but now it doesn't feel like such a big deal. It's kind of funny not to see you. Maybe they invented this so that you could pick your nose while you listen to patients. I feel like asking you again what I should talk about, but you will probably remind me to sort of look around and notice what came to mind. I wonder why I didn't lie down before. You know, I knew all along that I would. There's something kind of scary about it. You don't talk to anyone else but a psychoanalyst lying down.

A few weeks later John reported the following experience during the first analytic hour of the week. He had complained of feeling "groggy" and mildly confused following several previous analytic hours.

> JOHN: The weirdest thing happened to me on Thursday [the last hour of the previous week]. I got on the wrong train after I left the session and it turned out to be an express that went way north. I got real upset as it went through my home stop and I stood in the corridor where you get off the train. Suddenly I was absolutely furious and I kicked the door several times. It was very, very cold and the train just kept going and suddenly I noticed that the whole thing was made out of steel and that the steel was hard and cold and I thought about how if I asked the conductor to let me off he wouldn't do anything—he'd say something like "Sorry, son, but this train just keeps going and it follows its own route." The more I thought about it the angrier I got and I actually kicked the door several times. And then I thought, what if I don't have enough money to get the train going back, what happens then? I had the thought that I would get off in a fancy suburb. Then we rode past the street where there had been an amusement park where I had gone when I was a little kid and I remembered how nice it was, but now looking at it from the train it didn't seem nice at all. The neighborhood had deteriorated a lot in the last several years. And then I thought more about being in the suburb and I thought about going up to the door of some rich man's house, someone whom I knew, or maybe my father knew, and knocking on the door and

he would take me in and wait till I was warmed up and then he would give me money to go back home on the train, and all I'd feel was a little bit stupid for having acted that way. You know, I think getting on the wrong train was partly the result of that groggy feeling I was talking about here on Thursday.

I agreed.

JOHN: What comes to mind is the idea of going up to a rich man's door. You gave me the bill last Wednesday and I suddenly realized that you must make a lot of money. For some reason I don't think you live in the city, but you're much too cool to live in some place like Glencoe [a Chicago suburb]. I know what! You probably live in Evanston, or something like that, and you have a big house there.

ANALYST: The man in your fantasy had a big house in the suburb.

JOHN: What comes to mind about riding the train is some of the stuff I talked about last week about how passive I feel, about how I can't do anything about it. [Laughs] Do you know the expression "to be taken for a ride"? Sort of like being tricked into something. The worst part of the whole thing was how very alone I felt on the train and how cold everything felt and hard and like metal. It was really awful. And I thought about how I could be left out in the cold forever.

ANALYST: Maybe last week you began to feel sort of at home here, like it was a comfortable, safe place, and then with the end of the week you felt thrown out into a hard, cold world, and maybe even felt at the same time that I might help you and be kind like the man in the suburb. I also made it into a hard cold world by indifferently throwing you out of here.

JOHN: I think that's right. After I left here I had the thought, "What if I became really confused and upset, would he see me on the weekend, could I call him?" I really get very depressed sometimes. I don't like talking about it but there are times when I feel like crying all the time, and I can imagine I would call you up and I'd get your answering service or an answering machine and it would say something like "The doctor is busy. You can call him on Monday to make an appointment," and I'd be left all alone and by myself. Do you ever get bored with being an analyst?"

ANALYST: Maybe you ask that now because you're afraid that if you just begin to tell me about yourself and what's bothering you that you anticipate that I'll somehow lose interest in you before you have time to do what's necessary here.

JOHN: Oh, no, that doesn't bother me because you make so much money doing this that you'd listen to me no matter what. Father is always talking about his annoying colleagues. He is extremely good with people and he keeps them happy by kowtowing to them. He answers their phone calls in the middle of the night or over the weekends and everyone says how wonderful he is. Psychoanalysis is different though, I guess, because you can talk about that if it goes on. My father never talks about them making him angry, but sometimes he talks about how they make him tired. What would you do if I really got nasty to you? What would you do if I started making anti-Semitic remarks in here? Would you start thinking I was a Nazi because I'm blond and blue-eyed and hated Jews?

ANALYST: We'll see.

Interpretative efforts during this opening phase of the analysis were directed at understanding the anxiety associated with regression and especially with resistance to awareness of the transference. Such interpretations, along with John's experimentation about the limits of what he could say, resulted in a tolerable regression within the analysis.

With the arrival of the baseball season, John discovered that, contrary to his expectation, it was easily possible to both play baseball and be in analysis but insisted this was just a happy coincidence. He talked about how the analytic hours interfered with games and practice. When I said that he viewed analysis as interfering with his athletic prowess, he responded with a particularly intense set of rational statements and insistences on external reality. I was then surprised—John readily agreed with my interpretation. This was the first example of a character defense that John named "admit and go on" in which he agreed with an interpretation only to put it aside and avoid any further discussion of the idea.

There were many indications of the development of an intense transference. There were many less dramatic episodes similar to the one involving the train and a reluctance to speak of masturbation as masturbation was equated with homosexuality. The first manifestation of conscious irrational feelings toward the analyst took the form of "joking" remarks that Jews were weak, asexual, and always trying to curry favor with others. John soon understood that these depreciating remarks reflected his own worries about my responses to him. He feared I would be contemptuous of him for a variety of reasons. He was sexually immature, he was dependent on me, and I played a central role in his life, while he was only a small part of mine.

During the fourth month of the analysis, he reported many physical changes of puberty including a quite incredible growth spurt. He was defensive and quickly joked that the analysis was amazingly powerful.

With increasing sexual tension the theme of masturbation reemerged. John fantasied that the analyst had "made him a man," and his own impulses combined in ideas of being phallicly attacked. He shamefully remembered at age four masturbating by rubbing his sister's dolls between his legs. The activity combined the ideas of engaging in sexual activity with the dolls and of being given a gigantic penis by the sister.

Anticipating the first long break in the analysis, John was glad. Not having analytic hours would make him more like other guys. But he feared I might not return from my vacation. When, earlier in the analysis, I canceled a session, he fantasized that I had died. At the end of the analytic week, he often had similar feelings though of lesser intensity. He now recalled his grandmother's death and how, under the guise of not requiring him to be hypocritical, his parents discouraged his mourning. The memories led in turn to recollections of the death, when he was age five, of a housekeeper who had been one of his major caretakers.

On my return from my vacation, his feeling toward me continued to intensify. At the same time there was marked symptomatic improvement outside the analysis. John behaved more directly and aggressively with his parents and began to enjoy school and friendships. The analysis and the analyst had become central to his life and the focus of his symptomatology. His conflicts and neurosis centered on the person of the analyst. In other words, he had developed a transference neurosis.

John's conflicts about masturbation came sharply into the transference. Any reference by me to masturbation was understood as a recommendation that he masturbate. I first interpreted this idea as another example of his externalizing an internal conflict—he attributed to me his own erotic impulses and was aware only of his counterwishes—thus avoiding the experience of internal conflict. The interpretation reminded him of his sister's ongoing seductive behavior. For example, one day she brought him a copy of *Playboy* to read while he was taking a bath. He realized that he also used her behavior to represent one side of his conflicted wishes. He masturbated after his sister gave him the magazine, thinking it was her fault, not his. This led in turn to recollections of how, when he was three, his sister had encouraged him to exhibit his penis to her and a friend. He recalled, with affect, how at that time rather than express exhibitionistic wishes of his own, he felt instead the despised object of seduction and shame about his passivity.

John repeatedly returned to the idea that I wanted to control his genitals. I was old and wanted John's virility—my own penis now being inadequate. However, many of John's associations suggested I was not seen as an emasculated man but, rather, as a woman, the mother and sister who desired to have penises of their own.[3] John's protection against such malignant control was neither to masturbate nor to engage in other erotic activity. If he had no penis no one would take it away from him. The fantasy had clear anal aspects: he spoke of the amount of ejaculate and of the masses of free association that he produced. His masses of clever thoughts were to be admired but were also "just shit."

The idea that I wanted John to make up for missing aspects of myself took many forms. He thought that my interest in his studies reflected a wish to pursue academic disciplines vicariously through him. I wanted him to become involved with women so that I would vicariously enjoy the experience. It was possible to demonstrate repeatedly that these ideas represented fantasies transferred from his childhood experience of his mother and sister—of having his own instinctual wishes, both sexual and anal, be under their control and exist for their needs.

Let me describe an hour from this period in the analysis to give you a sense of what I mean.

> JOHN [beginning]: I feel sleepy and hungry. The last baseball game of the season was yesterday. There was lots of cheering but the game was disappointing. There are no dreams or anything. The night before I had a distinct dream but I don't remember it. Something about being worried about getting here. It can't be that important if I don't remember it.
>
> ANALYST: It's almost like you were saying our work here doesn't feel that important right now.
>
> JOHN: Maybe. Oh, the dream's coming back. You know, I thought with the end of the baseball season the analysis would once more become important. I'm working at a hospital this summer and the dream is that I was riding a bike between the hospital and here. I was fifteen minutes late and I had to leave there fifteen minutes early.

You complained so I kept the bike at the station, but that didn't work either—I had to padlock the bike and that didn't work out. There's a show at school that my sister put a lot of work into, but there's nothing left now. We have new bleachers. They're the old bleachers from another private school. They're secondhand. My right wrist hurts. Maybe I sprained it. My hand gets very sweaty when I pitch. My right hand sweats too much. I masturbated last night. I watched my penis become erect like a balloon. That's an inexact meaning. I was planning to do it, but I forgot. An image of Cupid shooting arrows, killing you, hitting you in the dick and you become impotent. If I masturbate too much, will I become narcissistic?

ANALYST: It sounds like your "narcissism" could lead to a lot of violence between us.

JOHN: A fairy tale comes to mind of a narcissistic woman who is made to fall in love with a man. A shabby middle-aged, I mean Middle Ages, peasant.

ANALYST: What do you think about the slip?

JOHN: He did actually have a beard [the analyst is bearded]. It was a cartoon, I saw. There were silver arrows shooting from the parapet.

John elaborately described the film.

ANALYST: You get away from feeling intensely.

JOHN: I'm thinking about girls, but something is stopping me.

ANALYST: Something you're afraid of.

JOHN: When I think about girls I get a better erection. I don't know why I think of this, but I think of the Pillsbury Doughman. I used to have fantasies about the Pillsbury Doughman and cutting off various parts of him. I'd cut off his head and throw it across the room. On "Saturday Night Live" there was a Jewish man who was talking about fancy food like his mother used to make. I have some fudge from grandmother. A very funny thought—a gigantic Pillsbury Doughman. I was thinking of something else but I forget it now. Think of how my grandmother made my father femalish, like the Pillsbury Doughboy. An image of how, in the commercial, they tickle him and make him laugh, but instead an idea of sticking a finger through him and him screaming in pain . . . blood all over the flour. My sister and I made cupcakes yesterday and followed a yellow-cake recipe, but we used peanut oil as shortening. They tasted absolutely awful. I resolved today to get a can of corn oil on my way to school. It's your fault that I'm thinking all these things about masturbation and corn oil.

ANALYST: How are they connected?

JOHN: You could use corn oil as a lubricant like vaseline for trying to screw.

He gives an elaborate discussion of how vaseline is made from petroleum.

ANALYST: Something frightened you away from the thoughts of corn oil as a lubricant.

JOHN: The term corn hole—for anal intercourse—comes to mind. But my abdomen is very firm. Besides the anus is in the rear. The Cubs played very well yesterday. My mother becomes skittish around her boyfriend. She can't remember phone numbers. I seem to be jumping from one thing to another.

ANALYST: Maybe what we're talking about makes you jumpy.

JOHN: But, but, but! [Laughs] That too could be a reference to anal intercourse, couldn't it? But it wasn't I who brought it up, it was a response to your interpretation. I feel like arguing with you. Like you attribute all sorts of things to me. My mother always does that. She is always making interpretations and I immediately defend myself. Yesterday that happened and she pointed out that she hadn't said anything, and indeed she hadn't.

We had many occasions to examine John's identifications with his father. Certain of these identifications had been obvious from the first—for example, John's professorial logic. Others emerged gradually. Both father and son employed sarcastic humor and disavowed the affective significance of experience by rapidly putting the experiences in intellectual terms. Yet these intellectualizing obsessional defenses had other important origins in John besides identification with his father.

John became ever more preoccupied with the volume of his ejaculate. This preoccupation became a focal point which led to the clarification of the obsessional defenses which involved both compliance and avoidance of compliance. When the anal quality of this interest was pointed out, John revealed a continuing mild symptom of constipation which was followed by copious and proudly produced stools. He was particularly pleased that on occasion he clogged toilets with his feces. In the transference John worried whether he masturbated properly and whether he produced enough associations. I told him he saw me as like a mother preoccupied with the question of whether he had produced enough stool and in the right place and at the right time. I said further that he expected me to take away his pleasure both in the actual physical experience and in his capacity to decide what he did for himself. This reconstruction of John's toilet training led to the affective recall of several occasions when he withheld feces as an expression of intense rage, particularly at his mother. A particularly convincing reconstruction concerned the patient's being given an enema which both interfered with his sense of autonomy and supported the fantasy of the phallic woman who dominated and controlled men.

Not only were women seen as owning and controlling John's bowels and genitals, but his father was seen as too weak to interfere. His father, like John, had a powerful mother who denigrated her own husband and constantly demanded that her son perform for her. John was humiliated that his middle-aged father was unable to stand up to either his ex-wife or to his mother.

As these ideas were worked over, another role for his father gradually emerged. His father's protective and benign functions were recalled and father's humor valued. John recalled how, in contrast to mother's wish to give him an enema, his father had suggested that his constipation might respond to coffee—a suggestion which combined a calmer view, less urgency about controlling the child, and an image of John as being a grown-up, not a passive infant.

These themes came into the analysis proper. In addition to the central maternal transference, a secondary important transference centered around the idea of the analyst as a benign, helpful figure who was not to be feared and with whom the relationship was free of anxiety. However, in this image the analyst (father) was weak and ineffective.

The actualities that father was enormously successful professionally and that the analyst was also doing well in the world led John to the realization that these views must be defensive against the image of the powerful and dangerous analyst-father. John gradually also discovered that the image of the phallic castrating mother, as important as it was in its own right, was also used defensively against anxieties about damage at father's hand.

Here are two hours from relatively late in the analysis which illustrate the interdigitation of these themes:

JOHN: My philosophy paper is due tomorrow and I haven't done any of it. I want it to be brilliant but I can't seem to get it out. Something blocks me. I worked on it for a while at the library. I hate studying at the library but my roommate plays the record player so loud I can't study in my room. Some thought about hairy Jews—his girlfriend is supposed to come visit at the end of the month—he has a great hi-fi set but he plays it loud all the time. You're sitting there saying "Oh, the poor stupid WASP kid can't even write his paper." My stepfather keeps talking about my mother as his "shickse." He's such an asshole. We were watching the football game and he never pays attention and then he says "What happened, what happened?" so I have to tell him—he never lets me alone.

ANALYST: You've often complained that I don't leave you alone.

JOHN: Yeah, but you are not an asshole like he is. Sometimes I really want to punch him. He never shuts up. Now he thinks he's a writer—he wants to write his autobiography—it should be real easy for him all he does is talk about himself anyway—he could just tape-record one of his dinner conversations and put it out on the market as "The Autobiography of the Great, Wonderful, and Profound Mr. ———." He calls his talking oral diarrhea but he's right, it really is shit.

ANALYST: Has he done anything in particular to make you so mad at him lately?

JOHN: No, not really. In fact, I haven't seen him for almost two weeks. But you're right, for some reason I'm going on and on about him today. I really don't know why.

ANALYST: I wonder if you don't feel ashamed about not finishing the paper and sort of cover your shame with an angry attack on your stepfather.

JOHN: I feel stupid about the paper. I've had two weeks to do it and I just can't seem to get to it. I keep going to movies and stuff instead of working on it. Maybe it's because of the homosexual theme in the book. It's supposed to be an example of Socratic method. Socrates teaches the boy the Pythagorean theorem. But all the boy ever says is "Yes, O Socrates." That's what I'll say to you after it's all over. "Yes, O Socrates." And then they go off and fuck under a tree. Maybe I should write an autobiography. "And then G-L taught me how to masturbate and I did it punctually at 7:32 P.M. each day."

You know, I really enjoy masturbating, but I still really sometimes think, "Oh, Dr. Levy would approve of this" or "What a good analytic patient I am for masturbating."

ANALYST: Like somehow the analytic work we've done makes it mine rather than yours.

JOHN: Yeah.

ANALYST: Do you think the same might apply to the paper?

JOHN: Maybe. You're the big intellectual who thinks this stuff is so important. When I told you I was taking the course you said "neat." And you do have an academic title.

The next day he began by reporting what he said was a straightforward dream.

JOHN: I was having intercourse with this girl in my philosophy class and it felt great—and then I came a huge amount. It wasn't really a wet dream.

ANALYST: What came to mind?

JOHN: A profound insight—the patient would like to fuck a girl—did you get that down?

ANALYST: You're mad at me.

JOHN: Sometimes this is so stupid. A seventeen-year-old kid comes in and says he has a dream about screwing some girl and you try to pull all kinds of meanings out of him. "What comes to mind?" "Shit comes to mind." I didn't get the paper done but I got a week's extension on it. I just couldn't get it out last night. All your brilliant interpretations didn't help a lot either. You're sitting there shaking your head and thinking "oy vey, I'm losing my power as an analyst—how will I support my wife and children—my interpretations don't work—oy vey, oy vey."

ANALYST: As we've seen many times before, you're saying jokingly what you mean quite seriously. Perhaps a motive for not producing the paper is precisely to show I can't force you to produce nor am I so powerful as I claim.

John experienced further improvements in his life outside analysis. He became comfortably aggressive, so that, for example, his baseball game, previously characterized largely by much trickery, became clearly aggressive, more straightforward, and more effective. For the first time since his eleventh year he was enthusiastic about academic work.

With these improvements, John considered leaving analysis at the end of his senior year of high school. To go away to school would be a good step in separating from his mother. This wish for a premature termination was not only a resistance to the continued unfolding of the transference. It also involved his father's wish. As long as John could remember, his father had hoped that he would develop by attending the right college. John shared his father's fantasy that athletic success would make him bold in other ways, though not with much conviction.

Externalization was again the major defense. The patient experienced the conflict between whether to attend college away from home or to remain in analysis as if it were between his father and me. As this defense was again analyzed, the patient's own motives could be examined. Gradually, John's wish to comply with his father's idea was recognized as an attempt to withdraw from a competition with both father and analyst. Though John had many natural athletic abilities, his greatest talents were intellectual. He came to realize that competition in the athletic sphere was safe precisely because it avoided this area of his greatest talent. John avoided reading in psychoanalysis with the conscious intent of not giving himself ammunition for his intellectualizations. At the same time he avoided competing intellectually with me. As this inhibition was analyzed, John discovered an intense interest in history and literature, as well as psychology and psychoanalytic ideas. He decided to attend a local university known for its intellectual rigor. To have interrupted the analysis at the end of high school would have served many purposes—almost all of which would have avoided competition with father and me. He would both have had an incomplete analysis and would have attended an intellectually inferior school. It is perhaps worth mentioning that, although the patient remained in geographical proximity to his parents, this, of course did not interfere with the psychological processes involved in separating from them but, on the contrary, clarified those processes.[4]

By the middle of his first year of college, John was increasingly enjoying his peers. Real friendships with other boys emerged. He enjoyed athletics and took pleasure in the vigorous competition and exhibitionism made possible by his ever-increasing athletic ability. He began dating. His masturbation fantasies involved a combination of affection and sensuous feeling toward the women he met, along with phallic exhibitionistic ideas. The continued role of a regressive position was evident in a masturbatory technique he sometimes employed in which he would rub his penis and testicles in a continuous smooth motion, often delaying orgasm for extended periods—all of which was reminiscent of his early childhood masturbation by rubbing the doll between his legs, the anal themes which had been so prominent earlier in the analysis, and feminine identification.

By the end of his freshman year in college, John and I seriously considered termination. I shall try to give an idea where we stood by describing the two hours when we agreed to finish up.

JOHN: Well, I got my grades—two A's and two B's. I guess I did better on the chemistry test than I thought. Everyone will say I didn't do as well as my sister, and that is true. This semester she got three A's and a B, but last year, when she was a freshman, she really screwed up royally. You're sitting there thinking, "The boy won't get into medical school with a B in chemistry." Well, in the first place, maybe I will, and in the second place, I don't want to go to medical school, and in the third place, thinking about it is really part of the same competitive business we've been talking about, and in the fourth place, I know it. [I laugh] And in the fifth place, I enjoy it. You know, the funny part of it is that that theory is all wrong. Men don't want to cut off their sons' dicks. Men like me better when I'm competitive and not so wimpy. Mom's husband, and Dad, and you, all seem to enjoy me more, and I certainly enjoy me more.

You know, maybe doing so well this semester gives me some confidence, but I think maybe it's time for us to stop. I still like coming here a lot but it doesn't seem like the most important thing in the world. I was thinking how it would interfere with the baseball season again this year, and I remembered how when I started the analysis I'd used the baseball season as a resistance to beginning the analysis, and I wondered if I was doing the same thing again, but I don't think so. You know, if anyone objectively looked at my life they would have said the most important thing was therapy, and now that's not so, I don't think. Maybe I should stay in treatment 'til I screw a girl, then we'd know I was cured—but of course we'd know nothing of the kind. What do you think?

ANALYST: Well, we've accomplished a whole lot together and we've largely succeeded in dealing with the things that brought you here—the depression and the inhibitions, and you seem now to be vigorously enjoying your life. It's worth talking seriously about termination.

JOHN: You know, every time you discuss the analysis you leave out one important reason I got into analysis—I was curious about myself. You know I probably would have done okay without the analysis—at least to the outside—but I wouldn't know about myself the way I do. It's weird to be lecturing your own analyst about that—I imagine Sigmund Freud shaking his head.

In the next hour there was a dream:

JOHN: There was this funny little animal in the road and I sort of teased it and it got angry and sort of bristled at me. Any good Freudian knows that the animal is my penis and bristling is getting an erection.

ANALYST: Sounds like you're the one who's angry.

JOHN: You sounded so satisfied and smug when you said you thought we could stop. I agree, but you kept referring to what "we" did and I thought you were carefully choosing your words. "Let the kid think I respect him." Maybe the little animal is a guinea pig. Whenever you referred to the controversy about adolescent analysis, I thought—"Oh, maybe I'm being used as a guinea pig." Why is there such a controversy? This analysis certainly has gone well. I hate to say this, it's stupid that it's so embarrassing, but the thought I had was that you're a very good analyst and maybe some analysts would find it harder to do. And then I think maybe you'll be embarrassed if I talk like this. How do you thank an analyst anyway—can you hug your analyst on the last day of the analysis? The animal in the dream was sure angry.

ANALYST: Maybe when you're thinking of leaving it's easier to feel the anger than to recognize your tenderness and gratitude toward me.

JOHN: Yeah, it is easier. You know the animal in the dream was arching its back—it had its back up—remember that thing with the train at the beginning of the analysis. I somehow feel like since I decided to stop here like I'm backing up—all of a sudden I feel way back there.

With the setting of a termination date for nine months later, a variety of topics emerged with intensity. It was repeatedly understood that whatever other meanings it had, the termination was partly a resistance to further analytic exploration. The patient was concerned that the analysis was incomplete and that, in particular, he would be left with residual symptoms. He was particularly concerned that he had as yet not had intercourse and that he might leave the analysis prematurely, remaining sexually inhibited. A new edition of the idea that the analyst, not the patient, wanted the patient to masturbate, appeared in the idea that now the analyst wanted the patient to have intercourse. John imagined himself compliantly having intercourse not from his desires but to please me and demonstrate his readiness to terminate.

For the first time manifestly homosexual fantasies appeared. For example, the patient became interested in his Jewish roommate's sexual activities and the size of his roommate's genitals. He was curious about what it was like to perform fellatio and concerned that a girl might choke on a penis. These ideas were understood in terms of the patient's wish and fear of incorporating the analyst, a wish stimulated by the anticipated loss at the end of the analysis.

Partly defensively against these homoerotic feelings, partly as a result of further working through of vagina dentata fantasies in the context of the patient's ideas about fellatio, partly in an attempt to find a replacement for me in anticipation of the loss of the analyst, and because of the success of the analytic work, the patient developed a warm relationship with a girl his own age and had intercourse with her. What was most striking was not only the patient's capacity to have a relationship with a woman but his ability to affectively understand the complexity of his motives.

At the same time his capacity for mature object relations with a variety of people became ever more evident. Friendship with other boys developed in depth. Particularly interesting was his relationship to his family. Fully aware of father's limitations, he felt an enthusiasm and appreciation for father that he had never had before. In contrast to the situation at the beginning of the analysis, when John had been afraid even to let father know of his depression, there was an opinionated and affectionate interchange between them about all sorts of things. There was a more ambivalent relationship with mother, who indeed seemed intrusive and often was critical of the patient—constantly urging him to improve but little pleased by his actual accomplishments.

As termination progressed, John discussed his wish to himself become a psychoanalyst. The fantasy of keeping me by becoming like me was closely examined. At the same time he wanted to be different from me.

He disliked the idea of medical training, which he saw as irrelevant and unpleasant. This very distaste involved a wish to remain a patient—for John thought his distaste for blood and guts was a neurotic symptom. He worried that the wish to become an analyst was again a kind of compliance. An additional theme emerged. The patient, in addition to the transference, had been observing the analyst over the years of the analysis and had perceived much about me. It appeared to him that I was more consistently happy and engaged in my work than either of his parents, so that it was not surprising that he might wish to take up my vocation, especially when it was so clear that he himself was very talented in psychoanalytic understanding.

During the final weeks of the analysis there was considerable mourning for the loss of the analyst and the analytic situation. Throughout the termination phase, repetitions and recollections of earlier phases of the analysis became ever more frequent. Now important and trivial episodes from the analysis were repeatedly recalled. Material about previous losses, the maid and the grandmother, as well as the parents' two separations, also emerged. The family prohibition on grieving once again came to the fore.

Let me describe two hours from the final week of the analysis.

> JOHN: I might be late to the next hour. I saw my girlfriend, and the big game is coming up. I didn't get laid last night. We'll do it once every other night. I think about my baseball playing, I don't run as fast as I should but I have really good moves, I'm able to dodge people. Thinking of sex and chastity. I worked real well, I'm not sure what to do with my dream. In it I felt normal and smallish. I went to my grandparents' apartment like it was a new apartment, as far as its design, but it was like the apartment they used to live in when I was a child. Something had to be set up for a party. I relished telling my sister about my new girlfriend. I let myself in, and I was alone, and I could masturbate if I wanted to. I was suspicious that grandfather would come in. I went into the kitchen. I thought I heard his walk and I left. I felt like leaving and debated whether to stay. He had an old man's walk. I went running down the stairs, but then I came back. I assume it was you I was running from. There were lots of heaps of garbage around. I had a choice of going upstairs or not. I felt sort of little. I decided to go back and talk to my grandfather because I liked him.
>
> There used to be huge hills at my elementary school. I never thought

of it but their being huge must reflect my point of view as a child. We used to like going up the hill and running down. Maybe it was a hill of garbage or compost or something. Analysis doesn't really get rid of all the garbage, it's still there in a way. You know, even though I've been through the analysis, at times I wish I didn't think of some of this stuff. Why am I having such a childish dream now? It reminds me of grade school. You know, I'll always carry a memory of this office. There's not a right way to end an analysis. I feel like it's the right time to be stopping, that there are lots of other things that I am interested in besides the analysis. Like in the dream, I'll always miss the analysis some, I think. I'll always imagine this room and you sitting in it. We talked a lot about grandfather before and how I am really like him a lot and learned a lot from him. But I could have learned more; and I think I'll always wonder about the analysis, if I could have learned more in the analysis. You know, the other day we were talking about how I started the analysis feeling very sad and that's true, but you never talk about how I want to know things about myself. Ending the analysis is resistance, just like running away from my grandfather in the dream, and it may be a stupid thing to do in a way. But there's no way to make it real simple and straightforward. It would be real nice to say it's just a resistance and continue the analysis, or it would be real nice to say that the analysis was all finished, but I don't think it would ever be finished. Sometimes I hate the analysis. It always seems to say things are real complicated.

He continued during the next hour.

JOHN: It's groggy weather. I still haven't really integrated the idea that the analysis is really ending. I worked for a couple of hours to do a chem test. Even that is the end of a section. It reminds me that the analysis is ending. Things come to a head at the end, idea of giving head. I'll get a paper back and worry that I'll get a B− and it'll say "well thought out" but I won't get a good grade. I don't like the idea that it would be possible to go back into analysis. It would simplify things to know it was all done. I may get to meet my sister's boyfriend. It would be funny. But, you know, I'll meet him this weekend and I won't be able to tell you about it. I have the idea of coming back here in a few years and filling you in on everything that's happened. I can imagine coming to see you maybe when I'm forty years old. You'll be almost sixty then. I'll be a tall, handsome, debonair associate professor and all sorts of college girls will have crushes on me, and I'll enjoy it, but I'll be happily married. You know, I feel like I'm really healthy. I feel really good about myself and it's very hard to say that directly. I think you probably feel the same way I do. You're happy with what's happened but you're sad that we won't be working together any more. The thing with my girlfriend was partly because I really enjoy her but I think it was two other things at the same time: I think I want to show you that I was ready to stop the analysis, and maybe show myself that; and also, I think maybe I feel real sad about ending the analysis, and talking about fucking and how much fun it is covers that over. I think it's all right to feel as big as you. You know, remember when I talked about the Sears Tower and how I was afraid of the rats in the Sears Tower and that was associated with feeling fuzzy and groggy. I think that has a lot to do with an idea of a kind of fake confidence that I used to feel, like this big phallic thing really had little dirty rats at its base, and I think I feel different about that now. But when I feel sad I worry about it some more. You know, I'll probably not be much taller than I am now and I still can't stuff a basketball. I'll have to work on my jumping. Is that all you get at the end of an analysis? That you know you're sad about ending it? I would never have believed when I came here that I would stay here for three and a half years. I got an A on my math quiz. I never thought I'd do anything like that. How do you end an analysis? Do you go over to the student bar and get drunk? Is it appropriate to celebrate? Or do you just go home and study for your chem test? You know, I don't know anyone but you whom I can talk to about what it's like to be ending an analysis.

Conclusions

I have tried to illustrate an "ordinary" analysis of an adolescent. I do not mean to imply that John, an extraordinarily bright, psychologically minded, and articulate adolescent, was an ordinary adolescent patient. Rather, he represents a member of a significant group of such adolescents for whom the usual methods of psychoanalysis are an optimal treatment. Of course, there are important differences between the analysis of adolescents and the analytic experience with adults and younger children. The emergence of the capacity for abstract and increasingly decentered thought, sexual maturation, the shifting of attitudes to parents and in parents' attitudes toward the child, all introduce elements into the analysis of adolescents not present in the analysis of children. On the other hand, the use of certain phase-appropriate defenses, particularly externalization and action, are more commonly important in the analysis of adolescents than in analytic work with neurotic adults. The intensification of countertransference experienced with children is often the case with adolescents, and adolescents are far more likely than adult patients to confront and stimulate the analyst's psychopathology.

However, as I have illustrated in this case report, neurotic adolescents are eminently analyzable by essentially standard analytic technique. The end result of successful analysis is the resumption of normal development and the emergence of the self-analytic capacity characteristic of successful analytic work at all ages (Schlessinger and Robbins 1983). The adolescent's relatively flexible character structure as well as his not yet having made neurotic marital and vocational choices places him in an ideal position to benefit from the developments in personality resulting from successful analysis.

So my tale is done. I hope I have conveyed some of the pleasure and reward of working with a patient such as John and that you will be encouraged to think about making such experiences available both to yourselves as therapists and to patients who may come to you.

NOTES

1. Externalization in its various forms is *the* characteristic defense of adolescents. It may be difficult to work with for a variety of reasons. When the analyst is engaged within it, countertransference responses are intensified. Parents are often engaged, as in this case, to enact some aspect of the externalization, which may lead to concrete difficulties in the analysis or shifting the analyst's attention away from the patient's psychological world. The defense is not only often ego-syntonic but also syntonic with the adolescent's social milieu. All these factors tend to lead the analyst away from the only stance I have found genuinely effective—that of interpretation.

2. The material presented in quotations is a paraphrase of the patient's and analyst's statements as recorded in my notes. The patient was very

articulate, and his actual statements did not differ widely from those recorded here.

3. Sam Weiss (personal communication) has described a group of transferences that may go unnoticed because they are dystonic with the analyst's image of himself. Thus, while most male analysts have little difficulty in experiencing themselves as a preoedipal mother in the transference, maternal genital transferences are far less syntonic and tend to be ignored.

4. The idea that children must march, lockstep, off to college away from home regardless of their developmental needs, including needs for treatment, is not only pervasive in the upper middle class but is even accepted by analysts (Blos 1983; Kaplan 1982), partly because it seems consistent with the idea that adolescence represents a second separation-individuation phase. The investigation of the social psychology of this imperative would be most useful, as many adolescents are done great harm by its blind acceptance.

REFERENCES

Blos, P. 1967. The second individuation process in adolescence. *Psychoanalytic Study of the Child* 22:162–186.

Blos, P. 1983. The contribution of psychoanalysis to the psychotherapy of adolescents. *Psychoanalytic Study of the Child* 38:577–599.

Eissler, K. 1953. The effect of the structure of the ego on psychoanalytic technique. *Journal of the American Psychoanalytic Association* 1:104–143.

Freud, A. 1965. *Normality and Pathology in Childhood: Assessment of Development*. New York: International Universities Press.

Harley, M., ed. 1974a. *The Analyst and the Adolescent at Work*. New York: Quadrangle.

Harley, M. 1974b. Introduction. In M. Harley, ed. *The Analyst and the Adolescent at Work*. New York: Quadrangle.

Kaplan, E. 1982. The dilemma of disposition: psychiatric decision making and the college-bound high school senior. *Adolescent Psychiatry* 10:469–483.

Laufer, M. 1981. The psychoanalyst and the adolescent's sexual development. *Psychoanalytic Study of the Child* 36:181–191.

Pearson, G. H., ed. 1968. *A Handbook of Child Psychoanalysis*. New York: Basic.

Sandler, J.; Kennedy, H.; and Tyson, R. 1975. Discussions on transference: the treatment situation and technique in child analysis. *Psychoanalytic Study of the Child* 30:409–441.

Schlessinger, N., and Robbins, F. 1983. *A Developmental View of the Psychoanalytic Process*. New York: International Universities Press.

Sklansky, M. A. 1972. Indications and contraindications for the psychoanalysis of the adolescent. *Journal of the American Psychoanalytic Association* 20:139–144.

24 PRINCIPLES OF RESIDENTIAL TREATMENT: STAFF GROWTH AND THERAPEUTIC INTERACTION

JACQUELYN SANDERS

Anyone who has worked with severely disturbed individuals is familiar with the onslaught of primitive, complex, and ambivalent emotions that such individuals present. How the therapeutic person deals with this onslaught can contribute significantly to both professional development and the patient's course of treatment. Therefore, helping staff members to cope with this emotionally trying phenomenon is a critical part of training them. While to do so seems important at every level of human services, it is perhaps most dramatically critical for those who work with groups of adolescents; that is, teachers, child-care workers, aides, and, at our school, counselors. These are the people who experience this emotional onslaught from several sources at the same time and for extended periods. Whether this is basically a depleting or rewarding experience is to a large extent determined by the way the staff member deals with the emotions stimulated in him or her by the situations. Whenever, for example, we "tolerate" behavior, we tend to feel depleted because emotions are aroused in us which we keep in check, thus requiring a large expenditure of energy. On the other hand, if we can use the experience of the arousal of these emotions as an opportunity to come to grips with issues raised and thus gain greater mastery, we tend to feel replenished.

At the Orthogenic School, we assume that those who are in the closest, most sustained contact with the patients are those who have the possibility of having the greatest therapeutic impact. We, therefore, devote as much teaching and support to the milieu staff (counselors and teachers) as pos-

0-226-24058-4/85/0012-0011$01.00

sible. We also assume that unconscious attitudes influence interaction and that the more aware the staff member is of unconscious issues and free of conflict related to the interaction, the more therapeutically effective he can be. Therefore, one aspect of our teaching, for the benefit of both staff and patients, is helping staff to recognize, accept, and understand the emotions that are aroused in working with these disturbed youngsters.

The Sonia Shankman Orthogenic School of the University of Chicago is a residential setting for the treatment of emotionally disturbed children and adolescents. It is technically under the Department of Education; the director traditionally holds an appointment in that department. Its purpose is threefold; service, research, and training. We can have as many as forty youngsters, divided into six living groups with three counselors responsible for the therapeutic milieu of each group, and five classroom groups with one teacher responsible for each. Counselors come to the school for training in psychoanalytically oriented milieu therapy. Requirements for this program are a bachelor's degree, commitment, and sensitivity. Beginning counselors have a wide variety of backgrounds ranging from bachelor's to doctorate and from no experience with children to extensive experience. They also vary in regard to prior experience with personal therapy, ranging from none to analysis.

A counselor will regularly be with a group of six or seven disturbed youngsters for at least four approximately eight-hour "shifts" per week and will also spend some time alone with the youngsters, attending to their needs, playing, or talking. The counselors are, thus, after a very short introduction, responsible for maintaining a therapeutic milieu. To accomplish this, they are involved in a very intensive training program. We have five formal staff meetings per week, led by either the director or associate director, who are psychologists, one of our social workers, or one of two consultants who are both psychoanalysts. Some meetings are organized around a particular child, and some are devoted to questions and problems about general practices or particular difficulties.

In their first year counselors are required to take staff meetings as a course for credit at the university. For this course there is an assignment of related readings. Written and oral presentations are required that demonstrate integration of the clinical work and the readings. Counselors are expected to take courses related to the work at the university, for which scholarships are provided. In the second year and after, counselors have individual supervision with a social worker. There is also a loan fund for psychoanalytic psychotherapy.

The staff who work on a given day meet for fifteen minutes before the shift begins to coordinate activities. In addition to these formal meetings, there are many informal meetings. The director or associate director is usually at meals and in the staff room evenings when the counselors get "off." Cocounselors talk with each other frequently, and senior staff are available for advice and discussion. Since counselors live at the school, informal contacts are easily made. Though people are encouraged to raise questions about the work publicly, the director and associate are available for individual consultation.

The examples of our approach will be from our general staff meetings. At these staff meetings anyone can bring up areas of difficulty. As the leader of two of these meetings, I use these periods both to help with particular problems and to teach an approach to the resolution of problems. Some of the essential components of this approach are the importance of the recognition of one's emotional reaction and the acceptance and understanding of that reaction; these, of course, are all prerequisites to a therapeutic action. Thus, in those meetings devoted to general problems, much of our effort is directed at encouraging the staff to recognize, accept, and understand the emotions aroused in the work and in helping them with those issues that interfere with the recognition, acceptance, and understanding.

Since the first issue involved in coping with emotions aroused is a recognition of them, we will often ask a staff member when he brings up a problem what his emotional reaction was to it. Though this seems fairly simple, it is quite striking that the question is often difficult to answer. I believe that the reason for this is that the emotions aroused, for a variety of reasons, are difficult to accept. Therefore, the staff member may misconstrue the question. For example, when I ask, "What was your reaction?" a staff member will often give an explanation of the child's behavior rather than a statement of his own emotional reaction. I also believe, however, that the very asking of the question in this situation—and persistently asking it despite such misconstructions—helps toward the acceptance of those emotions because it indicates that the staff member is expected to have an emotional reaction and that it is of great importance.

The following is an example of this initial resistance in which the staff member afterward was able to explain why she was evasive and then was able to examine her emotional reaction to the problem raised. We were discussing the issue of children's leaving the dormitories without permission. In response to the question regarding her feeling about it, one relatively experienced staff member first tried to remember the last time her girl had gone out and then attempted to trace the possible precipitating events. This was a valid approach to understanding the girl and, of course, an essential component of resolving the situation—but not an answer to the question. When I pointed this out, the staff member recognized what she was doing and explained that she thought that trying to figure out the girl's behavior was fortifying herself against my criticism. I then assured her that she was accurate in expecting criticism because it is characteristic of me to look for what was missed in a problematic situation. But while it was painful to sort these things out, my purpose was not criticism but clarification and finding solutions. She then was able to talk about her view that, when this particular girl went out of the dormitory, the smooth functioning of the group could be maintained—whereas if she had stayed in, this particular girl would have been likely to do something to disrupt the smoothness. Because of this, the counselor was relieved when the girl left. This staff member had not been aware of this reaction in herself and had thought, until she began to discuss it at this meeting, that she had simply wanted the girl to stay in the dormitory, since she knew that this was best for her. To feel that she did not want her in the dormitory was contrary to her idea of the way a good counselor should feel, and, therefore, particularly when questioned by the director, she had to avoid recognizing that aspect of her feeling. With the assurance that I would expect and accept such ambivalence, she could recognize it and begin to examine it. Furthermore, the staff member was sophisticated enough to realize that this girl was extremely sensitive and that her leaving the dormitory was usually an indication of some often unstated anxiety in the group—so that continued smooth functioning was a facade, an evasion of some issue. Though the counselor understandably liked a smoothly functioning dormitory, she had a deeper commitment to the resolution than to the covering up of problems. Therefore, she valued being able to view the running as a clue to her that she should look for some underlying anxieties in the group. The discussion enabled her to recognize her ambivalence and direct her energies to what she really valued most.

In this example both the advantage and the disadvantage of the director's position are apparent. It is likely that the counselor's anxiety about being criticized was much greater because of my being in the position of responsibility and power. At the same time, my acceptance and assurance that her having such emotions was to be expected could have a most powerful effect against her own self-criticism that a good counselor should not feel this way.

At times, such exploration leads to quite dramatic results. One of our psychotic boys was tearing his clothes. In our discussion of this it became clear that some of the staff had difficulty with the economy of the problem. This could be dealt with by pointing out that the cost of one week's treatment could replace many clothes, so that if tearing his clothes reduced the length of treatment it was economical. The staff member working with the boy most closely then talked about her personal reaction to his tearing clothes—how it was related to the significance of clothes to her as a child, that clothes were connected to a kind of loving care for her. After this discussion she felt much less distressed by his actions—she no longer experienced his actions as destroying her loving care. Immediately thereafter, the clothes tearing stopped.

The staff member who could discuss this at a staff meeting was very experienced, quite secure in the setting and with me, and had good results with personal treatment. However, such dramatic results from the exploration of feelings and attitudes can take place in less intensive settings. For example, when I served as a consultant to a nursery/day-care facility, there was an outbreak of obscenity that seemed inappropriate for such small children and was distressing to the nursery school director and some others. We called all the staff together and discussed everyone's reaction to the obscenity. There were a variety of feelings, including enjoyment of the children's ability to do something that the staff had never themselves been permitted to do. It became clear that the staff were all in agreement that swearing was a bad idea for the children, though their reasoning about it and emotional reactions to it were varied. Immediately after this meeting, the swearing stopped almost entirely.

In the ongoing work of residential treatment, the results are not often so dramatic, but the issue is persistent, as is the necessity for the support of the exploration and acceptance of the emotions of the staff. To demonstrate and examine this, I would like to present as examples (chosen more or less at random) three issues that happened to come before the staff in an arbitrarily selected three-day period: a boy wanted to start on a diet; two boys wanted to dress as Siamese twins for Halloween; and two boys wanted to watch a horror movie. On the one hand, a decision had to be made about each of these issues in terms of what would be "good" for the boys. On the other hand, the counseling staff had to deal with the boys in effecting the decisions. In dealing with these issues, the staff's own feelings have to be considered because they would affect the way the boys were handled and the staff's psychic economy. When I was discussing this presentation with one senior staff member, she said that recognition that her emotions are so important to the treatment gave her the feeling of having potentially great significance in the student's growth and that this helped to make the painfulness of facing unpleasant emotions worthwhile. For each of the three issues we, of course, considered the meaning to the boys, but besides and sometimes before doing so I asked the staff member involved what his reaction was to the issue.

The counselor of the boy who wanted to diet talked about the boy's desire to run, which related to the diet, saying that he thought it was a good idea. His reason was that the counselor himself felt good after running. Now, the boy did not always feel good about running but had, to this counselor, presented only his positive feelings about it. In the staff meeting I could point this out by citing my own and other people's different experience with this boy. To me, who never exercised at the time, the boy had complained. It seemed, therefore, that the boy was presenting to each staff member what was most acceptable to that staff member. I could also point out the danger in assuming that what one person likes another will also like. The counselor's assumption that diet and running were positive, because he himself is trim and likes to run, might interfere with his ability to see that others have negative feelings about running and positive ones about being fat. The counselor's readiness was such that just the suggestion of such a different perspective enabled him to realize how much the boy tried to respond to each staff member's feeling and that further consideration of issues involved was necessary.

The counselor of the proposed Siamese twins said that she had a negative reaction to the idea because of the deformity involved. In our discussion we reviewed the fact that both boys had some kind of deformity and her negative reaction could be related in their minds to their real deformities. The counselor had been wrestling for a long time with her own problematic reaction to the epilepsy of one of the boys. With the recognition of this connection she became more accepting of their costume choice. She then spent considerable time making a Siamese shirt for them, whereupon they decided to go as two of the "Kiss" ensemble. It seemed that as she was able to accept deformity they had less need to emphasize it.

The third counselor was very uncomfortable about the possibility of watching the horror movie with the two boys. She had herself seen the movie. She became noticeably embarrassed when I pointed out that she could not, without further examination, say that it was good for her but bad for them. Later she said, with what appeared to be some satisfaction in the realization, that there was some reassurance in watching such a horror film from a safe place. This, of course, was only a beginning for this issue. Since she could not fully recognize and cope with all that was involved in her interest in the horror films, the boys' disorganization in doing so would likely have been very threatening for her. I do not believe the situation was well resolved. The boys watched the film with another staff member and the following day had a fight.

The examples I have used show, I believe, that it is cogent that the staff member's recognition and resolution of his emotional reaction are beneficial to the patient. There are at least three issues raised from these examples that create difficulty in the accomplishment of this end: the staff member's guilt about having feelings that are not in the best interest of the patient; the staff member's ability in terms of his own psychic organization to recognize certain feelings; and the question of whether it is of benefit to the staff member to behave in the best interests of the patient.

As we have seen in the example of the counselor who was relieved when the disruptive girl was out of the dormitory, staff often have difficulty in accepting in themselves feelings that seem to be at cross purposes to their conscious intentions and that they feel are unacceptable to others. Since they may feel guilty about such feelings, they may resist acknowledging them and perceive any questioning about them as a criticism or an attack. This is sometimes made more difficult because the issue frequently comes up around something going wrong. I know very well that in helping staff I first have to contend with my own feelings of frustration and annoyance when something has gone wrong with a patient related to mixed feelings of a staff member. If I approach the staff member with annoyance this will contribute to guilt about feelings and make the worker less able to examine them. For example, a female counselor came into her dormitory on Halloween. A well-developed twelve-year-old boy put his hands over her eyes aggressively and tried to prevent her coming in. She picked him up and carried him to his bed. He, of course, became more stimulated and aggressive. In the end, she did something retaliative to him, putting her hands over his eyes. When she told me about it, she had recognized her own anger and retaliation—about which she felt bad. She did not, however, recognize the stimulation involved in her lifting him up. I myself at first felt angry at her for stimulating him to such a degree. However, I realized that she probably was unaware of her stimulation and that my anger was unwarranted and would make her less likely to be able to have access to her own feelings. I then explained to her that with his growing sexual development, such play could be overstimulating and therefore undesirable, but that she should not feel bad about her own desires for such play with the boys.

Much effort is necessary to help staff members believe that their feelings, particularly aggressive and sexual, toward the patients are not bad. Discussion of these issues at staff meetings can be very helpful in that staff members can see that others have these kinds of feelings. Some of the guilt associated with such feelings can be dealt with at this level with direct reassurance from other staff members. When the guilt is alleviated the staff are more able to recognize, accept, and understand their own feelings and have less need to act them out.

A second problem area relates to the timing of a staff member's readiness to deal with a particular dilemma. While it can be very valuable for a counselor to deal with the psychological issues stimulated by the patients, and, in general, the staff is usually quite intrigued and stimulated by this possibility, the psychic timetables do not always match. For example, the counselor of the costume issue had some grasp already of what deformity meant to her and could then interact with the boys constructively. The counselor of the horror movie watchers had only begun to explore the problem and so could not do much with her boys. When this is the case, contending with the emotional barrage is very stressful for the staff member. At times we are able to see a staff member gradually able to become more cognizant and accepting of unacceptable feelings. For example, one counselor would joke with me about her statement of several months earlier that she is not a person who hits. Since she works with a girl who does hit, her total rejection of her own aggressive inclinations, as revealed in this statement, both distanced her from the girl and made the stimulation of her aggressive feelings much harder to contend with in herself. When the girl was aggressive, the counselor would have to overly inhibit her own reactions because her own aggressive impulses were unacceptable to her; she then could not react in a reasonable self-protective manner. Furthermore, she would have no empathic response because to be empathic with someone who hits would mean that she was also someone who hits. It was several months and many conversations before the counselor was ready to recognize that she was a person who many times felt like hitting and occasionally might hit. With this recognition, she became much more able to deal with the student since she could have an empathic rather than a distancing response. Through such times it is important that the staff member have support. The rest of the staff needs to maintain a noncritical attitude while recognizing that the staff member who is having such trouble will be better able to deal with it by becoming aware of and accepting his own feelings. The staff member is under stress. If those working with him are critical for the nonacceptance of those feelings that are unacceptable, it will simply add another conflict or intensify the existing one. On the other hand, if other staff deny the importance of such acceptance, it will only support a nonproductive defensive stance.

A third and most difficult problem area is the arousal of emotional issues that are so intensely conflictual that the staff member feels unable to stay in the situation. For example, one staff member felt devastated by the students' derogatory comments directed at her. At times she was able to see that she did things to provoke such comments. When I assured her that the opinion of psychotic children was not a valid indicator of her worth, she could gain momentary security. However, at the next onslaught she would feel terrible about herself. She finally decided that it was bad for her to be continually putting herself in such a degrading position and resigned. Though it is possible that she had some need to put herself in such a position, her awareness of the conflict was not enough to enable her to be completely unprovocative to highly sensitive acting-out students or to not react with great distress to their intense provocation. She sought treatment, and her decision to remove herself from a situation in which she felt devalued was probably a healthy move. This decision, I believe, can become clearer the more one is aware of one's own emotional reactions.

Conclusions

This has been a discussion of some of our efforts to help staff members learn to deal with emotions aroused in work with severely emotionally disturbed children and adolescents. Examples have been presented mainly from some of our staff meetings, during which we try to transmit some attitudes that we believe to be significant. These meetings are those attended by all staff and led by the director. This arrangement has the advantage of supportive unity. It has the disadvantage of anxiety created by the director's various dimensions of both power and responsibility. It also has both the advantage and disadvantage of publicity. That is, while it is greatly reassuring to know that others have the same problems, it is sometimes difficult to be open in front of too many others.

It is possible from our work to identify at least four attitudes that are helpful in these efforts: (1) that the staff does have an emotional reaction; (2) that no matter what that reaction is, it is acceptable and somehow understandable; (3) that knowing about the emotional reaction will be helpful in further interaction; and (4) though it may be slow and painful to do so, it is really possible to sort out even the most chaotic emotional barrage. Our experience has given evidence that, with the proper support of these attitudes, the stimulation of our feelings in this kind of work can lead to empathic understanding and rewarding mastery.

25 MOURNING IN ADOLESCENCE: NORMAL AND PATHOLOGICAL

BENJAMIN GARBER

Although the mourning process of the adult has been studied extensively and the mourning work of the child has been well demarcated, the mourning process of the adolescent has been relatively neglected. Furman (1974) makes many astute observations on and comparisons between mourning in children and the mourning process of adults, but she makes no specific references, either descriptive or comparative, to the mourning of adolescents.

Since the parents of the adolescents are at least middle-aged, we can assume that a certain number of adolescents do experience the loss of a parent. A recent survey (Ewalt and Perkins 1979) of high school juniors and seniors indicated that many more students than might have been suspected had experienced the death of a loved one; their concerns and preoccupations with death did not emanate just from fantasies but from the death of close relatives, friends, and parents. Nearly 90 percent of students in this study reported that they had seen a dead person or had lost a grandparent, aunt, uncle, sibling, or someone else about whom they had cared. Approximately 40 percent had experienced the death of a close friend their own age, and at least one parent of 10 percent of the students had died. Again, although there has been extensive literature both on children who experienced parent loss and who were subsequently followed into adolescence and on adults who had lost a parent in adolescence, the psychoanalytic literature on parent loss in adolescence proper—that is, at the time of the loss—has been rather scanty.

Root (1957) makes some rather cogent observations on adolescent

0-226-24058-4/85/0012-0064$01.00

mourning. "When the adolescent attempts a shift in object cathexis which is associated with object removal, the result is painful grief if there has been a loss of a parent earlier, especially one of the same sex; for then the grieving is equated with letting the parent die." He concludes: "Every adolescent, as a part of normal development, must make a real psychical renunciation and then suffer the loss of childhood and its aims and objects; he must do this much more completely than in the more infantile earlier struggle with the oedipus complex. This task is hampered greatly when mourning for the lost object is evaded. By the same token the loss of the parent needs to be mourned before any kind of analytic process can proceed."

Laufer (1966), who was less pessimistic about the impact of parent loss on the adolescent, nevertheless agreed that it could become a prominent obstacle to normal development, stating that although the parental death itself is not necessarily pathogenic, object loss can become the nucleus around which earlier conflicts and latent pathogenic elements are organized. He concluded that "the extent to which the work of mourning will interfere with normal adolescent tasks is determined by the kind of defenses available to deal with the oedipal ambivalence and by the quality of the relationship to the object." Laufer is one of the few authors to appreciate the possibility that adolescent developmental tasks may interfere with the mourning process.

Wolfenstein (1966, 1969) has probably contributed some of the more definitive clinical findings as well as theoretical constructs on the subject of childhood and adolescent mourning. From studying 42 cases of parent loss, Wolfenstein arrived at a series of far-reaching impressions and conclusions. She felt that in those instances in which depressed moods emerged in adolescence, they were quite isolated from thoughts of the parent's death, thoughts to which reality testing had not yet been applied. She got the impression that the representation of the lost object was not decathected, that it indeed became invested with an intensified cathexis.

Wolfenstein (1966, 1969) as well as Laufer believe that the adolescent idealizes the dead parent and that the rage the adolescent feels is diverted toward the surviving parent. In time, reproachful feelings toward the abandoning parent emerge, and this ambivalence may represent the initial step toward reality testing. The fantasies of the parent's return are either more clearly conscious or more readily admitted in adolescence than at earlier ages. The readiness to admit such a fantasy, thus risking confrontation with reality, represents one of the steps in giving up the lost parent.

One of Wolfenstein's more astute clinical observations was that adolescents are deeply ashamed of having lost a parent, that they try to conceal that fact, and that they feel inferior to those from intact families. It would appear that the giving up of a major love object lost in childhood or adolescence requires many preparatory stages. Wolfenstein wonders if children and adolescents are capable of such "trial mourning."

Although Wolfenstein's work stands as a milestone in our attempts to understand mourning in children and adolescents, there are a number of additional questions that must be posed. One of the questions Wolfenstein raises is whether the strong impression of developmental unreadiness for the work of mourning observed in these children and adolescents might not indicate some type of limitation in subject selection, but a more disturbing aspect of her work is her willingness to draw conclusions from and make generalizations about such a heterogeneous sample, since some of the children were seen only diagnostically, some were in psychotherapy, and others were in psychoanalysis. Yet the most puzzling aspect of her work is that she mixes children and adolescents without bothering to recognize developmental differences either at the time of the loss or subsequently. The hypothesis that Wolfenstein proposes is as follows: adolescence not only resembles mourning but constitutes the necessary precondition for later being able to mourn the painful and gradual decathexis of the parents. The individual who has passed through this decisive experience has learned how to give up a major love object. It is only in adolescence that developmental imperatives require a radical decathexis of the parents.

Ever since Anna Freud (1958) described a type of mourning process as part and parcel of normal adolescent development, psychoanalytic researchers perhaps have felt that the study of mourning in adolescents may become an overly complex and relatively unproductive task. The clinician would be compelled to examine two intertwined mourning experiences, one an aspect of normal development, the other a product of a here-and-now traumatic event. To separate the two and focus on differences and similarities might indeed become superfluous and not clinically productive or useful.

Jacobson (1964) contended that in the process of decathecting the infantile image of his parents, the adolescent experiences an intensity of grief unknown in previous phases of his or her life. Blos (1962) indicated that the object loss that adolescents experience in relation to the parent of their childhood, a loss in relation to the parent image, contains prominent features of mourning and that this adolescent loss is more final and irrevocable than the one that occurs at the end of the oedipal phase.

Root (1957) spoke of the work of mourning as an important psychological task during the period of adolescence. This accounts in part for the seemingly larger number of depressive states occurring during this developmental period. Adolescents have a normal and healthy need to remove themselves from both parents, to stop being dependent, and to become more self-sufficient as they proceed on the pathway to mature adulthood. This so-called "object removal" continues ambivalently for years and ushers in a mourning reaction as described by Sugar (1968). The first phase of this process, which has been called separation-protest, is characterized by disequilibrium and corresponds to Bowlby's description of the urge to recover the lost love object. The second phase, labeled as one of disorganization, has as its hallmark a shift away from both parents that corresponds to the storm of adolescence; antisocial behavior is commonplace during this period. The final phase, one of reorganization, occurs in late adolescence and is one of relative calm. Throughout this three-phase process, the adolescent mourns for his parents, the lost infantile objects from whom he is separating. This postulated mourning reaction consists of sequential phases that correspond to Bowlby's (1960) description and theory of mourning.

The loosening of the ties to the parents is a difficult and protracted process often accompanied by genuine mourning. What the outcome of the mourning process will be, that is, whether it is a relatively normal or a pathological one, depends on many factors, one of which is the amount of aggression originally directed toward the parents, since this may be colored by aggression turned inward. Although mourning thus appears to be an expected and usual accompaniment of adolescence, the depressive affect is not necessarily the same as in depressive illness. Mourning in adolescence is often difficult to recognize, since it may be expressed through depressive equivalents or mood swings. In being alienated from the internalized parents, the adolescent has the pervasive sense of being intrapsychically alone. While this may be a valid description of an internal state, it does not necessarily follow that the adolescent is in a constant state of mourning.

The term mourning has been overused in recent years, with some analysts describing the reactions to disappointments, frustrations, loss of love, the experience of powerlessness, feeling injured, and so forth as mourning. This overuse of the term blurs the precision of a rather valuable and specific psychoanalytic concept (Lampl-deGroot 1983). Nevertheless, the psychoanalytic literature is consistent in contending that something approximating a mourning process occurs as an important component of normal adolescent development. Perhaps, then, the question is how this so-called normal mourning may relate to the mourning for a lost parent.

Before addressing this question, we must examine the more basic issue of whether the adolescent is capable of mourning. Fleming and Altschul (1963) discussed the effect of parent loss in adolescence as it was evidenced in the analysis of adults. In describing the case of a young woman who experienced parent loss in adolescence and who was analyzed at age twenty-nine, they concluded that, "this traumatic event had intensified the adolescent developmental task of emotional and social emancipation from childhood parent relationships. The mechanisms by which she adapted to this experience included denial of the reality of her loss and of the passage of time. This adaptive effort resulted in a prolonging of adolescent behavior patterns and a failure to complete either the mourning for her parents or the normal resolution of developmental conflicts."

Laufer (1966) and Root (1957) presented two cases of a parent's death occurring during adolescence. Both of their patients exhibited denial, inhibition of grief-related affects, idealization, identification with the lost parent, fantasies of restitution, and severe interference with the normal developmental processes of adolescence.

In Wolfenstein's (1966) view of the process of mourning, "that reaction to loss in which the lost object is gradually decathected by the painful and prolonged work of remembering and reality testing" does not become possible for the individual until he has successfully negotiated the major adaptive task of adolescence—that is, the giving up of the parents as the principal love objects and ego and superego adjuncts. The painful, gradual decathexis of the parents in adolescence is seen as an initiation into how to mourn. Where the work of adolescence has remained incomplete, the adult remains unable to accomplish the work of mourning in response to a loss.

The consensus from these researchers would imply that adolescents are not capable of mourning the loss of a parent. However, a vocal minority of researchers, such as Bowlby (1960), Furman (1964), and Kilman (1968), have proposed the view that since the responses to loss are similar in children and adults on a descriptive level, the processes should also be quite similar methodologically. Furman (1964) in particular has stressed that mourning does occur in children under specific circumstances, that if they have achieved certain developmental milestones, even three- to four-year-olds are capable of mourning. The main prerequisite is that the child be provided with an adequate adult substitute who will meet his needs and allow him to express his feelings about the loss.

Lampl-deGroot (1983) is also quite definite in her contention that a child who has achieved some structuralization of the mind is capable of mourning the death of a beloved person in a way that is not much different from an adult's reaction. Latency children, adolescents, and adults know intellectually that a dead person never returns, but emotionally they all more or less deny this fact.

Pollock (1977, 1978) proposed an alternate hypothesis to deal with this complex issue. He suggested that the differences between children and adults with respect to mourning can be reconciled if one considers the mourning process as phasic, with different developmental onset ages for each component. If one views the mourning process as sequential and intimately related to the maturation of the psychic apparatus, then the either/or dilemma becomes a spurious argument. Other workers in this area, especially Furman (1974), have recently suggested that there may be similar shifts in their own thinking.

If we accept the idea that the adolescent is cognitively and to some extent emotionally more mature than the latency-age child, then we can also assume that the adolescent may be capable of engaging in some type of mourning in response to a loss. Turnball (1980) observed that the adolescent showed a capacity to introspect with regard to feelings as well as thoughts about death. The adolescents' concepts of death were often concrete but based less on a ubiquitous causality and more on the uniformity of nature. There seemed to be an accommodation to the natural processes among adolescents.

In a very detailed study of adolescents' responses to bereavement, Gapes (1982) defined the typical adolescent response to a loss as escape. Although the usual responses of guilt, anger, depression, anxiety, and confusion were present, the adolescents frequently suppressed their emotional responses. They did this because they felt that such emotions frequently were unacceptable to their peers. They were much concerned about the expected normal response to the loss because they were overly concerned about being considered different or abnormal. Instead of risking such an exposure, they often chose to suppress any intense affects about their loss.

Inconsistency and unpredictability of behavior form a normal accompaniment of the adolescent state and one that may in some respects resemble narcissistic neuroses. Dynamic and clinical formulations seem to have far more difficulty explaining the adolescent than any other age group; with the constant danger of spontaneous regression, character formation is indeed precarious. By the same token, then, the adolescent perhaps presents a fluid and inconsistent picture of his mourning process.

It may well be that the adolescents' mourning does not necessarily follow one prescribed clinical pattern but manifests itself in multiple types of experiences, which are a function of the fluid state of the adolescents' psychic structure. Perhaps, then, the more specific question should be not whether adolescents mourn but just how they do mourn—or how adolescent mourning may be similar to that of the latency-age child and to that of the adult. Perhaps the more cogent and all-encompassing question concerns what is unique to the mourning process of the adolescent.

The recurrent association of adolescent acting out and depression has been described by a number of investigators. It has been suggested that adolescent acting out is likely to mask underlying depression and to take the form of temper tantrums, dropping out of school, truancy, running away, drug use, underachievement, and promiscuity. The adolescent's antisocial behavior may be a deliberate attempt to provoke parental condemnation, since it allows for both parties to focus on such behavior while ignoring long-standing hostilities and allows for the child to ward off the feelings of loss.

One of the ways in which adolescents have been seen as mourning the death of a parent is by means of some type of acting out. In the 1950s and 1960s, when psychoanalytic researchers were just beginning to come to grips with the psychology of adolescence, acting out was seen as the final common pathway for expression of a variety of traumatic events and their accompanying psychological states. Bonnard (1961) described two boys who had experienced the loss of a parent in preadolescence. Although the clinical data in these cases were rich and interesting, they did not offer any insight into how the acting-out behavior was a direct expression of the grief and mourning for the lost object. In both cases, the problems had been present before the parent died and were accentuated after the death. If anything, these cases seemed to support the ideas of the adolescent as being a delinquent from a sense of guilt. However, Bonnard dealt scantily with how the adolescent experienced the loss and whether internal changes occurred in response to such a trauma.

There have been occasional reports in the literature in which the adolescent's acting out was preceded by the death of a parent, but they have not been particularly convincing. In almost every instance there were problems prior to the death, and the adolescent experienced an inordinate amount of aggression toward the lost object. Clinical experience with parent loss through death tends to reveal behavior and symptomatology that is more inward directed, whereas the clinical picture in parent loss through divorce is more often that of a youngster who is in conflict with his environment (Garber 1982).

Since the adolescent considers it crucial to be part of a group and equally important to conform to the group, he is very conscious of anything that may set him apart from others. Whatever factors set him apart—physical, social, or emotional—the typical adolescent will try to diminish them. Consequently, the adolescent who has lost a parent will be acutely aware that he is looked at and treated differently and that in some ways he may even be different from his peers. As a result, the adolescent will feel very self-conscious and embarrassed whenever his loss and its implications are mentioned. He will go to great lengths to avoid talking about the loss or at least do everything possible to diminish its significance and importance. All of these efforts will be quite conscious and will be expressed in direct and indirect ways. However, unconsciously the adolescent will engage in something far more subtle and complex. Unconsciously, the adolescent who has experienced parent loss will exert much energy to appear as normal and as appropriate as he possibly can. He will persist in doing average work in school, participate in those activities that will make him appear a part of the crowd, and insist that he is just an average teenager. Any unusual interests or activities that may distinguish him will be hidden or discarded, whereas those activities that show him to be a part of the norm will be cultivated. It is this quest for conformity, stability, and predictability that serves as a powerful balance to the profound sense of shame and embarrassment that the adolescent feels about his loss.

Adolescent Reactions to Loss

CASE STUDY 1

Susie was an attractive, outgoing, and vivacious fourteen-year-old who talked readily about her various interests and activities. She discussed at great length her many friends, their importance in her life, cheerleading and track-team activities, and her acceptance by a prestigious choral group. She felt that her grades could be better, although she received Bs and Cs with an occasional A. She dated and wished to marry and go to college or maybe a junior college after graduation. She was unable to understand why her father was concerned about her schoolwork, since she received average grades in all of her subjects. The interviewer was so taken and impressed with how stable and normal this girl seemed to be that he neglected to ask about her mother's death, which had occurred two years previously.

Clinically, we have noticed a number of adolescents who have attempted and often succeeded in impressing the diagnostician with how normal and seemingly stable they were, in spite of their loss. Perhaps we need to recognize that this cultivated sense of normality and stability exists because of the loss. Although such a defense may have a here-and-now stabilizing potential, the long-range implications are unknown.

One of the recurrent struggles of all adolescents tends to revolve around the basic issue of just how mature the youngster really is. In certain situations, most adolescents can behave in an exceptionally mature and responsible manner; however, they are just likely to regress in response to such maturational forays. Clinicians accept such behavior as the norm and maintain the expectation that ultimately the periods of high-level functioning will exceed the regressions. Such a vacillation between progressive and regressive trends has a certain periodicity which is determined in part by environmental response as well as by each individual's internal timetable. More often than not this is a leisurely to-and-fro which is a developmental imperative and which some cultures promote, others restrict, and the majority probably learn to accept and tolerate.

When a parent dies, the surviving parent is usually depressed and anxious. The depression is related to the loss of the object as well as to the previous state of well-being. The anxiety is related to economic concerns, future hopes and aspirations, and one's own sense of well-being. Within such a highly charged interactional matrix, the regressive trends of the adolescent are not tolerated and in fact tend to be greatly discouraged. Because of the parent's regressive longings and pervasive anxiety over everyday and future concerns, the adolescent is not allowed to regress. In fact, the opposite occurs; the youngster is constantly urged to be more mature and to assume the responsibility of being the man or the woman of the house. Such demands and expectations will indeed lend themselves to the adolescent's assumption of a hypermaturational cast. The adolescent will do this not necessarily to please the surviving parent, but primarily because such a demand dovetails with his own need to prove to both others and himself just how grown-up he can become. Thus, the adolescent will tend to assume inordinate responsibilities, and there may even be a reversal of roles such that he or she will become the parent to the parent. Although perhaps not totally comfortable within such an arrangement, the parent will have an obvious sense of pride in the child's seeming maturity. Although such a maturational stance will to some extent address the needs of both parties, it does tend to short-circuit the leisurely back-and-forth movement that is such an essential component of normal development. Such an accelerated impetus to becoming an adult may deprive the adolescent of the opportunity to experience the necessary regressions that serve in his or her mastering of progressive developmental positions. Consequently, the clinician may be faced with a youngster who is exceptionally mature under stress or in the daily self-caretaking activities but who may regress and even decompensate when all is well or during periods of solitude. The result may be a personality structure in which areas of competence and achievement coexist with islands of primitive defenses and unacceptable regressive trends. Psychodynamically this may portend a situation in which there is a striking imbalance between hypermaturity and the concomitant infantile longings. Sensing both of these aspects to the extreme, the adolescent may often wonder if he or she is growing up in comparison to his peers. It is also just such an imbalance between hypermaturity and regressive wishes that will contribute to the adolescent's feeling—and perhaps even being—different from his or her peers.

The hypermature teenager will often elicit a sense of awe and admiration from the clinician, not so much because of a lack of awareness but rather because we tend to be impressed with the orphan who seems to be doing well. The countertransference response most common in the therapy of youngsters with parent loss is one in which the basic elements of the treatment contract are overlooked and special allowances are made for the patient. These will frequently distort and even derail the therapeutic process.

Since the adolescent's personality is in constant flux, he or she is both subject and prone to experimentation with various identificational styles. Whether such identifications are with entertainment figures, athletes, political radicals, or admired teachers, they emphasize the adolescent's receptivity and need to test various identifications and then to either discard them outright or retain whatever in them is inherently useful for further development. Although identification is part and parcel of any reaction to the loss of an object, we have noticed a particular type of identification in response to the death of a parent.

Although the adolescent may identify with the absent parent as a totality, we have also seen instances of the adolescent's identification with specific ambitions, hopes, and aspirations of the dead parent. If the absent parent was intensely invested in a particular achievement or goal, either for himself or herself or for the child, the adolescent feels compelled and at times almost driven to pursue and even complete the unfinished task of the lost object. Although such a quest may have an obviously unrealistic quality, the goal is often well thought out, planned, and pursued with diligence and tenacity. Some clinical examples may illustrate this point.

CASE STUDY 2

A thirteen-year-old boy engaged in an intensive physical conditioning program in pursuit of his goal of becoming a football player ran several miles every morning and lifted weights at night to attain peak physical condition. His father, who had died two years previously, had been a good football player in high school but had not played football in college. The father had blamed his lack of further athletic success on his inability to stay in shape because of commitments to his studies and work. The boy's mother supported her son's program with a sense of pride because he had apparently inherited his father's determination.

CASE STUDY 3

A twelve-year-old girl decided to become a fashion model after her mother's death the previous year. The mother, who died of leukemia, had always wanted to be a model but did not achieve this "because of an early marriage and pregnancy." The daughter sent away for various modeling catalogs and beauty aids and embarked on a controlled weight-loss program to attain a model's slimness.

CASE STUDY 4

> A fifteen-year-old girl, who had always been an average student, proceeded to show a dramatic improvement in her school performance following her father's death. The father had suffered from a chronic heart condition, and while he was confined they had spent much time together while the mother worked. During many of these periods, the father had helped the girl with her schoolwork and encouraged her to do well in her studies. He often reminisced about how well he had performed in high school and in college. Although the mother was somewhat uneasy about her daughter's staying up late to study, she also understood that this was the latter's manner of dealing with the loss.

Although the behaviors in the examples may be multidetermined and subject to a variety of dynamic interpretations, they do show a striking identification not only with the absent parent but, even more so, with the parent's accomplishments and hopes, dreams, and ambitions. Although these phenomena manifest an obvious constructive pattern, there is a certain driven and self-propelled quality about them and a seeming lack of both closure and integration into the total personality. Which aspects of these identifications eventually will be retained and which discarded is difficult to assess. It may well be that under stress such a defensive system will collapse and that the underlying pathology will then emerge.

CASE STUDY 5

> Carla was a bright, ambitious, conscientious fifteen-year-old whose mother had died two years previously. While Carla was in junior high school, she and her mother had fought constantly about her poor grades, poor atttitude toward school, and absence of extracurricular interests. After her mother's death, Carla's grades began to improve. She also became involved in student council, choir, and a school dance group. In addition, she worked part-time at a drug store. Soon after her father announced that he was getting married again, Carla began to lose interest in her schoolwork. She felt bored and apathetic, had numerous physical complaints, and repeatedly commented that all of her activities did not serve any useful purpose.

It is important to note that many of these cases' identifications and associated behavioral patterns were supported overtly and covertly by the surviving parent. However, these behaviors were also recognized as phenomena unique to each adolescent in the process of dealing with his or her loss.

If one discounts the occasional extremes of severe psychopathology on one end of the behavioral spectrum and relative contentment and maturity on the other, these adolescents' responses to a parent's death seem for the most part to fall somewhere in between these two poles. Some of these youngsters had the ability to discuss their loss fairly directly and openly. Although they were not overwhelmed with powerful affects, there was a certain somber tone and an underlying tension to their personalities. These cases were usually mid- to late-stage adolescents who were functioning adequately both in school and in other situations. Conflicts with the surviving parent were present but not outstanding. They were quite definite in their future hopes and plans and seemed realistic in their hopes of attaining these goals. Nonetheless, they were seen in consultation, and although there was no specific problem and/or conflict, there was the definite impression that something was amiss.

These youngsters indirectly conveyed a kind of drivenness and a certain sense of restlessness. This was evident from the content of the interviews as the adolescents detailed the various activities and numerous trips that composed their busy and frantic schedules. The more one listened to such details the more it became apparent that, in spite of their doing many things and doing them rather well, these adolescents derived little pleasure and satisfaction from these pursuits.

The process of the interviews also conveyed a certain tension and restlessness, as if the adolescents were searching for something but not quite finding it. They indirectly transmitted a demanding quality, and when this was responded to with interpretations, the latter were rejected with a sense of disappointment or with a "well that sounds OK, but. . . ." There was always the "but," as if there were a sense that something very basic was missing.

Such youngsters do not accept treatment, even though they know that all is not right, that something is missing that then has to be searched for, replaced, or compensated. They often reject treatment while simultaneously proposing a plan of action that will alleviate their uncomfortable state. Yet they know that such action will not be the answer, for they realize that the feigned enthusiasm is based on previous experiences of a similar nature. Although such individuals continue to function effectively and achieve various measures of success in their personal and professional lives, one must wonder if they ever succeed in mastering this pervasive sense of drivenness and restlessness.

Much of what we understand about adolescence and adolescent psychopathology has come from our insights into child development and adult psychopathology. Since psychoanalytic understanding of the adolescent has been a relative latecomer to the subjects of scientific literature, such extrapolations are plausible and to some extent acceptable. Nevertheless, there is the danger that we might adapt to the adolescent what we know about the child and the adult, even though such knowledge may not necessarily fit the adolescent's behavior.

Because of the fluidity of the adolescent's psychic organization, his mourning for the lost parent may be expressed in a number of differing ways. There are numerous adolescents who deal with their loss in the manner described by Wolfenstein (1966). They do hypercathect the image and the memory of the absent parent. They overidealize to defend against their ambivalence, and they form a split between a conscious awareness of the loss and an unconscious fantasy of reunion. There may also be other adolescents who are quite competent and skillful in dealing with their loss in the sequential mourning process that we assume to be characteristic of the adult. One could also postulate multiple combinations and variations of these extremes.

There are also certain characteristics unique to adolescent development that may either interfere with or facilitate the work of mourning. The adolescent's powerful amnesia regarding earlier life experiences is a natural developmental phenomenon and a viable deterrent from that integration of one's historical past that is such an integral part of the mourning process. The adolescent's ever-present fear of regression may manifest itself in an inability to experience certain affects, especially in an inhibition of crying and a blocking of anger.

In adolescence, one's sexual urges may impel one to detach oneself from one's beloved parents and from one's childhood. The intensity of sexual feelings may heighten the ambivalence and so interfere even further with mourning for the lost object. However, the adolescent's advanced cognitive development as well as the experience of trial mourning for the infantile objects can be seen as facilitators of an adult-like mourning process. The simultaneous longing for an idealized past and the conviction that it can never return may usher in a sense of hopelessness just as easily as it may promote a more realistic acceptance of the present.

Conclusions

In an attempt to understand the mourning of the adolescent in response to the loss of a parent, we have considered a number of interconnected possibilities. The existence of these various possibilities may be due to the multiple clinical observations that indicate that there are basically two concomitant processes for the adolescent to accomplish. One is the mourning for the parent as the infantile object, whereas the other is the mourning for the parent as the here-and-now real parent and as the internalized current object of the adolescent's attachment and ambivalent feelings.

To complete the so-called normal work of mourning requires much time and repetition. In the course of this work there may be a profound difference as to whether the mourned image of the childhood parent can be transformed gradually into a more reality-scaled image of the still-existing parent or whether such transformations have to be completed in fantasy alone, as in the case of the parent who died.

While recognizing those components of the child's response that are to be seen in the adolescent mourning, we have also attempted to highlight some of the latter's unique features. If we can succeed in recognizing what constitutes both the child's and adult mourning, we have only partly succeeded in understanding mourning in adolescence, for it is only with an appreciation for the integration of those components that make the adolescent unique that we can say something about that complexity that we call adolescence.

NOTE

I would like to thank Dr. Ann Petersen, head of Individual and Family Studies at Pennsylvania State Universiity, whose research on normal adolescent development stimulated many of the ideas in this paper. I would also like to thank Mrs. Nan Knight-Birnbaum from the Barr-Harris Center of the Chicago Institute for Psychoanalysis for allowing me to use her clinical material.

REFERENCES

Blos, P. 1962. *On Adolescence: A Psychoanalytic Interpretation*. New York: Macmillan.

Bonnard, A. 1961. Truancy and pilfering associated with bereavement. In S. Lorand and H. I. Schneer, eds. *Adolescence*. New York: Delta.

Bowlby, J. 1960. Grief and mourning in infancy and early childhood. *Psychoanalytic Study of the Child* 15:9–52.

Ewalt, P., and Perkins, L., 1979. The real experience of death among adolescents: an empirical study. *Social Casework* 19:547–551.

Fleming, J., and Altschul, S., 1963. Activation of mourning and growth of psychoanalysis. *International Journal of Psycho-Analysis* 44:419–432.

Freud, A. 1958. Adolescence. *Psychoanalytic Study of the Child* 13:255–278.

Furman, E. 1974. *A Child's Parent Dies: Studies in Childhood Bereavement*. New Haven, Conn.: Yale University Press.

Furman, R. 1964. Death and the young child: some preliminary considerations. *Psychoanalytic Study of the Child* 119:377–397.

Gapes, C. 1982. A study of bereaved adolescents and their church group. Unpublished manuscript.

Garber, B. 1980. The effects of the death of a parent and divorce on the child: a clinical comparison. Unpublished manuscript. Presented at Parenthood Conference, Michael Reese Hospital, Chicago, 1980.

Jacobson, E. 1964. *The Self and the Object World*. New York: International Universities Press.

Kilman, G. 1968. *Psychological Emergencies in Childhood*. New York: Grune & Stratten.

Lampl-deGroot, J. 1983. On the process of mourning. *Psychoanalytic Study of the Child* 38:9–13.

Laufer, M. 1966. Object loss in adolescence. *Psychoanalytic Study of the Child* 31:269–293.

Pollock, G. H. 1977. The mourning process and creative organizational change. *Journal of the American Psychoanalytic Association* 25:30–34.

Pollock, G. H. 1978. Process and affect: mourning and grief. *International Journal of Psycho-Analysis* 59:255–276.

Root, N. 1957. A neurosis in adolescence. *Psychoanalytic Study of the Child* 12:320–334.

Sugar, M. 1968. Normal adolescent mourning. *American Journal of Psychotherapy* 32:258–269.

Turnball, H. 1980. The concept of death in bereaved and non-bereaved latency and adolescent children. Master's thesis, University of Newcastle, New South Wales, Australia.

Wolfenstein, M. 1966. How is mourning possible? *Psychoanalytic Study of the Child* 21:93–123.

Wolfenstein, M. 1969. Loss, rage, and repetition. *Psychoanalytic Study of the Child* 24:432–460.

PART V

PSYCHOTHERAPEUTIC ISSUES IN ADOLESCENT PSYCHIATRY

EDITORS' INTRODUCTION

For most adolescent psychiatrists, the principal professional concern is their efforts to heal troubled patients with psychological—or at least psychosocial—interventions. Psychotherapy in its various forms is their primary technical instrument and they continue to seek ways of testing and improving its efficacy. Experience in varied settings leads to new advances in technique and the evolution of new strategies in applying and teaching them. The following chapters explore issues of training and administration as well as difficult psychopathological challenges.

John E. Meeks discusses inpatient management of the violent adolescent. In a comprehensive overview, he reviews contributing organic factors, life experiences (abuse), impaired ego functioning, pseudocompetency (grandiosity), and life-cycle heroic motives, as well as human reactions to real intimidation and a very rational fear of violence on the part of staff. Meeks outlines an approach to the treatment of violence in adolescents that first accepts the legitimacy of anger and desires for violence but then provides a wide range of sublimitory defenses, including a redefinition of heroes.

Norman R. Bernstein considers psychotherapy for the mentally retarded to be effective and discusses indications and goals along with the bias among professionals against this group. He examines the idealizing anaclitic transference of the retarded patient and the complicating negative countertransferences of therapists because they believe that the potential of these patients is minimal. Bernstein believes a therapist may alter the potential of the retarded more dramatically than patients with normal intellect and discusses establishing the atmosphere for treatment, conflict resolution, and use of the positive transference.

Dennis L. McCaughan reflects on the training experiences of the adolescent therapist as an object of the delinquent adolescent's disturbed and disturbing reactions to developmental crises. A principal assumption is that the adolescent therapist's response to the clinical setting often parallels the delinquent's reaction to the structure of the therapeutic milieu. The author illustrates the various ways therapists deal with problems of engagement and describes two patterns of adaptation and defense; flight from therapy and flight into therapy. A number of areas are discussed with specific recommendations regarding teaching, learning, and clinical goals: institutional and program philosophy, previous training attitudes, reactions to adolescents, perceptions and expectations, principles of supervision, and reactions to the developing therapist and the training experience.

Mary Davis and Irving A. Raffe describe the administrator-therapist team approach as used in inpatient psychiatric treatment of adolescents. Using Winnicott's and Lang's concepts of holding and containing, the authors clarify how the treatment environment can reduce fragmentation, provide consolidation and organization, and allow psychotherapeutic efforts to be more utilizable. The authors recommend that the clinical director serve the administrative role that then contains and metabolizes staff, patient, and parental conflict and allows the therapeutic process to proceed.

26 INPATIENT TREATMENT OF THE VIOLENT ADOLESCENT

JOHN E. MEEKS

Although violence is a common behavior among psychiatrically disturbed adolescents, there is a relative paucity of clinical studies on the topic in the psychiatric literature (Madden 1977; Nadelson 1977; Penningroth 1975; Richmond and Slagle 1971; Stine, Patrick, and Molina 1982). There are many excellent discussions of violence as an instinctual behavior and of the political meanings of violent behavior, and many reviews of the frequency of violence occurring in the psychiatric population (Halleck 1980; Kalogerakis 1971; Sosowsky 1978; Zitrin, Hardesty, and Burdock 1976). The use of medication to calm and quieten the acutely disturbed patient and the techniques through which staff can be trained to deal with threatening behavior in the psychiatric hospital are topics that have been covered (Madden 1977; Penningroth 1975; Shevitz 1978; Wilson 1976).

Perhaps the reason why there is so little in the way of comprehensive discussion about the inpatient management of the violent patient is related to the behavior itself. First of all, violence occurs in patients over the entire diagnostic spectrum. Psychotic, brain-damaged, intoxicated, and even severely anxious patients on occasion erupt into violence. In addition, the behavior itself is episodic rather than constant, so that in a real sense the question is, not how we should treat violence in the inpatient setting, but how we could prevent it and modify its origins for the future. Acute treatment of the violent actions of a patient are basically limited to efforts to contain that behavior in the safest manner possible utilizing humane restraint and/or a variety of medications. Aside from the still unproved possibility that lithium carbonate or carbomazapine may be ef-

0-226-24058-4/85/0012-0017$01.00

fective therapy for episodic dyscontrol, medications are important primarily as emergency measures of chemical restraint. Physical restraint may be essential since violent adolescents are, paradoxically, frightened by their own potential loss of control. They need reassurance that the environment will control them safely and without excessive counterforce. However, these measures, while important, help little in understanding the basic issues in inpatient treatment of the violent adolescent.

We are here faced with an episodic event, one that we can predict only inaccurately since there are too many causes—first, the entire range of contributing organic factors that, even if one excludes temperament, includes overt brain damage resulting from perinatal cerebral insults, infection, or injury (Elliot 1978; Lewis, Shanok, Pincus, and Giammarino 1982). In addition, most studies (and I would say the overall thrust of research findings) suggest that more subtle defects in cognitive functioning, such as learning disorders, also predispose to violent delinquency (Karniski, Levine, Clark, Palfrey, and Meltzer 1982). Drug intoxication, particularly with alcohol, phencyclidine, and secobarbital, strongly increases the possibility of violent outbursts (Rinklenberg and Stillmen 1970; Simons and Kashani 1979; Tinklenberg, Murphy, and Pfefferbaum 1981). Reactions from withdrawal from these drugs, particularly the amphetamines, may include violent behavior as a component.

To further extend our already long list of important factors, we must now look to the life experiences of the adolescent. There are extensive data to indicate that youngsters who have been the victims of violent physical abuse themselves are more likely to show violent behavior later. Even if violence in the home has not been directed personally toward the child, merely observing the habitual utilization of violence as a problem-solving technique encourages the adolescent to adopt this behavior as part of his or her coping armamentarium.

One common quality which unites all of the causative factors that we have described is their impact on the individual's adaptive skills. Generally speaking, all of the etiological elements that we have discussed act to impair ego functioning and the successful development of self and secondary narcissism. In various ways these conditions or events interfere either with the structures that determine coping skills or with the learning experiences necessary to encourage proper development.

It is a commonplace observation that delinquent adolescents, as well as adolescents with episodic dyscontrol and most youngsters with paranoid problems, demonstrate low self-esteem and generally feel helpless and driven by the winds of fate. They do not believe that they possess the ability to control their own lives. Clinical evaluation of their capacities often confirms a deficient level of skills in interpersonal relationships, study and learning habits, and techniques of problem solving.

Given this state of affairs, the tendency to develop Erikson's negative identity patterns and to embrace life-styles which permit achievement of a pseudocompetence is very understandable. Pseudocompetence is gained, for example, through that spurious sense of well-being. Pseudocompetence may also be gained by joining subcultures with value systems that confer prestige and a sense of accomplishment to those who cannot gain such prizes in the more conventional world. For example, in the delinquent subculture, impulsive daring and shortsighted bravado as well as physical violence may gain one a reputation for bravery and leadership. Rebellion against standard measures of success, such as academic performance, in this subculture would be applauded rather than condemned. In such a world a prudent measuring of risk and consequence may be viewed as simply a lack of courage.

Violence plays a very important role in the world of pseudosolutions. Violent acts are clear-cut and simple as well as rapid and easily seen. To make the point through an oversimplification: a latency child in the playroom can spend frustrating extended periods of time attempting to build a tower from blocks. If he has some problems with coordination or in his capacity for visual conception, the effort may be attended by a variety of failures as blocks tumble down or refuse to rise in the directions of the child's dreams. Even when the task is successfully completed, the structure may or may not please the youngster, or he may fear that it is not good enough for others. He will worry about what others think since construction is always at least partially done to please, impress, and reward others. On the other hand, with a single decisive, powerful swipe of the hand, the largest tower of blocks can be reduced to instant shambles. The resulting sense of mastery, total control, and strength is highly satisfying. Often it is accompanied by a sense of triumph over the play therapist and a gleam in the child's eye that says he is happy to be relieved of the burden of trying to please. This satisfying piece of violence toward an inanimate object carries a sense of finality which makes one feel that a problem has been *solved*. No more fumbling around! The destructive action also provides a sense of self-sufficiency and independence that I have called pseudocompetency and that can be at least temporarily reassuring. Trying to build a tower can be slow and frustrating if one's skills are poor or if one is subjected to harsh criticism or expects to be, based on one's previous experience. In the effort one feels weak, ineffective, oppressed by the demands of others, discouraged, and frustrated. In contrast, knocking the tower across the room is quick, makes one feel strong, and sweeps away the demands of others in one carefree and triumphant moment. Pseudocompetence is the silver lining of self-doubt and servitude.

The leap from our example to the complex topic of violent behavior is a large one, and we shall lose something in the transition. However, I think if we expand our definition to include not only violence toward other people but also extreme outbursts of violence toward property, and if we keep in mind that the complexity of the topic will always defeat any efforts toward excessive generalization, I think we may gain from applying some of these ideas to the violent adolescent and young adult. Let us begin with two well-documented examples reported outside the clinical literature.

In the first example, a nomadic young adult, attempting to stabilize what had reportedly been a somewhat turbulent youth, was employed by a farmer. The drifter formed a warm relationship with the farmer's family, especially a latency-age son, and seemed content in his new position. However, the farmer faced a number of economic difficulties, many of which clearly resulted from unfair business tactics practiced by a major competitor whose goals for development in the area were quite different from those held by the farmer. As a result of his employment by the farmer, the drifter also experienced considerable harassment and even humiliation at the hands of the competitor. Eventually, the tactics engaged in by the villainous competition became so reprehensible and threatening that the drifter, apparently in a fit of white rage, armed himself, went into the home territory of the competitor, and in the course of a gunfight killed the competitor and his associates.

A second example involved a washed-up ex-boxer (probably with some degree of brain damage secondary to that experience) who became gradually convinced that the union with which he and his relatives and friends were involved was wicked and grossly oppressive. Ignoring all realistic caution and using only his bare fists, he eventually erupted into violence against that group of individuals.

Both of these examples illustrate some of the common characteristics of the violent person. According to Halleck (1980), two of the common motives for engaging in violent activity are to escape oppression and to increase self-esteem. In our examples both of these motives seem predominant. Some readers may have recognized our first example as the behavior of the character Shane in the movie of the same name and our second example as the character played by Marlon Brando in the famous film *On the Waterfront*. In these two films one is gradually led to identify with a sympathetic character who encounters escalating frustration at the hands of villainous and violent opponents. Gradually, both the character and the viewer are forced to conclude that the only solution is a violent one. I think it is safe to say that almost everyone who sees these movies experiences the final scene of violence as justified, satisfying, and very logical. Shane and Brando were heroes, their violence heroic.

Halleck also notes three other common motives for violent behavior: (1) to gain power or control over others; (2) to gain territory or wealth previously held by others; and (3) to gratify emotional needs such as sadism or revenge. If the motives we ascribed to Shane, namely, to escape oppression and to increase self-esteem or at least to avoid humiliation, are heroic motives for violence, then the three reasons might be considered to be the villain's motives for resorting to violence.

Now, with our oversimplified model, let us look at the nature of violent behavior in the adolescent inpatient. Are they villains or are they heroes?

To some extent, the answers to this question depend on one's perspective. The staff often feel that the adolescent patient is threatening violence or engaging in violent behavior in order to gain power and control over them and to satisfy an unhealthy desire to feel triumphant over staff and staff rules. In the case of some adolescent patients, the staff feel that the youngsters do gain a pathological emotional thrill from intimidation and violent behavior. Villains for sure! Since I no longer have to seclude aggressive adolescent patients, I feel that these opinions are obviously distorted. They are understandable countertransference reactions to the threat of violence. In fact, it may be incorrect to refer to these staff attitudes as countertransference. They may be just human reactions to real intimidation and a very rational fear of violence.

While I say that I do not agree with the staff's opinion about the nature of most violence in adolescent inpatients, I do not mean to suggest that we do not get any villains admitted to our unit. Since our program includes a unit which specializes in treating youngsters with a combination of psychiatric and drug problems, we admit and evaluate a number of antisocial youngsters who regularly utilize violent action to gain power and control over others. They use force to secure and maintain their drug-dealing territories, and they use violence and threats in outright extortion for financial gain. Many of these young people are convicted criminals who have been involved in armed robbery and other violent acts designed to gain villainous ends. Some of them embrace this view of themselves with considerable comfort and enjoy thinking of themselves as tough, streetwise "enforcers."

The point is, for the most part these youngsters are not usually violent in the hospital setting. Since they are basically entrepreneurs who somewhat voluntarily and consciously utilize violence to gain fairly rational ends, they are similar to the individuals in organized crime or the professional "hit man" or assassins who utilize violence not out of passion but from a conscious decision that it will gain them certain practical objectives.

In the hospital setting, these genuine villains recognize quickly that there is little to be gained by open shows of force since they are unlikely to emerge victorious. They may secretly engage in a variety of intimidating activities in order to gain special privileges among the patient group as well as to enjoy the sense of power that may come from being feared. However, when directly challenged, they rarely explode into violence toward the staff but engage instead in negotiation, subterfuge, conning, and other techniques that are more likely to be successful. In my experience, at least, our villainous adolescents may frighten and intimidate the staff but, in fact, rarely erupt directly into violent activity—at least as long as the overall milieu remains constructive. These individuals can become quite dangerous under riot conditions, as reports of a number of uprisings on adolescent units have confirmed. However, in the normal course of events, almost all of our problems with violence come not from our villains but directly from our heroes.

Clinical Example

Bobby was seventeen years old when he was admitted to the hospital because of uncontrolled polydrug use, inability to accept any limits from his mother, uninterest in getting a job or pursuing any occupational goals, and an increasingly dangerous tendency to become involved in violent fights. In the three months prior to admission Bobby had been in numerous fights, two of which were very serious. In the first one he received a massive laceration of his face and head which had already required one episode of plastic surgery and appeared to require a second to avoid serious scarring. He emerged from the second fight with two broken fingers and an injured leg. In addition, Bobby had been in trouble with the law, having been arrested once for breaking and entering and on another occasion for possession of a switchblade. Bobby was opposed to hospitalization and insisted that he had no serious drug problems. He did admit, however, that he had been feeling depressed since his graduation from high school and was concerned that he did not seem able to develop any interest in his future. He agreed, somewhat ambivalently, to give the hospital a chance.

Over the first few weeks of hospitalization, psychotherapy sessions with Bobby were characterized by a steady diet of opposition, negativism, and disputation. He questioned the basic therapeutic philosophy of the hospital program, which he regarded as Pollyannaish and unrealistic. He was afraid we would turn him into, as he put it, "a pussy." It should be noted that Bobby engaged in these argumentative activities with considerable skill. Unlike many youngsters we see, Bobby had no evidence of brain damage aside from one febrile seizure in early childhood. He had no learning problems, and his IQ was a sparkling 135. He was a worthy opponent on the verbal battlefield.

Bobby particularly objected to the efforts of the staff and the psychiatrist to convince him that his involvement in violent fighting was part of his difficulty. In fact, even after he began to recognize that drugs presented more of a problem for him than he had originally admitted and that they did play a major role in his chronic depression, he still argued for the necessity in his world of frequent violent response. It should be noted here that Bobby was not a ghetto child but in fact lived in a lower-middle-class to middle-class neighborhood that was not characterized by massive social disorder or ridden with crime. Bobby's predilection for fisticuffs was socially deviant in his environment.

Bobby did not claim that his violent behavior was purely self-defense. He saw it instead as directed toward assuring social justice and maintaining his own good name and self-esteem. Gradually Bobby described his peer interactions and the role that fighting played in them. In his depressive view of himself, Bobby did not really expect to be liked. In some ways his situation with peers was a reaction to his place in his family. Bobby's mother had been twice divorced. In her opinion neither husband had been particularly fond of Bobby. Bobby's younger brother had a congenital heart defect and was overprotected and doted upon by mother and the maternal grandparents. Bobby's older brother was adored by the grandparents—who rationalized his cruel physical domination of Bobby. Bobby's mother worked all day so that Bobby was often left at the mercy of his big brother, who taunted and beat him regularly throughout much of his early childhood. When the mother would come home she would feel sorry for Bobby and take up for him, but this seemed only to increase his brother's anger at him. This annoyance tended to be expressed on the following day when mother was no longer around to provide protection. Bobby soon learned not to complain about his brother and, instead, gradually became more effective at fighting back. By the time adolescence was reached, the older brother's intimidation was greatly reduced because Bobby could hold his own in a fight. However, the two brothers occasionally still fought and had to be separated to prevent the possibility of bodily harm to one or the other.

In any case, Bobby's friends encouraged Bobby to see himself as unusually brave and tough. They called on him as a bodyguard whenever any of them was bothered by other youngsters who were regarded as bullies. When they had a problem they would sic Bobby onto the offender. Bobby would taunt and provoke the enemy until he either fought or backed down publicly and promised not to bother Bobby's friends again. Naturally, this position in the peer group marked Bobby as the modern equivalent of a gunslinger. Those who wished to make a name would periodically challenge him since, if they were able to beat Bobby, they would have proved their mettle. Bobby was quite paranoid about the possibility of being hurt in this way and was very worried that hospitalization might lower his physical skills, which he kept finely honed by working out regularly in a community gymnasium. Bobby was also willing to consider giving up drugs because he recognized that on several occasions he had lost fights and, indeed, had been badly hurt because some of his enemies simply waited until he was sufficiently under the influence of drugs that he would not be effective in combat. On the other hand, Bobby was convinced that a moderate amount of alcohol greatly increased his effectiveness in battle since it raised his pain threshold, removed anxiety, and raised his enthusiasm for the fight. Naturally, in the small society of the psychiatric treatment unit, Bobby was tempted to utilize his skills as a fighter. There was absolutely no doubt that he saw himself as a hero. His near-fights occurred when he defended the honor of some of the girls on the unit, stood up for a youngster whom he saw as oppressed and unfairly treated, and, of course, most often when he felt the yoke of oppression was settling on him.

There were some near-scrapes with the staff around the highly structured and somewhat strict controls of the unit. As noted, Bobby was not accustomed to rules and generally ignored those placed on him by his mother. He experienced the inpatient restrictions as demeaning and frequently saw the staff as simply trying to, as he put it once, "prove they had the keys."

Bobby's management in treatment was extremely complex and proceeded on a number of fronts. Family therapy was quite active and had to include his brothers. Since his mother had received a diagnosis of bipolar affective illness, Bobby was carefully tested for any biological evidence of endogenous depression. These tests were negative. There were many other issues, too. However, it may be more truthful than poetic to say that most of Bobby's treatment centered around two goals. The first was to help Bobby see that he had the basic equipment and many basic attributes of genuine heroism. The second was defining his previous behavior and his natural inclinations toward violence as less heroic than he previously had thought. We tried to convince Bobby that he could be competent, that he did not need pseudocompetence.

First of all, the entire staff worked to understand Bobby's view of the world. They decided together to avoid power struggles with him as much as possible by carefully orienting him to all the rules before he was in a position of conflict with any of them and by offering him options and choices whenever possible. They made the decision to accept and indeed to praise verbal opposition, labeling it as honesty and independence of thinking. This acceptance was always accompanied by a reminder that behavioral compliance with the rules and expectations of the unit would still be required even when Bobby disagreed with them. Every effort was made to encourage Bobby to become active in the student government and to learn the acceptable approaches to changing rules and practices on the unit. The staff realized early that, like many potentially violent people, Bobby required a good deal of physical space. Bobby seemed to experience people standing close to him and particularly people touching him as an invasive provocation. He even evaded extended eye contact not out of embarrassment but out of a fear of being controlled or dominated—as though he thought everyone had the power of the evil eye.

While accommodating some of Bobby's defenses, the staff decided that his fear of backing down would be addressed as a weakness—an understandable weakness, but a weakness nonetheless. In Bobby's psychotherapy, every possible example of when it took courage to avoid a fight or provocative comment was noted and underlined to him. His tendency to be used by others to fight their battles was pointed out sympathetically as an understandable insecurity rather than as a noble knight-errant mission. This was first addressed around his interactions with youngsters on the unit who used him to gain their ends but was gradually expanded to help him look at his peer interactions at home.

Bobby never agreed verbally with any of these new versions of reality that were presented to him. In fact, he continued to argue, verbally defend the underdog, and describe his plans to wreak physical havoc on almost everyone who made him angry. However, his actual behavior changed in many ways, both overt and subtle. Bobby became pleasant to be around. He smiled and relaxed and in obvious ways sought out the company of the male staff whom he admired, with only the expected transparent adolescent denial of dependency and desire for approval. More important, when important treatment issues arose with other patients, Bobby almost invariably came through with good advice, human supportiveness, and sensible compromises. He was clearly a constructive leader and was elected representative to the student government from his treatment team. Finally he was discharged to outpatient treatment, still verbally promising nothing, indeed, suggesting that he might well continue extensive contact with his old friends and with drugs, but at the same time demonstrating entirely different interactional patterns within his family and with the treatment team, which he left with appropriate affectionate regret.

I hope that by telling the story of Bobby I have illustrated that the inpatient treatment of a violent adolescent can be largely a matter of the redefinition of heroes. In addition to some of the individualized elements that I described, there are general approaches which are also important. First, there should be an explicit statement that violence will not be permitted in the inpatient program, accompanied by a clear explanation for the necessity of this position. It must be made clear to each patient that, although the staff does not wish to be hurt, that concern is not the only reason why violence is forbidden in the inpatient treatment setting. The treatment process is defined as an effort to learn to deal with one's feelings and with other people in such a way that there can be a satisfaction with life, no disabling symptoms, and sufficient comfort and happiness to avoid the temptations of crippling drug abuse. To achieve these goals, the patient will need to learn to deal with intensely angry feelings as well as many secret feelings of shame and inadequacy that cause him or her to feel highly vulnerable when exposed. It is obvious that it would be utopian to try to create an atmosphere where anger could be discussed openly, where differences between people could be addressed honestly and directly, and where people would feel safe to reveal uncomfortable secrets about themselves if the environment included the possibility of physical violence. In other words, violence is not permitted because violence would destroy the very hope that brought the youngster to the hospital, namely, the hope that he can be treated and will be able to help himself gain a more satisfactory life.

Now, there are some unstated assumptions here. Obviously, the sense of oppression felt righteously by many of our patients is seen as very unrealistic by the rest of the world. A treatment program tries to make the patient feel more rationally powerful, therefore less vulnerable to oppression. Treatment also tries to redefine malice and oppression. For example, limits and controls are shown to be beneficial organizers of life rather than arbitrary attacks on autonomy. If paranoia distorts benign interiors or if detoxification produces pathological sensitivity, these issues are addressed with medication, explanation, and any other interventions that may help to constructively redefine the situation. Phantom enemies can be dispelled. However, the entire sense of reality of the youngster cannot be challenged.

Conclusions

In the inpatient treatment of violent adolescents, the legitimacy of angry feelings and even desires for violence that the patient feels must be accepted. Legitimate alternatives must be presented that include such things as assertiveness training, symbolic outlets like art therapy, opportunities for supervised confrontation of conflict between patients and between patients and staff, and a willingness to understand the origins of anger and to assist the patient in resolving internal chronic hostility. Finally, as I think we could see in the treatment of Bobby, the treatment program needs to espouse convincingly a value system that insists that it is more heroic to avoid violence than to inflict it on even the most deserving villains. It is probably impossible to extend this value system of total pacifism to all people. For example, in the rural area where I grew up, a total unwillingness to fight under any circumstances was virtually a provocation, whereas the ritual and relatively harmless scraps engaged in by the various youngsters established an accepted pecking order and a comfortable interaction. However, at least in the treatment milieu, the adolescent can learn that it is possible to find solutions without violence and for many, perhaps, with a gain of honor and respect through building competence in positive interactions with others. The lesson may not hold in all situations throughout all time, but it is still worth learning that there is more genuine satisfaction in the laborious and intricate task of building a tower than in the illusory triumph of destroying one.

REFERENCES

Elliot, F. A. 1978. Neurological factors in violent behavior. In R. Sadoff, ed. *Violence and Responsibility*. New York: Spectrum.

Halleck, S. 1980. Social violence and aggression. In H. I. Kaplan, A. M. Freedman, and B. J. Sadock, eds. *Comprehensive Textbook of Psychiatry*. 3:3149–3155. Baltimore: Williams & Wilkins.

Kalogerakis, M. G. 1971. The assaultive psychiatric patient. *Psychiatric Quarterly* 45:372–381.

Karniski, W. M.; Levine, M. D.; Clark, S.; Palfrey, J. S.; and Meltzer, L. J. 1982. A study of neurodevelopmental findings in early adolescent delinquents. *Journal of Adolescent Health Care* 3:151–156.

Kinzel, A. F. 1970. Body-buffer zone in violent prisoners. *American Journal of Psychiatry* 127:62–63.

Lewis, D. O.; Shanok, S. S.; Pincus, J. H.; and Giammarino, M. 1982. The medical assessment of seriously delinquent boys: a comparison of pediatric, psychiatric, neurological and hospital record data. *Journal of Adolescent Health Care* 3:160–164.

Madden, D. J. 1977. Voluntary and involuntary treatment of aggressive patients. *American Journal of Psychiatry* 134:553–555.

Nadelson, T. 1977. Borderline rage and the therapist's response. *American Journal of Psychiatry* 134:748–759.

Penningroth, P. E. 1975. Control of violence in a mental health setting. *American Journal of Nursing* 75:607–609.

Richmond, A. H., and Slagle, S. 1971. Some notes on the inhibition of aggression in an inpatient psychotherapy group. *International Journal of Group Psychotherapy* 21:333–338.

Rinklenberg, A., and Stillmen, W. 1970. Drug uses and violence. In D. Daniels, M. Gilula, and F. Ochberg, eds. *Violence and the Struggle for Existence*. Boston: Little, Brown.

Shevitz, S. 1978. Emergency management of the agitated patient. *Primary Care* 5:625–634.

Simons, J. F., and Kashani, J. 1979. Drug abuse and criminal behavior in delinquent boys committed to a training school. *American Journal of Psychiatry* 136:1444–1448.

Sosowsky, L. 1978. Crime and violence among mental patients reconsidered. *American Journal of Psychiatry* 135:33–137.

Stine, L. J.; Patrick, S. W.; and Molina, J. 1982. What is the role of violence in the therapeutic community? *International Journal of the Addictions* 17:377–391.

Tinklenberg, J. R.; Murphy, P.; and Pfefferbaum, A. 1981. Drugs and criminal assaults by adolescents: a replication study. *Journal of Psychoactive Drugs* 13:277–286.

Wilson, J. G. 1976. A program for the prevention and management of disturbed behavior. *Hospital Community Psychiatry*. 27:724–729.

Zitrin, A.; Hardesty, A. S.; and Burdock, E. L. 1976. Crime and violence among mental patients. *American Journal of Psychiatry* 133:142.

27 PSYCHOTHERAPY OF THE RETARDED ADOLESCENT

NORMAN R. BERNSTEIN

There is a good deal of evidence that psychotherapy has been effective with the retarded, and yet there remains a strong bias against this group by psychiatrists, psychologists, and social workers. DSM-III acknowledges the realities of the mental retardation dilemma by permitting a diagnosis of both the developmental handicap and the behavioral psychopathology. The wide range of disorders that may be seen encompasses the whole of the nomenclature of psychiatry.

In treating retarded patients, it is important to make an accurate diagnosis and not to dismiss behavioral manifestations simply as part of some vague concept (Adams 1975; Bernstein 1970, 1978, 1979a). The strategy of treatment should be laid out with goals stated by Jakab (1982): (1) to alleviate the symptoms painful or uncomfortable to the patient; (2) to improve behavior which is socially unacceptable; (3) to accumulate positive affective experiences of love, gratification, and acceptance for the intellectually handicapped patient; (4) to help the patient realize his or her intellectual potential, meaning to remove psychological disturbances which impair the utilization of the patient's already diminished faculties; and (5) to enable the patient to accumulate social and factual knowledge consistent with the level of the retardation.

A major factor in dealing with retarded people is the transference. The dependence of the retarded tends to make for an idealizing and anaclitic type of transference that, overall, can be an aid to therapy since these patients are so eager to please and work toward treatment goals for approval. One of the major handicaps of therapy is the negative counter-

0-226-24058-4/85/0012-0027$01.00

transference which is often demeaning about what can be done and dismissive about what the therapist wants to do. Many therapists dislike working with this group because one of the shibboleths of psychiatry is treating patients with potential. In referring normal IQ patients for therapy, it is always more positive to talk about their unrealized skills or unleashed creativity—even if it never comes to pass. In fact, one may alter the potential of the retarded more dramatically through psychotherapy than one does for patients of normal intellect. Szymanski (1980) wrote that, in the psychotherapy of emotional disorders of mentally retarded persons, there are several features that must be attended in terms of the style of the therapy (Bernstein 1979b); the directness of the therapist is very important, and the language level of the therapist needs to be congruent with the level of functioning of the patient.

Retarded people are able to verbalize much more than they are given credit for. If someone is functioning on the level of a nine-year-old in terms of intellectual or mental age, this is a level that is consistent with good expression of emotions, hopes, and fantasies—as is seen in the therapy of more intellectually normal children. Nonverbal techniques which are suitable to younger children may also be applied. Techniques such as drawing, model making, and doll play may be helpful. The body language from sitting close to the patient, shaking hands with the patient, and patting the patient reassuringly is useful in communicating affection and support.

Establishing the Atmosphere for Treatment

Many of the things that are taken for granted in treating adolescents of normal intellect need to be underscored, verbally stated, and clearly contracted with the parents of the retarded. The patient needs to hear in the presence of his parents what will be done, what will be kept secret, and what accusations of misconduct and claims of emotional disturbance will be worked on (Loft 1970; Parish, Baker, Arheart, and Adamchak 1980). The role of the doctor needs to be restated as being one of a helping friend rather than of a punitive agent of society who is punishing the patient. Retardates do not have structurally more rigid superegos but, rather, a life experience in which crude standards of good and bad are imprinted.

Entry into the world of the retarded child follows easily if the contract for treatment has been described as a working, friendly, helping matter in which the patient has a right to some privacy. The therapist must clearly make the atmosphere a friendly one while encouraging the patient to express inner doubts, fears, and concerns verbally as well as in pictures and play. However, for the mildly retarded, words remain the basic vehicle if they are encouraged along this line. Retarded adolescents are even more sensitive than the regular adolescent patient in fearing the criticism or negative attitude of the therapist, and this needs to be carefully and constantly watched in the course of the treatment.

Storr (1979) wrote, "Psychotherapists seem to be best at treating the inhibited, the frightened, the shy, the self-destructive, the fragmented, the overdependent, and the overcontrolled. They are far less successful with those who lack control over their impulses and who act out their emotional conflicts." This presents an immediate paradox in mental retardation because the social structuring of the role of the retarded is one that permits retarded people who are very disturbed but quiet to be left alone. The retarded person who is withdrawn and obedient may bear in isolation an enormous amount of pathology. People, however, are not concerned about it until the patient does something that causes social embarrassment or problems of management; then he or she is referred with alacrity. Storr goes on cogently:

> The first duty is to provide a secure, reliable background of personal concern against which the patient can develop. Just as a child may be assumed to develop toward maturity in the best way if he is fortunate enough to live in a stable home in which continuing care is taken for granted, so it is assumed that neurotic patients are more likely to learn to understand themselves and to cope better with their personal problems if they are provided with a secure base in the shape of a therapist to whom they can turn as a caring, concerned person.

In terms of the overall matrix for mounting therapy for the retarded, Cytryn and Lourie (1975) stress that psychotherapy must be effectively integrated into a plan for the whole life of the patient, including family treatment along with the work of the treatment center or school. Parental attitudes influencing treatment are often different from those of parents with physically handicapped offspring. The anger of parents about their plight is often a major issue which must be attended to in establishing and maintaining a therapeutic environment. The parents of the retarded are often enraged, frustrated, and unhappy about what has been their fate, and this is coupled with the reality that they often do not get good care for the retarded from any professional group.

Intellectually retarded children usually suffer acutely from archaic fears. Owing to the immaturity of their ego functions, they lack orientation and mastery of their inner and outer worlds alike; the very intensity of this anxiety in turn prevents further ego growth. In successful child therapy of the retarded, this vicious circle is interrupted, with the result that the child can proceed gradually along the development scale mastering apprehension over annihilation, separation anxiety, castration anxiety, fear of loss of love, and guilt. But the therapeutic element responsible for improvement in these cases is more the therapist's reassuring role, not his analytic one (Freud 1965; Sternlicht 1965).

CASE EXAMPLE 1

A twenty-year-old male with an IQ of 62 had been dismissed from his job carrying cartons in a supermarket when the market went bankrupt. He began to wander in the streets and was picked up by the police, who suspected that he was following young women or children with sexual intent. He was terrified by the experience and withdrew to his room where he was preoccupied, less interested in eating, truculent with his mother, and frequently found masturbating.

Patient had two siblings and two working parents who consistently brought him for special help as he was growing up. As he reached adulthood his family became fearful of his sexual impulses and dreaded that these might lead to catastrophe for himself and harm to some innocent victim. The patient himself was fearful of his desires, though he had never done anything beyond staring at girls and fantasizing conventional sexual activities, stimulated by television and sexual content in magazines.

In interviews with his therapist, he was impressed through repeated reassurances in front of his family and while alone that his therapy was not a punishment but a place for him to talk and work out his feelings. Efforts were made to find another job. He was given permission for, and his parents were told not to interfere with, his masturbation. In his sessions he began to explore two salient areas: the loss of the job and all the social contacts which went with that and his sexual fantasies. While he did produce some incestuous fantasies about his married sister, there had been no overt activity, and he was relieved by telling about it. He was cautioned that incest was something he should not ever do but that sexuality was something that he could experience. He began to come out of his room to deal in his more usual way with the family. As independent work jobs were hard to find, he was placed in a sheltered workshop and efforts continued to find another job. The therapist kept in contact with him on an as-needed basis for about eight months after the end of their twelve interviews, and he was not in further difficulty.

Retarded patients sustain more reality loss than other patients. The retarded commonly lack a varied social input, and they are delighted to have an interested adult in the therapist explore their personal world with them. When, however, this opportunity is terminated they feel it intensely and find it hard to replace. For this reason, many who work with the intellectually handicapped will continue supportive sessions over a long period of time and exchange cards and Christmas letters and remain available for an extended period after active treatment has ended. An occasional phone call to or from the family helps maintain this relationship.

Conflict Resolution

One of the reasons therapists devalue therapy of the retarded is that many feel they cannot accomplish the kind of conflict-resolving, exploratory psychotherapy that they find most creative and satisfying. On the contrary, psychotherapy should be undertaken with retarded people because, since the conflicts they face are likely to be more simple and direct, they are more readily accessible to resolution. The alliance is tied also to the willingness of the patient to please the therapist, and the positiveness of the transference helps enhance the self-image of the patient by showing he is a worthwhile person for examination and treatment even though he is slow. As Zigler (1966) has pointed out, the retarded person frequently, in contrast to the normal young person, does not get his major gratification from doing the job; he gets it from the praise he receives from the person overseeing the job. The style of the therapist must be a more active one. He needs to say things to introduce subjects, to make bridges for the patient to finish some of his fragmentary comments, and he must actively demand that the patient not lapse into passivity and silence when fully capable of delineating his personal and private feelings in many events.

CASE EXAMPLE 2

A fifteen-year-old retarded girl was brought for evaluation because she had been "acting crazy" in her residence. She became moody and combative and said silly things to the staff after having been a generally cooperative child with a tendency toward hypermotility. Recently she had begun talking to herself, looking for fights, and being preoccupied with her body and posture. At the assessment interview, she presented herself as a pubertal, well-developed black female. Her IQ was reported as 55. Exploration with her in interviews about her changing body and her fears of sexuality began to quiet her down in her day-to-day behavior. She also required work with the staff; they were told that what actually was happening was not a deterioration into schizophrenia but the reaction of a handicapped, ill-equipped child who was caught among her sexual impulses, her fear of changes in her body, her desire to attract people, and her wish for attention of all kinds. She was seen supportively by a female therapist who helped sort out with her hobbies and interests that could involve her and also clearly laid out the rules by which the patient had to live in her residential environment. They reviewed sexual rules of conduct and reviewed reproductive information numerous times. In doing so, the therapist helped the patient explore and clarify conflicted attitudes toward sex and her bodily changes.

Some patients do not appear retarded and can manage well in life because of this. Two-thirds of the retarded disappear into the general population without any professional help.

CASE EXAMPLE 3

An anxious, fourteen-year-old girl had been referred to a community health clinic for treatment for her multiple phobias of streets, elevators, storms, the dark, and animals. She was a pretty and compliant girl who seemed more like a latency-age schoolchild than an adolescent, but, as she came from an immigrant background, retardation was not diagnosed in the referral to the community clinic. She responded very quickly to psychotherapy that involved active support and environmental manipulation to get her to go out, to go into elevators, and to accompany the therapist while talking out her fears. It was only when psychological testing was done to prepare the patient for conference presentation that the level of her IQ (67) was made evident. This is in keeping with the experience of many clinicians and research workers that attractive-looking children are much less likely to be considered retarded and that people who are treated as more intelligent will behave appropriately even if they are intellectually handicapped (Rosenthal 1968).

Conclusions

The biggest handicap in treatment remains the negative countertransference that psychiatrists feel in dealing with people of low intellectual potential. The best antidote to this is clinical experience—seeing the retarded quickly and gratefully responding to treatment. When this is observed by psychiatrists, they rapidly become enthusiastic about therapy with this group. The limits of intellectual competence no longer seem as handicapping. The transference of retarded patients is quickly shown by their trust, passivity, and dependence. They hunger for attention, especially that of teachers and doctors. Once the manifestations of positive transference become evident, the patient can be given clear directives about behavior and taught the limits of friendly interaction in therapy. The patient needs to be shown that the interest of the therapist is not seductive but, rather, energetic supportiveness. Modest environmental manipulation of work and sleep arrangements can be very effective in therapy of this type, with significant improvement in the patient's functioning. The best tactic is to tell and teach repeatedly what is being done, and why.

Therapy of the retarded is both challenging and rewarding. The therapist of the retarded adolescent patient must come across as friendly, active, and real to his patients. An experienced therapist will require very little shift in style to be able to help intellectually handicapped adolescents. Help can be direct, short term, and enormously significant in the life coping and long-term adjustment of these patients.

REFERENCES

Adams, P. 1975. *A Primer of Child Psychotherapy*. Boston: Little, Brown.

Bernstein, N. R. 1970. *Diminished People*. Boston: Little, Brown.

Bernstein, N. R. 1978. Mental retardation. In A. Nicholai, ed. *The Harvard Guide to Modern Psychiatry*. Cambridge, Mass.: Harvard University Press.

Bernstein, N. R. 1979a. Special therapeutic considerations, mental retardation. In J. Noshpitz, ed. *Basic Handbook of Child Psychiatry*. New York: Basic.

Bernstein, N. R. 1979b. Psychiatric consultation in mental retardation X. Formulated by the Committee on Mental Retardation Group for the Advancement of Psychiatry, New York.

Cytryn, L., and Lourie, R. 1975. Mental retardation. In A. Freedman and H. Kaplan, eds. *Comprehensive Textbook of Psychiatry*. 2d ed. Baltimore: Williams & Wilkins.

Freud, A. 1965. *Normality and Pathology in Children: Assessment of Development*. New York: International Universities Press.

Jakab, L . 1982. Psychiatric disorders in mental retardation. In I. Jaleb, ed. *Mental Retardation*. New York: Karger.

Loft, G. 1970. Psychotherapy of the mentally retarded: values and cautions. In F. J. Menolascino, ed. *Psychiatric Approaches to Mental Retardation*. New York: Basic.

Parish, T. S.; Baker, S. K.; Arheart, K. L.; and Adamchak, P. G. 1980. Normal and exceptional children's attitude toward themselves and one another. *Journal of Psychology* 104:249–253.

Rosenthal, R. 1968. *Pygmalion in the Classroom: Teachers' Expectations and Pupils' Intellectual Development*. New York: Irvington Press.

Sternlicht, M. 1965. Psychotherapeutic techniques useful with the mentally retarded: a review and critique. *Psychiatric Quarterly* 39:84.

Storr, A. 1979. *The Art of Psychotherapy*. New York: Methuen.

Szymanski, L. 1980. Individual psychotherapy with retarded persons. In L. Szymanski and P. Tanguay, eds. *Emotional Disorders of Mentally Retarded Persons*. Baltimore: University Park Press.

Zigler, E. 1966. Research on personality structure in the retardate. In N. Ellis, ed. *International Review of Research in Mental Retardation*. New York: Academic Press.

28 TEACHING AND LEARNING ADOLESCENT PSYCHOTHERAPY: ADOLESCENT, THERAPIST, AND MILIEU

DENNIS L. McCAUGHAN

The psychotherapeutic process with delinquent adolescents is widely acknowledged to be difficult and challenging. The range of problems associated with their treatment is magnified when the intensity of their antisocial, disruptive, and often life-threatening behavior requires admission to an inpatient setting. While the clinical literature in the field offers rich opportunities for reflection on developmental and therapeutic processes, issues related to the training of the adolescent therapist remain relatively unexplored (Offer and Masterson 1971). Adolescent themes of identity, autonomy and authority, self-esteem and competence, activity and passivity are reflected in, and at times seem to dominate, the experience of the novice psychotherapist. These lingering, never fully resolved issues are reanimated as the student/therapist struggles with the intellectually demanding and emotionally charged experience that characterizes both professional socialization and personal development. The therapist is responsible both for the care of others and for learning how to provide that care. This experience is intensified as the therapist becomes the object of the delinquent adolescent's disturbed and disturbing reactions to maturational and developmental crises. The inevitable conflicts thus generated both influence and reflect the character of the clinical and teaching setting.

The purpose of this chapter is to explore a potentially significant dimension of the teaching and learning process in the psychotherapy of

0-226-24058-4/85/0012-0005$01.00

delinquent adolescents by focusing on the interaction between the adolescent therapist and the clinical setting. A principal assumption is that the adolescent therapist's response to the clinical setting often parallels the delinquent's reaction to the structure of the therapeutic milieu.

The adolescent and the therapist confront similar problems in that both have to master a complex social system that initially places great emphasis on containment and limit setting. The delinquent often feels persecuted, manipulated, and controlled on the basis of the circumstances surrounding his or her admission to the inpatient unit as well as his own internal structure and experience. The psychotherapist, new to the ward, invariably tends to identify with the persecutory aspects of the adolescent's experience. This not only reflects the therapist's initial attempts at empathy with the adolescent, who is often confused and enraged, but also derives from the therapist's own perceptions of the structure and philosophy of the milieu. Given the need to contain the delinquent's disruptive behavior through limit setting, the milieu inevitably seems rather harsh, demanding, and infantilizing. This conflicts with the therapist's conceptualization of his role as caring and giving. Hence the therapist and the patient tend to ally in feeling somewhat victimized by the environment. These kinds of responses are evoked in large part by the situation and, therefore, cannot be simply reduced to the psychotherapist's theoretical stance, personal conflicts, or previous training or experience.

Prior to conceptualizing and documenting an approach to this particular dimension of the therapist's training, I shall describe the characteristics of the setting from which these observations were drawn. The ward is a fifteen-bed, closed treatment unit at a state mental hospital. The unit serves adolescents between the ages of thirteen and seventeen who suffer from various personality disturbances (Marohn, Offer, Ostrov, and Trujillo 1979). The unit is an outgrowth of a model clinical research program developed by Marohn and his colleagues (Marohn, Dalle-Molle, McCarter, and Linn 1980; Offer, Marohn, and Ostrov 1979). The average length of stay on the unit is six months; many patients remain hospitalized for two years or longer. Within the last year the program has undergone an extensive administrative reorganization, with the result that adolescents are now referred exclusively by state mental health, child welfare, and corrections agencies. It has been our impression that recent admissions tend to be somewhat more disturbed and have long treatment histories characterized by foster care placements, incarceration for varying periods of time in correctional facilities, and multiple psychiatric hospitalizations. The therapeutic program emphasizes a highly structured and controlled setting in which the therapeutic task is to contain acting out, assist the adolescent in tolerating and regulating painful affects, and ultimately create the kinds of internalized conflicts amenable to psychotherapy. This approach is similar to those developed by Masterson (1972) and Rinsley (1968).

A common theme that has characterized the literature on the hospital treatment of adolescents is that of behavorial control (Beskind 1962). Programs that attempt to provide immediate and consistent responses to the adolescent's behavior often become divided in terms of "good" and "bad" behavior and "good" and "bad" interventions. As Crabtree (1982) has observed, staff groups can become quickly polarized along the lines of those who are "nurturant" and "understanding" and those who are "firm" and "set limits." In the treatment of these kinds of patients, fluctuations in the psychological and social integration of patients and staff are to be expected (Levinson and Crabtree 1979; Rapoport 1956). The tendency to externalize conflict and to reify these bipolar attitudes reflects both the psychopathology of these patients as well as the treatment staff's capacity to contain these externalizations. While these system-wide disruptions may be inevitable, it does not follow that staff participate in the adolescent group externalizations. Staff members respond with varying degrees of intensity to the behavior of the adolescent group. In an earlier study, it was found that, while the staff as a group were consistent in their ratings of patient psychopathology, they varied considerably in terms of the intensity of their individual perceptions (McCaughan 1982). It is within this affectively charged context that the novice psychotherapist must learn to navigate.

The Adolescent Therapist and the Delinquent Adolescent

Psychotherapy of the antisocial adolescent is a demanding task. The initial encounter with these adolescents is fraught with complications requiring endurance and commitment. The confusion and chaotic relating that surround these patients threaten to engulf the therapist. Reactions of anxiety, despair, intense frustration coupled with fantasies of retaliation, and loss of self-esteem are not idiosyncratically determined as much as they reflect the objective nature of the clinical situation and the kind of therapeutic ambience these patients create (Berman 1964; Giovacchini 1974). The character-disordered adolescent's need to act out as a defense against the recognition of a painful and often tormented inner world runs counter to the therapist's reflective orientation derived from psychoanalytic models of psychotherapy. Many of these adolescents simply do not want treatment. They resist its frustrations, having organized their lives around the immediate gratification of drugs, promiscuity, and a range of antisocial acts. What it means to be a "good enough" therapist with these adolescents is highly problematic for experienced clinicians and at times acutely stressful for therapists in training. Novice psychotherapists must contend not only with the emotional responses generated by the adolescent's hostility and impulsiveness but also with the devaluation of a psychotherapeutic orientation that they have come to prize both professionally and personally. While various techniques exist for developing an alliance with these patients, beginning therapists often feel so uncertain about themselves and the nature of the problem that their interventions lack conviction and therefore tend to fail.

The first session confronts the therapist with a serious dilemma: the adolescent denies any and all problems and demands immediate discharge. The therapist is forced to consider this emotional and value-laden decision concerning the patient's autonomy and the nature of the psychotherapeutic relationship. The therapist feels compelled to choose between the ideal of collaboration and the necessity of coercion in the form of supporting the adolescent's incarceration. For some, this dilemma reverberates throughout the initial phase of their psychotherapeutic work and parallels a central issue in the inpatient treatment of adolescents: control. I shall illustrate the various ways in which therapists attempt to deal with these problems of engagement and then describe two patterns of adaptation and defense which in my view typify what Keith (1968) has evocatively termed "unholy alliances."

The initial task in the treatment of the antisocial and behaviorally disruptive adolescent is containment that enables the adolescent to gain some degree of control over destructive and self-destructive actions. Beginning therapists often confuse this initial goal with the long-term goal of insight. They experience this immediate emphasis as contrary to their own therapeutic orientation and struggle to conceptualize their relationship with the adolescent during this phase of treatment. In reaction to a preoccupation with the adolescent's behavior, the therapist often adopts a position counter to the kinds of reactions that characterize adult perceptions of adolescents and their behavior (Anthony 1969). The therapist criticizes the staff, saying, in effect: "You are concerned only with the superficial, with behavior, while I am concerned with meaning." The problem is that the adolescent has become adept at isolating the psychological significance of his behavior through his chaotic relating. The novice psychotherapist, both through prior training and often through personal treatment experience, becomes preoccupied with the symbolic significance of the adolescent's verbalizations while ignoring the patient's overt behavior. The therapist often adopts a passive stance and relies on interpretation rather than active clarification of the meaning of behavior. The therapist unwittingly colludes with the adolescent's attempt to suppress meaning and deny responsibility for actions, and he becomes increasingly frustrated since efforts to conduct a psychotherapy consistent with his orientation are thwarted. This caricature of analytic listening is perceived by the adolescent as reflecting the therapist's passivity and impotence and often results in fears of loss of control both inside and outside the session. Overwhelmed and increasingly preoccupied with aggressive fantasies that undermine their compassionate and concerned self-concept, therapists disavow the adolescent's aggression and empathize selectively with the patient, utilizing the patient's often traumatic life history as a rationale for the adolescent's hostility. The adolescent presents himself as a long-suffering victim of failed caretakers and a repressive and retaliatory adult world. To the extent to which the adolescent's perceptions reflect reality, the therapist becomes increasingly identified with the adolescent and alienated from staff support.

The tendency of these adolescents to perceive adults in stereotypic ways, in a confused attempt to ward off the realistic dimensions of the psychotherapeutic relationship, is often misunderstood by the therapist (Kernberg 1979). The therapist identifies with the persecutory aspects of the patient's experience and attempts to convince the adolescent that he is "different" from other adults. Treatment falters since the therapist cannot realistically meet the adolescent's irrational and escalating demands. The therapist empathizes quite correctly with the helpless and persecutory aspects of the adolescent's experience but fails to understand the enraged and sadistic features of the adolescent's character. The adolescent begins to devalue the therapist on the basis of the therapist's inability to meet his unrealistic expectations. The adolescent begins to feel that the therapist is exploiting him for the therapist's own purposes and often becomes increasingly disruptive, fearing that the therapist is unable to contain his own as well as the adolescent's impulses.

Unholy Alliances: Patterns of Adaptation and Defense

The first alliance—or misalliance, following Langs's (1975) use of the term—can be described as "flight from therapy." Here therapists become overwhelmed by the adolescent's hostility and excessive demands and by their own discomfort with fantasies of retaliation fueled by frustration with the therapeutic task. Therapists who adopt this stance view the hospital milieu as hostile and uncaring while also questioning the usefulness of psychotherapy with these patients. They become advocates for the patient and assume the burden of responsibility that should be shared with the adolescent and the milieu staff. Supervisors of psychotherapy hear little about the therapeutic interaction but a great deal about the adolescent's disintegration and nursing staff errors, which are often viewed as a reflection of the unit's philosophy rather than as clinical mistakes. The psychotherapy becomes a time for the therapist to mollify the patient, reassure him, and deflect his anger and sense of deprivation. In the clinical team, the therapist attempts to convince the staff that various forms of gratification are necessary to communicate the hospital's concern for the patient. This becomes increasingly difficult because the adolescent's behavior is viewed as deteriorating. The therapist begins to assume the posture of a martyr to the treatment process and often appears depressed and long-suffering. While the therapist sees the wisdom of attempting to help the adolescent understand the treatment and develop some capacity for behavioral conformity, he is unable to work effectively with the nursing staff since this identification conflicts with his alliance with the patient.

The second type of misalliance represents a "flight into the therapy." This is a more subtle but potentially more destructive form of misalliance. The therapist feels strongly not only that the therapeutic environment is hostile and uncaring but also that psychological treatment in general and psychotherapy, in particular, are devalued. The therapist's investment in his own therapeutic powers moves him to proceed with an approach whose purpose the adolescent usually fails to comprehend since a relationship based on collaboration is absent. A cocoon-like structure is erected around the psychotherapy, and for a time this fragile alliance is maintained, although the patient continues to act disruptively, threatening the continuation of treatment. The supervisor hears little of the patient's problems in living on the unit, and the therapist's accounts of the psychotherapy are often couched in symbolic terms which rarely refer to the patient's immediate experience. Generally, there is little clarification of meaning at the verbal level and none in terms of behavior. The distinction between manifest and latent content is lost. In the clinical team, the therapist feels misunderstood and persecuted, reflecting in part an identification with the adolescent. A kind of paranoid atmosphere infects the team process, with the result that the therapist becomes increasingly isolated (Searles 1968). In one highly charged team meeting following a patient's vicious assault on a staff member, the therapist argued that the attack represented how desperately this adolescent was in need of human contact. The air of unreality about the assault bordered on pathological denial. While this is an extreme example, it represented a therapist who struggled to maintain a personal and professional identity in an affectively charged and chaotic clinical situation.

The adolescent therapist working with severe character disorders must tolerate a high degree of personal discomfort and professional uncertainty. Cohler (1981) has argued that, in the psychotherapy of developmental arrests, the therapist's task is principally to contain the patient's disruptive affects by employing his greater understanding of psychopathology and the structure of the therapeutic setting. The therapist of antisocial adolescents must learn to tolerate the affects that these patients generate, structure the psychotherapy in a manner that is consistent with the initial aims of hospitalization, and, most important, become an integrated member of a therapeutic staff group which can provide the kind of understanding, structure, and support that both the adolescent and the therapist require.

The Adolescent Therapist and the Therapeutic Milieu

The structure and ethos of the therapeutic setting form a crucial ingredient in the treatment of antisocial adolescents whose behavioral turmoil and lack of integration threaten the integrity of the staff and the stability and cohesion of the milieu. As the therapeutic milieu attempts to provide a secure framework and bring some degree of coherence to the adolescent's disruptive actions and inner turmoil, so must the setting provide conditions in which the therapist can achieve a higher level of personal integration and professional competence. Bettelheim (1974) has written: "While psychiatric hospitals generally realize that patients' needs demand cohesion of the institution, even very good hospitals fail to recognize that, to function best in their own and the patient's interests, the staff needs the institution's cohesiveness every bit as much as the patients." This is difficult even when the institution has been consciously organized to achieve this purpose. In our experience, it is essential that the adolescent therapist during the course of his training become an integral member of the milieu. The philosophy of the milieu must encourage the therapist's involvement, and, equally important, the therapist must have the motivation and capacity for such involvement. The acculturation of the therapist within the milieu has several aims: (1) development of a consistent and cohesive approach to the adolescent's treatment; (2) establishment of clearly defined roles and boundaries leading to mutual support and collaboration with members of the treatment staff; (3) enhanced opportunities for teaching and learning involving the student/therapist and senior staff. The achievement of these aims rests on an adequate understanding of both the constraints and the opportunities of inpatient psychotherapy.

The role of the psychoanalytically oriented psychotherapist within a highly structured therapeutic milieu poses problems not usually met in the standard psychotherapeutic setting (Druck 1982). While the therapist is not afforded the relative protection and anonymity of the outpatient setting, the milieu provides varied opportunities for productive encounters with patients that can result in positive therapeutic gain. This is especially so with hospitalized adolescents who benefit from a therapeutic relationship initially focused on here-and-now events and actions. Therapists who have been trained and oriented toward outpatient and private practice models often are fearful that their participation with patients in unit activities will contaminate the psychotherapy. For example, a very talented therapist became defensive when her patient began a session following a softball game in which they had both participated by asking whether she enjoyed being the catcher. Rather than allow this line of inquiry to develop, the therapist felt compelled to move on to more important matters. This reflected not only a potential countertransference problem in terms of exploring the relationship but the therapist's concerns with revealing aspects of her own experience and personality.

Similar problems develop outside the psychotherapy. For example, therapists often become concerned when their patients discuss the content of psychotherapy sessions with nursing staff. While these kinds of interactions can and often do have multiple meanings, it can be more helpful to view them as opportunities rather than as obstacles. Adolescents who have successful experiences form significant ties to other staff members. Adolescents often make excellent use of related staff to resolve impasses that develop in the psychotherapy or rehearse with nursing staff conflictual material prior to bringing it to the therapist.

Therapists are equally concerned about their participation in the clinical team. Here they are often asked to provide insight into an adolescent's potential response to a change in treatment plan or other clinical-administrative decisions. Particularly during the initial stages of treatment, the therapist feels inadequate to the task since the relationship tends to be somewhat chaotic and confused. Equally problematic for the novice psychotherapist is the expectation that he not only participate in the clinical and administrative decision-making process but that he also shoulder the responsibility for decisions with which he may not fully agree. A conflict of loyalties tends to develop. This conflict is reinforced by both the staff and the adolescent, who in their own ways demand the therapist's allegiance.

It can often be extremely helpful for senior staff to assist the therapist in understanding these kinds of dilemmas and to view their resolutions as a part of the therapist's professional development and personal growth. Equally important is that the therapist recognize that the milieu is not simply a context for psychotherapy but a therapeutic modality in its own right that can employ interventions designed to soothe, support, and structure the adolescent's experience in a variety of significant ways. This kind of shared understanding can promote an atmosphere of collaboration and common purpose.

The Therapist, the Adolescent, and the Milieu

In previous sections, the kinds of problems that confront the therapist both in the initial encounters with the delinquent adolescent and in integrating the role of a psychotherapist within the therapeutic milieu have been described. While an analysis of various aspects of the novice psychotherapist's experience may have heuristic value, it is necessary to develop a conceptualization that allows for the integration of the therapist, the adolescent, and the milieu. Without such a conceptualization, attempts at treating the adolescent and teaching the therapist are compromised.

Studies that have confirmed the influence of complex transactions occurring within the social field of the hospital milieu on the social and psychological integration of patients are relevant to the kind of conceptualization required in the training of psychotherapists (Caudill 1958; Kobler and Stotland 1964; Stanton and Schwartz 1954). Of particular interest in this regard are those studies of "special patients" whose psychopathology and disturbed and disturbing patterns of interaction disrupt the inpatient setting and evoke powerful emotional responses in staff members (Borowitz 1970; Bourne 1960; Main 1957). Conceptualizing the impact of overt and covert disturbances on both patients and staff is essential to an understanding of the novice therapist's experience. While the role of the therapist on an inpatient ward is often thought to be well defined, nevertheless each therapist must struggle to achieve an integration of the role with his own personality. Coser (1979), in her study of psychiatric residency training, described what she terms the "structural ambivalence" of the trainee's role in that the demands both to learn and to do are experienced simultaneously. The therapist must therefore contend not only with the disruptions associated with the initial engagement with the adolescent but also with the explicit and implicit expectations of the inpatient service and the training program.

One way to approach the problem is to conceptualize the therapist as representing but one point in a triadic relationship involving the patient and the treatment staff, particularly clinical administrators. While the therapist as a member of the clinical team shares responsibility for decision making, ambiguities and conflicts remain; the adolescent is "present" in treatment team meetings much like the "ghosts in the nursery" described by Fraiberg, Adelson, and Shapiro (1975). Delinquent adolescents are often quick to identify the authority structure of the setting and where decisions affecting their treatment are made. It is not unusual for an adolescent to speak of "my team" and demand that his therapist represent him. It is equally true that the milieu staff are represented in the therapist's individual sessions with the patient. This is made explicit when therapists are expected to explore in the psychotherapy the adolescent's "problems in living" as they arise in the milieu (Marohn et al. 1980). Therapists are often reminded both informally by milieu staff and formally in team meetings to discuss with the adolescent various "problem behaviors." Since the psychotherapeutic relationship is, unlike other treatment interventions, insulated from direct observation, fantasies about what is or is not occurring are easily generated. This concern was illustrated in the remark of an experienced milieu worker who stated, in the presence of a therapist, "If the therapist will not or cannot treat the kid, then the milieu staff will do so." These kinds of structural and interpersonal tensions can have a decided effect on the therapist's experience.

Clinical administration provides the conditions under which psychotherapy can progress. This is critical during the initial phase of treatment with antisocial adolescents as well as with borderline and psychotic adult patients (Gutheil 1982). Since clinical administrative decisions involve the exercise of power and authority through action, they can become a vehicle for acting out and a reflection of the kinds of triangulated relating involving the therapist and his patient. There is often the suspicion, shared by both the therapist and the nursing staff, that certain administrative decisions are designed as much for the therapist as for the patient. That is, they become communications in action. For example, certain privileges requested by the therapist for his patient are denied by the unit chief and the clinical team. The explicit rationale is that the adolescent is not ready to assume certain responsibilities. The implicit communication to the therapist is that these requests reflect a pathological alliance and are a form of countertransference acting out (Schneider 1963). While these administrative decisions are rarely viewed as acting out, they show a remarkable resemblance to the ways in which the disturbed adolescent communicates. It is not unusual, therefore, for the therapist to feel devalued and impotent about certain decisions that, in turn, act to reinforce the therapist's identification with the adolescent.

There is a tendency for senior staff to view the therapist's failures to adequately conceptualize the therapy and to act in concert with the milieu as resistances which reflect the therapist's own individual psychopathology (Spiegel and Grunebaum 1977). As an illustration, a senior clinician once observed that the novice psychotherapist goes through a process similar to that of mourning, beginning with denial and protest and resolving itself with despair and finally acceptance. It is interesting to note that this conceptualization parallels similar accounts of the therapeutic process with borderline adolescents (Rinsley 1981). While this interpretation has merit and indeed may be useful in understanding the novice psychotherapist's experience, it remains incomplete since it focuses on the therapist's intrapsychic experience without taking into account the context that sets this experience in motion. Again, this kind of limited conceptualization acts to reinforce the therapist's identification with the adolescent, so that both therapist and adolescent are "joined" and perceived as sharing delinquent and pathological object relations.

Communications in Action: Some Thoughts on Parallel Process

The concept of parallel process can be usefully employed in analyzing the triadic relationships previously described. However, it is necessary to broaden our understanding of this phenomenon. While the literature has been primarily concerned with parallel process occurring between individual psychotherapy and supervision, these identifications are not confined to the supervisory situation but emerge in a variety of interactional contexts (Sachs and Shapiro 1976). Parallel process phenomena are not unidirectional, derived exclusively from problematic interactions occurring between patients and therapists and "flowing upward," but multidirectional, with various points of origin (Doehrman 1976; Gediman and Wolkenfeld 1980). The following example may prove helpful in illustrating the multidirectional nature of parallel process and the ways in which such events can be utilized in teaching.

A difficult and disruptive adolescent assaulted a staff member. The chief of service called a special meeting to review the event and to discuss possible administrative actions with the clinical team, the therapist, and the patient. The meeting was held, but the chief was unable to attend. Both the therapist, who was new to the service, and the patient, recently admitted, were upset, having expected and wished for the chief to be present. The therapist was angry with the chief and felt that his position with his patient was undermined since he had led the patient to expect that the chief would lead the meeting. Further, the therapist feared that the milieu staff would want the patient discharged since the assault was on a member of the staff. He perceived the chief as an ally in preventing this outcome. The adolescent patient who felt compelled to test the milieu's capacity to contain and pacify his destructive impulses had located this capacity in the idealized chief and, to a lesser degree, in his therapist. The therapist was concerned that he would be quickly devalued by his patient since he failed to produce the chief. Following the meeting, in which it was decided that the patient would not be discharged, the therapist made known his anger and disappointment with the chief. The therapist's reaction was interpreted, although never directly, by the chief and other staff as the therapist's overidentification with the patient. While this interpretation was in many respects true, it failed to take into account the chief's absence and the transference and countertransference dimensions involving the therapist, the chief, the patient, the anxiety caused by the event, and the possible implications of the administrative meeting for the therapist. Like most therapists, he was concerned that the patient might be discharged with consequences not only for the patient but for his own sense of competence and self-esteem.

In the author's view, the therapist's response was overdetermined in that it reflected influences stemming from the patient, the chief, and the milieu itself. By examining the various contributions of all participants, the therapist could have learned something of real value about himself and about the therapeutic process. Since the initial interpretation was directed toward the therapist's intrapsychic experience and since the other points of origin were not considered, the event passed without adequate comment. If the event had been analyzed in terms of the contributions of all relevant participants, not only would the therapist have benefited in terms of learning but also the staff as a group would have better understood both the adolescent's behavior and what motivated it as well as something about themselves as a staff. In the initial phase of treatment, these kinds of disturbances occur with some frequency. If they are viewed as causes for concern as well as opportunities for learning, the therapeutic process can be enhanced. Unfortunately, these events are often reacted to with a kind of shock and surprise that leads the therapist to believe that he has committed some destructive error. Of course, an adequate analysis of such events would consider issues of responsibility. However, if conducted along the lines suggested, the outcome for the therapist as well as the rest of the staff might be a recognition of shared responsibility and involvement. This might enhance the sense of common purpose and mutual support. Certainly assisting the therapist to recognize the limitations of exploration and insight-oriented approaches in the initial phases of treatment would serve an important goal of teaching.

Implications for Teaching and Learning

It is argued that an adequate conceptualization of the education of psychotherapists in their work with delinquent adolescents requires an integration of the therapist, the adolescent, and the therapeutic milieu. There are a number of areas where specific recommendations regarding teaching, learning, and the aims and organization of the clinical setting can usefully be articulated.

1. INSTITUTIONAL AND PROGRAM PHILOSOPHY

Clinical service and education are not incompatible aims. While this may seem obvious, particularly in child and adolescent work, this relationship is often poorly articulated and narrowly defined in terms of professional education. By developing an approach to treatment that emphasizes staff development, both trainees and staff are encouraged to view their mutual involvement as leading to higher levels of professional and personal competence. Clinical care can only be enhanced with this kind of cohesive philosophy and orientation. Institutions and programs which lack commitment to training and staff development often reveal weaknesses in their conceptualization of treatment. While each program must determine how best to integrate training within a clinical framework, failure to consciously work through this relationship can result only in the erosion of the therapeutic experience for all concerned.

We have found it helpful where possible to have trainees spend a year with us. In our experience, it takes from three to six months for a therapist to develop an adequate understanding of the treatment approach and to become an integrated member of the clinical team. This alone, however, is insufficient in that a commitment to the educational process, broadly defined, must be reflected in staff attitudes and in the provision of related learning experiences.

2. THE TRAINEE'S PRIOR EDUCATIONAL EXPERIENCE

It is important not to assume that previous professional training has prepared the student to undertake psychotherapeutic work with delinquent adolescents. One of the most difficult tasks for the therapist is developing a sense of conviction in terms of the adolescent's psychopathology and character structure. As with most severe psychopathology, there is a tendency to minimize its significance and impact both for the adolescent and the therapist. To a degree the liberal *Zeitgeist* has reinforced this tendency by simplifying the process of behavioral and personality change. Similarly, there is emphasis on theoretical conceptualizations that tend to view the patient as a passive participant in the process of development. This attitude gives rise, in part, to the mythology of the psychotherapist as hero. An unfortunate aspect of this myth is the search for the "good" and "worthwhile" patient who can sustain such expectations (Ekstein 1966). While selection of trainees who are academically well prepared is important, it is not enough and can result in a disappointing experience for all concerned. In explaining our work to candidates, we emphasize the difficult nature of the work in terms of the adolescent's psychopathology and also in terms of the personal and professional demands it makes upon the therapist.

3. ADOLESCENT ASPECTS OF THE THERAPIST'S EXPERIENCE

As clinicians interested in adolescence, we need to recognize the range of adolescent issues evoked in ourselves and in the student-therapist. It is interesting to note that, while those who work with children describe themselves as child therapists, rarely do those of us who work with adolescents describe ourselves as adolescent therapists. It may be that adolescent has become a pejorative term. To my knowledge there has been no comparable discussion in the literature of the therapist's responses to adolescent work as in the literature on children (Ekstein 1966). While many of the issues are similar, the problem that both the adolescent and the therapist face is that adolescence is a transitional phase with few clear boundaries separating childhood and adult life. Anna Freud (1958) observed that the adolescent experience is rarely revealed fully during the analysis of adults. This may suggest that, for some of us at least, the adolescent experience evokes uniquely painful and conflictual associations. However, some recognition of its continuing influence may prove helpful to trainees. For example, when the author mentioned the parallel between the role of student and aspects of the adolescent experience in a seminar for residents and psychologists, there was spontaneous laughter reflecting both recognition and anxiety. However, what followed was an interesting discussion of significant aspects of their clinical work.[1]

4. THE TRAINEE'S PERCEPTIONS AND EXPECTATIONS

Therapists in training bring to their work a variety of expectations and perceptions. In conceptualizing the training experience, it is necessary to take seriously their perceptions of the clinical setting and their expectations concerning the psychotherapeutic work. Since none is completely free from fears of madness, it is essential to help trainees recognize their own fears as well as how frightening psychiatric hospitalization can be—especially for adolescents. Working with disruptive adolescents whose controls are such that they at times require physical restraint is a dimension of the hospital experience that often troubles therapists in terms of concerns both for the adolescent and for themselves. Workshops in patient management, principally designed for nursing and child-care staff, can assist the therapists not only in understanding a significant aspect of the ward staff's experience but also in becoming more competent in assessment, limit setting, and physical restraint as well as less fearful of their own and the adolescent's aggression. This kind of experience is offered even though we do not expect trainees to assist in the physical restraint of patients. The expectations that therapists bring to their work are equally important to identify. For example, a trainee after six months finally was able to verbalize how she had thought that the hospital was a psychoanalytic rather than a psychiatric institute. This distortion helped us to understand many of the problems she had been experiencing, particularly in self-esteem regulation. It served to remind us how powerful and potentially disorganizing the experience could be for some therapists.

5. TEACHING SEMINARS

Few, if any, of our trainees have been exposed to course work in milieu therapy. This, as Zeldow (1977) observes, is indeed a “blind spot” in clinical training. There is clearly a need for therapists to develop a conceptualization of dynamic milieu therapy and the kinds of possibilities as well as problems posed by working with hospitalized adolescents. We have tried various approaches to teaching this material both in seminars designed specifically for this purpose and through group supervision on the ward. It is most helpful when readings are combined with clinical examples drawn from the therapist’s observations of milieu interactions. Since every milieu will provide numerous examples of interventions that succeed as well as those that fail, the therapists are better able to understand the kinds of complex interactions to which they often make significant contributions. This kind of discussion also has the beneficial effect of demystifying clinical work by demonstrating that there is rarely, if ever, one right way to intervene in any and all situations. In addition, therapists are able to clarify the difference between clinical errors and the conscious application of a particular philosophy. Trainees are often surprised to discover transactions operating outside their awareness—knowledge of which helps them to examine their own involvement.

6. SUPERVISION

As Marohn (1981) has observed, supervision which recognizes the kinds of transferences that delinquent adolescents develop is essential in helping the therapist understand the negativism and devaluation that can characterize the therapeutic relationship. Equally important is supervision that helps the therapists conceptualize their role during the initial phases of treatment. Since management tends to be the focus, tensions inevitably develop between the therapist’s psychotherapy supervisor, who may be a consultant or someone not involved in the daily clinical work, and the ward’s senior clinical staff. Clinical disagreements between supervisors and administrators, in our experience, are less often the issue than the ways in which these differences are understood, integrated, and communicated. While there are no easy solutions to these kinds of problems, we have found that we can minimize their potential disruptive effects by providing weekly supervision with the unit chief or other senior person to discuss the integration of clinical and administrative issues. Impasses that do develop can be resolved by involving a consultant who understands the clinical, administrative, and training aspects of the conflict and who can provide an objective assessment of the situation particularly in clarifying responsibility rather than assigning blame.

7. THE THERAPIST AND THE TRAINING EXPERIENCE

While this chapter has emphasized the need to provide various opportunities for therapists to understand their roles, conceptualize the psychopathology of delinquent adolescents, and integrate their work within the context of a dynamic milieu, it is equally important for staff to respect the kinds of problems that therapists encounter during the course of their training. The tendency to pathologize the therapists' errors and to bemoan their lack of competence only serves to alienate the therapists and reduce their sense of mutual involvement and shared purpose. It is essential to recognize that the kinds of problems that therapists experience are an essential part of their learning, both personally and professionally. We can be too quick to rescue the therapists from difficulties which they need to struggle with and to work through with our support (Ekstein and Wallerstein 1958). As Bernfeld (1925) reminds us in *Sisyphus, or the Limits of Education*, there are indeed limits to the educational process as there are to the therapeutic process, and our acknowledgment of these limits can enhance our experience as teachers and the experience of our students.

Conclusions

The psychotherapy of the severely disturbed and delinquent adolescent is a challenging and demanding task. Therapists whose training involves work with these adolescents are confronted with personal and professional dilemmas requiring a clinical and teaching setting that provides them with a framework for understanding their experience. Such a framework acknowledges the complex transactions involving the therapist, the adolescent, and the milieu. The involvement and integration of the therapist within the milieu are an essential first step in the process of teaching and learning the dynamics of delinquent adolescents. The therapist's initial engagement with the therapeutic milieu and with the adolescent in psychotherapy provides rich opportunities for teaching and learning.

NOTES

An earlier version of this paper was presented at the panel "Teaching the Dynamics of Delinquency," annual meeting of the American Society for Adolescent Psychiatry, New York, April 30, 1983. I am grateful to the many colleagues associated with the Adolescent Program, Illinois State Psychiatric Institute, who over the years as teachers and as students contributed greatly to my education and therefore to this paper.

1. Therapists' reactions to the problems their patients experience in the hospital school are intriguing from the point of view of therapists' own transference to the school setting heightened by their roles as students.

REFERENCES

Anthony, E. J. 1969. The reaction of adults to adolescents and their behavior. In G. Caplan and S. Lebovici, eds. *Adolescence: Psycho-Social Perspectives*. New York: Basic.

Berman, S. 1964. Techniques of treatment of a form of juvenile delinquency, the antisocial character disorder. *Journal of the American Academy of Child Psychiatry* 3:24–52.

Bernfeld, S. 1925. *Sisyphus, or the Limits of Education*. Berkeley: University of California Press, 1973.

Beskind, H. 1962. Psychiatric inpatient treatment of adolescents: a review of clinical experience. *Comprehensive Psychiatry* 3:354–369.

Bettelheim, B. 1974. *A Home for the Heart*. New York: Knopf.

Borowitz, G. H. 1970. The therapeutic utilization of emotions and attitudes evoked in the caretakers of disturbed children. *British Journal of Medical Psychology* 42:129–139.

Bourne, H. 1960. Main's syndrome and a nurse's reaction to it. *Archives of General Psychiatry* 2:526–581.

Caudill, W. 1958. *The Psychiatric Hospital as a Small Society*. Cambridge, Mass.: Harvard University Press.

Cohler, B. J. 1981. On being therapeutic: issues of person and setting in the psychotherapy of developmental arrests. Paper presented at the annual meetings, American Orthopsychiatric Association, New York, March.

Coser, R. L. 1979. *Training in Ambiguity: Learning through Doing in a Mental Hospital*. New York: Free Press.

Crabtree, L. H., Jr. 1982. Hospitalized adolescents who act out: a treatment approach. *Psychiatry* 48:147–158.

Doehrman, M. J. G. 1976. Parallel processes in supervision and psychotherapy. *Bulletin of the Menninger Clinic* 40:3–104.

Druck, A. B. 1982. The role of the psychoanalytically oriented psychotherapist within a therapeutic community. *Psychiatry* 45:45–58.

Ekstein, R. 1966. *Children of Time and Space of Action and Impulse*. New York: Appleton-Century-Crofts.

Ekstein, R., and Wallerstein, J. S. 1958. *The Teaching and Learning of Psychotherapy*. New York: Basic.

Fraiberg, S.; Adelson, E.; and Shapiro, V. 1975. Ghosts in the nursery: a psychoanalytic approach to the problems of impaired infant-mother relationships. *Journal of the American Academy of Child Psychiatry* 14:387–421.

Freud, A. 1958. Adolescence. *Psychoanalytic Study of the Child* 13:255–278.

Gediman, H. K., and Wolkenfeld, F. 1980. The parallelism phenomenon in psychoanalysis and supervision: its reconstruction as a triadic system. *Psychoanalytic Quarterly* 49:234–255.

Giovacchini, P. L. 1974. The difficult adolescent patient: countertransference problems. *Adolescent Psychiatry* 3:271–288.

Gutheil, T. G. 1982. On the therapy in clinical administration. III. *Psychiatric Quarterly* 54:18–25.

Keith, C. R. 1968. The therapeutic alliance in child psychotherapy. *Journal of the American Academy of Child Psychiatry* 7:31–43.

Kernberg, O. 1979. Psychoanalytic psychotherapy with borderline adolescents. *Adolescent Psychiatry* 7:294–321.

Kobler, A. L., and Stotland, E. 1964. *The End of Hope: A Socio-Clinical Study of Suicide*. New York: Free Press.

Langs, R. 1975. Therapeutic misalliances. *International Journal of Psychoanalytic Psychotherapy* 4:106–141.

Levinson, D. F., and Crabtree, L. H., Jr. 1979. Ward tension and staff leadership in a therapeutic community for hospitalized adolescents. *Psychiatry* 42:220–240.

McCaughan, D. L. 1982. The impact of hopelessness on adaptation in the milieu therapy of delinquent adolescents. Ph.D. diss., University of Chicago.

Main, T. F. 1957. The ailment. *British Journal of Medical Psychology* 30:129–145.

Marohn, R. C. 1981. The negative transference in the treatment of juvenile delinquents. *Annual of Psychoanalysis* 9:21–42.

Marohn, R. C.; Dalle-Molle, D.; McCarter, E.; and Linn, D. 1980. *Juvenile Delinquents: Psychodynamic Assessment and Hospital Treatment*. New York: Brunner/Mazel.

Marohn, R. C.; Offer, D.; Ostrov, E.; and Trujillo, J. 1979. Four psychodynamic types of hospitalized juvenile delinquents. *Adolescent Psychiatry* 7:466–483.

Masterson, J. F. 1972. *Treatment of the Borderline Adolescent: A Developmental Approach*. New York: Wiley-Interscience.

Offer, D.; Marohn, R. C.; and Ostrov, E. 1979. *The Psychological World of the Juvenile Delinquent*. New York: Basic.

Offer, D., and Masterson, J., eds. 1971. *Teaching and Learning Adolescent Psychiatry*. Springfield, Ill.: Thomas.

Rapoport, R. N. 1956. Oscillations and sociotherapy. *Human Relations* 9:357–373.

Rinsley, D. B. 1968. Theory and practice of intensive residential treatment of adolescents. *Psychiatric Quarterly* 42:611–638.

Rinsley, D. B. 1981. Borderline psychopathology: the concepts of Masterson and Rinsley and beyond. *Adolescent Psychiatry* 9:259–274.

Sachs, D. M., and Shapiro, S. H. 1976. On parallel process in therapy and teaching. *Psychoanalyltic Quarterly* 45:394–415.

Schneider, I. 1963. The use of patients to act out professional conflicts. *Psychiatry* 26:88–94.

Searles, H. F. 1968. Paranoid processes among members of the therapeutic team. In S. H. Eldred and M. Vanderpol, eds. *Psychotherapy in the Designed Therapeutic Milieu*. Boston: Little, Brown. Reprinted in *Countertransference and Related Subjects: Selected Papers*. New York: International Universities Press, 1979.

Spiegel, D., and Grunebaum, H. 1977. Training versus treating the psychiatric resident. *American Journal of Psychotherapy* 31:618–623.

Stanton, A. H., and Schwartz, M. S. 1954. *The Mental Hospital*. New York: Basic.

Zeldow, P. B. 1977. Outline for a seminar in milieu therapy: a blind spot in clinical training. *Professional Psychology* 8:109–115.

29 THE HOLDING ENVIRONMENT IN THE INPATIENT TREATMENT OF ADOLESCENTS

MARY DAVIS AND IRVING H. RAFFE

The administrator-therapist team approach to inpatient psychiatric treatment is not new, although there is little written about it in the literature. It is used, perhaps, most often in institutions where psychoanalysis or psychoanalytic psychotherapy is the primary treatment modality. In the 1930s, Chestnut Lodge, in Rockville, Maryland, began using this technique because psychoanalysts found it disadvantageous to be involved in decisions regarding privileges and restrictions for patients they saw in analysis. They developed a system whereby one psychiatrist acted as administrator for a twelve-bed unit, while other psychiatrists treated those patients in psychoanalysis or psychoanalytic psychotherapy (Stanton and Schwartz 1954). More recently Cowan (1980) described a similar technique used in both in- and outpatient psychotherapeutic treatment of individuals with such diagnoses as psychosis, borderline or narcissistic personality disorders, and drug addiction. Cowan considers the case manager–therapist team approach as analogous to the situation in child psychotherapy: in both situations the third party (either case manager or parent) serves to safeguard the treatment setting by dealing with extraanalytic management difficulties, while the psychotherapist is free to deal with transference and other intrapsychic issues.

When one talks about safeguarding the treatment setting, the question immediately arises of what is being safeguarded from what threat. Two diverse theoretical concepts seem applicable in addressing this question: Winnicott's (1965) ideas about the "holding environment" and Langs's (1979) concept of psychotherapist as container and metabolizer of affect.

0-226-24058-4/85/0012-0019$01.00

Winnicott describes the "holding" in the parent-child relationship as the "total environmental provision" prior to the child's development of object relations. The holding environment "includes the management of experiences that are inherent in existence." During the holding phase of infant development, the ego "changes over from an unintegrated state to a structured integration, and so the infant becomes able to experience the anxiety associated with disintegration." The "holding environment has as its main function the reduction to a minimum of impingements to which the infant must react with resultant annihilation of personal being"—that is, with ego fragmentation. In order to achieve this goal—the screening out of overwhelming/overstimulating/fragmenting experiences—the mothering person must be able to experience a reliable empathy, to tolerate and contain tension herself without fragmentation or undue anxiety. She must also allow the child to do as much tension management as possible while she is unobtrusively available when the child's ability fails. In other words, she must be a "good enough mother" who meets the child's needs empathically, thus providing an environment which allows for separation-individuation and microinternalizations of ego functions.

Brown (1981) applies Winnicott's concept to inpatient treatment, writing that, in that setting, a holding environment provides structure, consistency, and a routine that helps to filter out excessively stimulating occurrences. These aspects of treatment have in themselves a consolidating and organizing effect. With such external structure, which prevents fragmentation of the patient's internal world, psychotherapy can proceed and, through interpretation of primitive defenses, repair ego weaknesses. Provision of a holding environment for the inpatient provides a type of auxiliary ego which takes care of ego maintenance functions, allowing the patient's energy to be reserved for and used in resolving conflictual and developmental crises so that the necessary tension-management skills, such as adaptive defenses and other ego functions, can develop.

Langs's concept of the psychotherapist as container and metabolizer of projective identifications seems similar. He sees one major therapeutic function as the maintenance of the therapist's receptivity to projection, together with the "ability to metabolize and detoxify pathological interactional projections." The therapist then turns this pathological interaction into conscious insight and imparts it to the patient. The "therapeutic hold," to Langs, is modeled on the maternal hold and implies a background of safety and no "impingements." The patient who is flooded and overwhelmed by affect cannot reflect on or understand either affect or behavior. The psychotherapist can allow the affect to be "given" to her or him by projection and can then act to reduce the level of stimulation, to soothe the patient much as a mother soothes her overstimulated infant, until both patient and therapist together can understand the source of the affect and rechannel the energies. If the patient is unable to contain the tension until the therapy hour, he or she may resort to acting out to discharge tension.

For the child patient, parents contain this acting out and maintain tension at a tolerable level until the therapy hour; they take over the ego function of tension containment for the patient. The adult borderline or narcissistic personality may also need someone to take over that function for him. Many therapists, of course, do this through "crisis" phone calls from the patient that moderate the crisis enough to allow the patient to wait until the next appointment. For the patient who lacks this self-soothing capacity, the acting-out patient, one of the therapist's functions is as container/metabolizer of affect in order to reduce acting out. This provides a basic, stable, consistent holding environment within which the restructuring of ego though interpretive work can proceed, safeguarded from crises induced by the patient's acting out.

In the inpatient setting, the unit staff provides a similar holding environment by offering a residence outside the stream of daily stresses. It is, of course, also necessary that any disruptive, overstimulating behavior of patients and staff be contained and modulated in order to ensure the therapeutic hold.

Let us look at one way that such a holding environment can be achieved. We shall describe one setting for the inpatient treatment of severely disturbed acting-out adolescents that closely fits this model of a holding environment: it attempts to reduce the number of potentially fragmenting experiences to which the adolescent must react without adequate ego structures. In this setting the administrator/therapist split is a major factor in maintaining a holding environment.

A Holding Environment

The adolescent treatment center (ATC) is an eleven-bed inpatient adolescent unit in a general psychiatric hospital. It uses a psychodynamic understanding of adolescents and their families combined with a flexible level system based loosely on behavior modification principles (i.e., the privileges and passes of each patient depend on his level, which in turn depends on his behavior on the unit and his involvement in treatment). All environmental management decisions, including passes, privileges, medication, and discharge, are made by the multidisciplinary treatment team, which is headed by the unit's clinical director. Individual psychotherapy is conducted by an outside professional, usually a child psychiatrist. The individual therapist, of course, is a member of the treatment team but does not write orders or make unilateral management decisions. Family therapy is conducted by a full-time family therapist; daily group therapy is conducted by the clinical director and ATC staff.

The separation between individual psychotherapeutic function and case management function has been seen to have a significant impact on all individuals involved in the therapy. The interaction of individual therapist, clinical director, nursing staff, activities therapy staff, social work staff, educators, and patient is complex, especially as it emerges in the patient's transference issues and in staff countertransference. This chapter deals primarily with countertransference issues in staff because those emerge more clearly in this system than in systems where the roles of individual therapist and administrative psychiatrist are mingled.

Most of the time, separation of individual psychotherapeutic and management functions works smoothly; patients deal with ATC staff and peers in reality-based incidents where maladaptive behaviors are identified, while the individual psychotherapist examines with the patient the underlying determinants for those behaviors. Most ATC staff/patient interactions focus on overt, task-oriented, interpersonal issues: for example, which behaviors achieve their conscious purpose and which behaviors defeat themselves. The unconscious motivations and conflicts which direct the self-defeating behaviors are often touched on briefly, but their exploration in depth is left up to the individual therapist, while ATC staff deal with the interpersonal effects of the behavior.

Not infrequently, a particular patient arrives whose hospital course requires frequent conscious attempts to look at and understand the individual therapist/ATC staff interface because that interface becomes a focus of difficulty. There have been rare patients whose pathology enabled them to set individual therapist and clinical director at loggerheads so thoroughly that it ended in a raw exercise of power. With other patients, there was little disagreement but a strong need for frequent conferences to clarify joint perceptions of dynamics and to share concerns and frustrations.

Resistance and Projective Identification

The patients for whom the individual therapy/ATC interface becomes an area of concern are, as one would expect, those patients whose primary mode of functioning in response to internal tension (anger, anxiety, sadness, etc.) is to act on the environment rather than to change themselves. This response, of course, occurs to some extent in all adolescents, but some are more difficult to contain and redirect than others. These latter patients require a more structured "holding environment" because of their deficits in internal control. The action of these patients on the environment may take the form of counteracting their internal tension by the excitement of drug use, truancy, fighting, rebelliousness, or other symptomatic behaviors. If such macroscopic forms of acting out are contained and prevented by the environment, the patient must then turn to such defenses as projection: for example, the internal hostile, abusing maternal imago is projected onto staff, and staff are responded to as if they are in fact hostile, abusing mothers. Staff may, in turn, respond to this projection in one of two ways: they may become the re-created negative maternal imago and be themselves altered by taking in the adolescent's tension, or they may take in the tension and alter it ("detoxify," "contain and metabolize," in Langs's phraseology). This allows the adolescent the opportunity to join in and gradually internalize the ability to regulate his tension instead of being overwhelmed.

This is, of course, a parallel to the functioning of the "good enough mother" who (usually) soothes her infant and relieves his tension instead of joining him in his howls of overwhelming discomfort.

Many of the difficulties with individual therapists versus ATC staff, like those between parents and ATC staff, revolve around competition for the place of "good parent": who knows best what is needed, who understands the patient best. Perhaps this reflects the parents' sense of themselves as failed because their child is disturbed and the child's view of himself as so bad as to be unmanageable and unlovable. The adolescent experiences internal discomfort arising from his negative self-image and the failure of the supposed-to-be-omnipotent parents. When he is not allowed, because of the daily routine of the ATC, to discharge this intolerable tension in accustomed behaviors, he turns to projection. The staff then are seen by him as the omnipotent parents, and the adolescent attempts either to prove their omnipotence by inducing them to control him or, failing that preferred solution, to establish that he is in control, unmanageable, and omnipotent, and therefore not in need of parents. If staff are aware of the ways in which patient behavior evokes feelings in staff and are prepared to tolerate the tension aroused in them and use these feelings to understand the patient, they tend not to allow themselves to become the projected failed parent: they do not participate in the projective identification. Instead, they are able to stay the "good enough" mother and allow the individual therapist to explore with the patient the origins of the expectations that parental figures will be incompetent/rejecting/abusing. That expectation is now demonstrably false, since staff remain their "good enough" selves, and the pathological interactional projection can be given back to the patient as conscious insight.

Two patients seen at different times on the ATC illustrate this process. The first, Ann, was a fifteen-year-old juvenile-onset diabetic who had been admitted after a suicide attempt. Much of Ann's acting out took the form of misadministering her insulin or cheating on her diet. She experienced several hypoglycemic seizures. She also, at one point, was discovered to be causing herself to vomit in an attempt to lose weight. For many reasons, the ATC staff were unable to maintain the crucial empathic stance and experienced much anger at Ann as they became entangled in the struggle to force her to "behave." For a period after the self-induced vomiting was discovered, Ann was not allowed in the bathroom without an escort. The life-threatening nature of Ann's behavior, of course, heightened the tension in nursing staff and made that tension more difficult to contain and metabolize. The inability of staff to contain this tension resulted in a replication of the family's intrusive, controlling style of nurturance.

Beth was a sixteen-year-old girl with anorexia nervosa. The same control issues and invitation to intrusive overcontrol were present as during Ann's treatment. Early in Beth's treatment, however, staff met as a group to plan their approach. Their inability to force Beth to stop exercising and to eat was acknowledged openly, and this was considered in establishing a plan of approach. The plan established was one which allowed for confrontation of Beth about the inappropriateness and danger of her behavior but avoided involvement in or repetition of the family's control struggle. By refusing to allow Beth's projection of the intrusive, abusive parents to develop into a projective identification, staff were able to be helpful to Beth in finding behaviors other than exercise, purging, or fasting to relieve her internal tensions.

So far, the discussion has focused on the difficulties of ward staff in dealing with acting-out adolescents. The factor that permits this treatment model to provide a more secure "holding environment" than other models is the functional split between individual psychotherapist and administrative psychiatrist. The individual therapist, although usually a physician, is not involved in daily management decisions. Since he is a member of the treatment team, his understanding of the patient helps to shape the team's approach to the patient. His direct contact with the patient, however, is directed at understanding the patient rather than containing behaviors. This reduces the narcissistic trauma experienced by the therapist when the patient acts out and staff become the failed omnipotent parents. Since it is not the therapist's failure, he can more easily maintain his therapeutic stance, resist projective identification, and be available to help the patient examine his behavior.

The Role of the Clinical Director

The clinical director of the ATC serves multiple functions: monitor of group process for both patients and staff; healer of potential splits among staff; screen for projections from patients, staff, individual therapists, and families; interface with the hospital and the community; and so on. All these functions can be considered a part of a more general function, that of providing a holding environment for the ATC as a whole. If parents are intrusive, demanding, and abusive to nursing staff and/or adolescents, they can be referred to the clinical director and their contact with other staff limited. If the unit's integration with the rest of the hospital is problematic, the clinical director hears the criticisms and negotiates for the ATC. The director functions as team leader who makes no unilateral decisions but facilitates the group decision-making process and identifies the presence or absence of a consensus and its content. When the treatment team is experiencing tension of any kind, either projected from a patient or from any other source, the process of tension regulation follows much the same pattern as within individuals. If internal regulation—intrastaff tension regulation—fails, an attempt is made to get rid of the tension by acting on the environment: extruding the patient, arguments within staff, and so on. If this behavior is prevented, the mechanism of projective identification comes into play, and the clinical director may be perceived by staff as the omnipotent mother who has failed. This arouses the murderous rage which we experience when our fantasies of omnipotent nurturance fail. The clinical director must, in this situation, be able to contain and metabolize the pathological interactional projection and return it to the staff as insight. If she can help them to contain their own tension and modulate it, they can do the same for the patients, and the patients can then explore the origins of the tension with their individual therapists.

The cases of Ann and Beth illustrate this process. In Ann's treatment, staff were unable to avoid participating in the projective identification, and they behaved much like the patient's intrusive, overcontrolling, but impotent parents. The tension aroused by experiencing themselves as impotent in a life-threatening situation was intolerable. Attempts were made to extrude the patient by asking for her discharge. They also projected the intrusive impotence they felt onto the clinical director when, late in her admission, Ann had several seizures which were clearly not hypoglycemic and were felt to be hysterical. Nursing staff told the clinical director, first, that a decision about whether to send Ann to a pediatric emergency room was a nursing decision (i.e., that the director's concern about that decision was intrusive) and, second, that they felt the director was not competent to manage Ann's diabetes appropriately (i.e., that the director was impotent and incompetent). These issues were not resolved until Ann was discharged because the clinical director was also caught up in the parallel process of layers of projective identification.

In the case of Beth, the parallel process was one of tension regulation rather than of projective identification. Beth's parents were very intrusive and overcontrolling in response to their own perceived impotence, as is the case with many parents of anorexics. They attempted to be equally intrusive and controlling with the ATC staff; they called four or five times daily to question what was being done, asked for multiple special exceptions to the program, and on one occasion attempted to dictate the use of medication. As part of the early attempt to establish a useful approach, Beth's parents were instructed that they were not to speak to ATC staff more than once daily and then only for a brief report of the day's events. Any other questions, and especially any disagreements with Beth's treatment, were to be directed to the clinical director. The clinical director found it necessary on several occasions to set firm limits about who made treatment decisions; but a change in Beth's behavior on the unit was noticeable within a week of the establishment of this policy. The clinical director was able to tolerate the intrusiveness of Beth's parents and prevent it from impinging on Beth or on staff. This allowed staff and Beth to learn new ways of interacting and allowed Beth and her individual therapist to examine the intrapsychic aspects of her behaviors.

The clinical director is assisted in her difficult task by several factors. First, and perhaps most important, is the quality of the staff. A good cohesive staff is able most of the time to maintain its "good enough" position and not be overwhelmed by tension from any source. In situations where the natural high tolerance for tension fails, a great deal of the tension has nevertheless been "detoxified" before it finds its outlet in projection onto the clinical director.

The clinical director's position on the unit may also help to siphon off some of the tension that otherwise would be directed at staff. Often the patient's projections of parental omnipotence or impotence are made directly onto her and remain projections (the patient's pathologic perceptions) rather than projective identifications (when she enters into the pathological perceptions) because of her relative distance. This may reduce the intensity of the projective identifications onto frontline staff and make it more possible for the tension to be contained at that level.

In addition, the majority of the clinical director's contacts with patients are in either group psychotherapy or in task-oriented contacts, such as around physical illness. This means that her exposure to the projective identifications is more distant and dilute, and therefore she is less likely to be caught up in the pathological interactional process. The contact of nursing staff and individual therapist with the patient is less structured and more ambiguous, and, therefore, their behavior is more open to distortion. The extra distance allows the clinical director to function as observing ego and container for the patient/staff/therapist triad. In essence, tension flows from patient and family to staff (including here the individual therapist) and thence to clinical director; it may be contained and used productively at any point. If tension and maladaptive behaviors are not contained and transformed into insight at the lower levels of the hierarchy (family or staff) and if the system is working well, that transformation occurs with the clinical director and then flows in the opposite direction, from clinical director to staff to family.

The clinical director's position as (in part) observing ego for the ATC complex is also facilitated by dual identification with staff and with the individual therapist; the director identifies both with staff, since the director is a member of and spokesman for the treatment team, and with the individual therapist, since she is herself a psychotherapist. As long as she is able to tolerate the ambiguity, she can assist others in healing any competitive splits that may arise.

Conclusions

This model of the ATC as a "holding environment" for the patient seems to be especially applicable to those patients, such as adolescents in general, borderline personality disorders, and other characterologically disordered individuals, who tend to act out conflict rather than to experience it internally. Individuals with a high degree of internal structure and ego/superego function would most likely not need such a "holding environment" since they already possess the ability to deal with internal tension by acting on themselves rather than on the environment.

REFERENCES

Brown, L. J. 1981. The therapeutic milieu in the treatment of patients with borderline personality disorder. *Bulletin of the Menninger Clinic* 45:377–394.

Cowan, N. N. 1980. The manager-therapist team approach. *National Association of Private Psychiatric Hospitals Journal* 12:60–74.

Langs, R. J. 1979. *The Therapeutic Environment*. New York: Jason Aronson.

Stanton, A. H., and Schwartz, M. S. 1954. *The Mental Hospital*. New York: Basic.

Winnicott, D. W. 1965. *The Maturational Process and the Facilitating Environment: Studies in the Theory of Emotional Development*. New York: International Universities Press.

PART VI

COUNTERTRANSFERENCE RESPONSES TO ADOLESCENTS

INTRODUCTION: COUNTERTRANSFERENCE RESPONSES TO ADOLESCENTS

PETER L. GIOVACCHINI

For those clinicians who work primarily with patients on an individual basis and utilize the relationship between patient and therapist as the pivotal element around which the therapeutic process revolves, countertransference elements have achieved increasing importance in a fashion paralleling our ever-deepening understanding of the transference. As recently as fifteen years ago, many therapists were reluctant to discuss their own feelings about patients, fearful that they might be criticized for them and that they were indicative of bad therapeutic practices. The situation today is completely different. If anything, it is sometimes difficult to get therapists to discuss their patients' material because they are talking about themselves and what they feel about the patient, rather than the reverse.

The chapters in this section strike a good balance between revelations from the therapist and revelations from the patient. They represent honest discussions of how most clinicians will respond when facing situations that, for the most part, are difficult to deal with. Adolescents have a propensity for creating problems within the treatment setting because of their reticence about becoming engaged or their inclination to express themselves through action rather than words and feelings. Our responses to the various impasses adolescents typically produce, interestingly enough, have become our most valuable asset in giving us technical guidance to deal with what at first seem to be impossible situations. True, some impasses may, in fact, be difficult; but if we make a frank and nonanxious examination of our feelings, many may prove to be resolvable.

The chapters in this section are rich with examples of delicate and sensitive clinical interactions that stress the use of countertransference responses for both understanding and the reestablishment of psychic equilibrium in therapist and patient, enabling the treatment process to be set in motion once again. Giovacchini outlines a variety of situations that often occur, especially with adolescent patients, that are threatening to the therapist. The countertransference responses described are, for the most part, expectable and would be likely to be evoked in the majority of therapists. Natasha Wallace and Marquis Wallace discuss a type of treatment impasse that is familiar to most clinicians, especially those who treat adolescents. The therapist had absorbed the patient's deepest vulnerabilities and isolation as she was reacted to in the same way that the patient had experienced her mother. W. W. Meissner extends his concept about the paranoid process as he observes it in his interaction with adolescent patients. He emphasizes special features and sensitivities that are stimulated by a particular characterological constellation. Feinsilver extends Meissner's area of inquiry by discussing schizophrenic patterns and interactions, as he observes parallels in his responses and sequences of thoughts, attitudes, and behavior with those he notes in the interactions between various family members and the patient. Zaslow recounts his experiences in the context of very basic and sometimes poignant feelings that have surfaced and that he heeded as warning not to repeat destructive psychopathological interactions.

These articles cover a comprehensive range of countertransference responses, but, inasmuch as the human mind is so diverse, there are many other interactions that could also be profitably shared. Therapists who rely heavily on countertransference responses tend to be more open in reporting their experiences with patients as they are willing to face disruptive and emotional elements within themselves. This is an enriching experience for the therapists, the patient, and the reader.

30 COUNTERTRANSFERENCE AND THE SEVERELY DISTURBED ADOLESCENT

PETER L. GIOVACCHINI

In the treatment relationship, the study of countertransference reactions has become as important as the understanding of transference projections. This applies especially to the treatment of severely disturbed patients, patients with characterological problems. Inasmuch as adolescence represents a developmental phase in which character consolidation occurs, psychopathology during this period of life tends to involve defects in character structure. Therefore, countertransference factors assume special importance when we attempt to deal with adolescents therapeutically.

It is generally assumed that the more disturbed or primitively fixated the patient is, the harder he is to treat. There is supposedly a direct relationship between the severity of psychopathology and difficulties inherent in psychotherapy. I raise the question whether this is true. If it is, is it intrinsic to the psychopathology itself, or do primitively fixated patients with structural defects provoke disruptive countertransference reactions that create therapeutic impasses?

In addition to the degree of psychopathology, there are other, perhaps more important, variables that determine how difficult it will be to treat a patient. I recall hysterical adolescents who had been sent to me as classical examples of well-integrated, oedipally centered psychoneuroses who were so resistive to becoming engaged in a therapeutic relationship in spite of constricting symptoms such as agoraphobia that treatment never really got started. In contrast, I have seen severely disturbed adolescents in the throes of an identity crisis that sometimes resembled an acute schizophrenic episode who eagerly sought the holding environment that therapy could supply for them.

0-226-24058-4/85/0012-0010$01.00

Perhaps diagnostic categories are not as precise as we have believed, nor do they inform us about the intensity of the psychopathology. Hysterics frequently reveal a psychotic core underlying the superficial hysterical organization and symptomatology. The patients we encounter who are obviously disturbed may be less defended but not more pathological than other patients who appear to be better integrated. Possibly because they are less defended, they are more accessible to and better motivated for treatment.

Thus patients are more or less difficult to engage in treatment, and the intensity of psychopathology is not a decisive factor. Some therapists can treat patients others cannot. No one can treat all patients, and our personal orientation and reactions figure prominently in our capacity to conduct psychotherapy. Rather than view treatability only in terms of the patient's limitations, it is more realistic to consider the patient-therapist relationship as the axis that determines treatability. A patient may not be treatable by a particular therapist, but that does not make that patient untreatable.

Today the acknowledgment and discussion of countertransference responses have become respectable. This is in sharp contrast to the analytic ideology of even just a decade ago. Freud (1910) had warned us about the need to do away with our feelings toward patients since they interfered with analytic neutrality and would inevitably disrupt the course of analysis. Perhaps the analyst would have to seek further analysis for himself to achieve this objective.

With the increasing realization that analysis is a very personal experience for the analyst as well as the patient, it was concluded that the analyst's feelings cannot be swept away, nor should they be, by further training analysis. We have learned also that much can be learned about the patient through our countertransference responses (see Epstein and Feiner 1979). Indeed, in many instances—and this is especially true of patients suffering from relative fixations on primitive mental states—a favorable turn of events which preserves the analytic setting from chaotic collapse may well depend on the recognition of how a relationship based on the interaction of transference and countertransference elements repeats infantile trauma.

Thus, countertransference can be both good and bad for analytic resolution. Obviously, if it is unrecognized, the analyst will lose his analytic orientation, and, as Freud (1910) insisted, it will lead to deleterious effects. More often than not the therapist becomes intrusive and subtly blames the patient because the analysis is not proceeding as it should. He may make interpretations that are really criticisms, the purpose of which is to give the analyst relief rather than furnish the patient with some insight about his mental processes. In extreme instances the analysis is terminated, either because the patient can no longer stand it or the therapist has dismissed the patient because he is too sick and should never have been accepted for treatment in the first place.

These reactions are familiar examples of the destructive potential of unconscious orientations and impulses if they do not become subject to ego-integrative forces. Are countertransference elements always useful for analysis if they become subject to conscious awareness? Of course, more than mere recognition is required. The analyst's feelings have to be understood in terms of various frames of reference. The therapist must know what has happened to his feelings and why, in terms of his development and infantile past. He also has to learn how the patient's psychopathology threatens some of his characterological adaptations.

Before enumerating instances of specific countertransference responses, I must first mention what I mean, that is, how I define countertransference. I believe countertransference is ubiquitous; it is found in every analytic interaction in the same way transference is. Everything a therapist or a patient thinks, feels, or does can be viewed as being on a hierarchal spectrum, one end dominated by unconscious, primary process elements and the other end dominated by reality-oriented, secondary process factors. When a patient directs his feelings toward the therapist, the primary process elements of the spectrum represent transference, and in a similar fashion that part of the analyst's responses that stem primarily from the more primitive levels of his psyche can be viewed as countertransference. These assessments are quantitative.

Although every reaction in the analytic setting has either a transference or countertransference element, it may not be significant or useful. Patients may present us with material that is so reality oriented that we cannot discern its unconscious transference component, or if we can discern it, we are unable to interpret it. Nevertheless, it is still there, as the principle of psychic determinism has taught us. Regarding countertransference, we may have to be even more alert to the primitive infantile elements within us so that they do not interfere with our analytic objectivity, as Freud (1910) has warned us. Equally important, not being aware of our countertransference may cause us to miss an opportunity that could become a turning point for the analysis.

There have been various classifications of countertransference responses. Racker (1968), for example, distinguishes two types of countertransference, one based on concordant identifications and the other on complementary identifications. In the former, the therapist is empathic and identified with some portion of the patient's id or ego, whereas, in the latter, the analyst is the receptacle for an unwanted projection. Other authors (see Epstein and Feiner 1979) consider countertransference responses to be direct reactions to the patient's transference, whereas some clinicians would consider any irrational response of the analyst, not just those stimulated by transference projections, as countertransference. I divide countertransference into two categories: (1) homogeneous and (2) idiosyncratic.

By homogeneous, I mean reactions that we might expect from most psychoanalysts. If a patient becomes murderously threatening, most of us would feel afraid. This is a realistic response, but it still has its unconscious roots. In a more subtle fashion, patients may produce certain types of material which would cause us to be somewhat disturbed. For example, a patient may project devalued parts of the self into us or he may withdraw and shut us out. A large number of analysts want to pursue the withdrawn patient. It is not that they are overwhelmed or that they will in fact react, but feeling some discomfort, even only transiently, is common under these circumstances. These are human sensitivities which are manageable as the therapist maintains his analytic perspective.

Idiosyncratic responses also need not be disruptive, but they often are. The unique qualities of the analyst's background and his particular character makeup are responsible for disturbing reactions to clinical material that could be taken in stride by another analyst. An analyst not wanting to treat a patient because she is in many respects like his mother is an especially clear and simple example of an idiosyncratic response. In some instances, this type of countertransference reaction is the outcome of the analyst's unresolved psychopathology. However, idiosyncratic orientations can be particularly favorable for the analytic treatment of some patients. In these instances, the analyst's tolerance is greater than that of the majority of analysts.

Clinical Examples of Countertransference

What follows are, for the most part, examples of the homogeneous type of countertransference. However, when one deals with human responses, absolute distinctions are neither possible nor desirable. As discussed, there will always be an unconscious personal element, no matter how rational our responses might be.

COUNTERTRANSFERENCE AND THE NEED TO BE UNREASONABLE

I will begin with one of the most difficult situations I can think of, that is, the patient who refuses to leave at the end of the hour. The patient knows he or she is being unreasonable and intruding on someone else's time, but this makes no difference. He does not care about other persons, just himself.

There are several ways in which we might respond to such a dilemma, but none is guaranteed to work. Of course, it is best to keep matters in an analytic context, but there are inherent problems. For example, we might attempt to interpret the meaning of such behavior, but when we do, we are doing it more to seek relief for ourselves rather than to make an unambivalent observation about the patient's mental processes. Our interpretation is either a prohibition or an appeal for the patient to leave. In extreme cases, I suppose we could call the police or security guards to have the patient ejected. It would be especially unpleasant physically to throw the patient out, even if the therapist were able to do so, but it has been done, especially with children. None of these alternatives is satisfactory, and some may permanently impair the capacity to continue the analysis, although the analyst may not particularly care.

Fortunately, I have not had this problem often. The first time I was faced with such a dilemma I told the patient, a young college freshman, that I wanted him to leave so I would not get further upset. I did not want to be put in a position in which I would not want to see him on his next appointment. I did not want to be analytically useless, since, if he persisted in such behavior, I would sit there worrying about the end of the hour rather than listening to him. This patient understood and left.

Years later, I had a similar encounter with a middle-aged woman. I said exactly the same thing to her that I had said to the previous patient. She surprised me when she sarcastically replied that she did not have any interest at all in my feelings, all she was concerned about was herself. Furthermore, she had heard from a friend who attended one of my seminars that I had said the same thing to another patient, and she was fully prepared for what she labeled as a ploy. I felt helpless and told her so. I then added that I was leaving. The appointment was in my home office, so I could move to another section of the house. When I returned, I expected her to be gone; otherwise, I would terminate the treatment. The patient angrily left, but I was not pleased with myself for having threatened to break off the analysis. However, I did not know what else I could have done, and I still do not know.

Another patient, a young lady in her late teens, is being treated by a psychiatrist who comes to see me periodically for supervision. Briefly, she is a primitively fixated person who has little in the way of adaptive techniques to relate to the external world. She made demands of her therapist, but there was little substance to them. What gradually became apparent was that she needed to have constant contact with him. She called frequently during both day and night. At first this irritated him, but on occasion he was able to tell her that he did not want to talk to her any longer and he hung up.

The situation in the office was another matter. She refused to leave at the end of the hour. The first time this happened, it had no particular consequence, since the psychiatrist had no other patient scheduled. He simply left and asked her to make certain the door was locked when she finally decided to leave. He felt uneasy about the situation but vainly hoped it would not happen again.

The inevitable occurred the next session when again she firmly stated that she wanted to remain there forever. This time, the therapist picked her up and carried her into the hall. He did not want to do this and felt humiliated and guilty for having abandoned his professional decorum.

He reached the following unorthodox conclusion. He would see her in a place where he could be mobile and terminate the session without being dependent on her acceptance. Instead of meeting in his office, they held their sessions early in the morning in a booth in the restaurant of his office building. This arrangement has been in effect several months and has turned out to be comfortable for both therapist and patient. It might be stretching the point to consider this an analytic relationship, but it is based on an understanding of the patient's needs, psychodynamics, structural defects, and transference demands. In any case, the treatment continues, and it seems to be progressing as it should.

Demanding that our patients see us in a particular setting can be considered rigidity. I know that I have this kind of rigidity, and because I am comfortable in my consulting room and happen to treat patients who accommodate themselves to the setting I provide, I do not feel at all impelled to become more flexible. In part this is due to the many years

I have spent working in this fashion, having become a creature of habit. Furthermore, we also have to realize our limitations. No one can treat all types of patients. However, I believe it is important to recognize that some patients cannot be treated in a conventional setting, and if the therapist is not totally tied to that setting, many of these patients could have an analytic experience in surroundings in which the therapist is not vulnerable to infantile demands.

This lack of vulnerability creates a calm, secure setting in which the patient's anxieties can be contained. The analyst maintains an observational frame of reference and does not become personally enmeshed in the content of the patient's feelings and associations. These are essential features of any analysis. The unreasonable patient's demands interfere sufficiently with what we might consider the formal elements of analysis. Analytic sessions for some patients recapitulate certain infantile rhythms. The routine frequency of the interviews is perceived as a nurturing or soothing experience. Tension accumulates during the time between sessions. If some mental representation of the analyst can be sustained, then waiting for the next session becomes tolerable, since the patient can obtain some gratification, or at least relief, from the analytic introject and the anticipation of the next session. The unreasonable patient finds this in-between time intolerable.

These patients' lack of psychic structure does not permit such variability of symptomatic manifestations. Freud (1915) discussed how sexual drives can be directed toward many different objects. They have considerable flexibility, whereas the ego or self-preservative instincts do not. They can be expressed in only a limited fashion, and there are no substitute objects of gratification. In the treatment setting, most patients can modulate their symptoms, the expression of their psychopathology, in such a fashion that they can be contained in the consultation room. Adolescent patients, especially, often fear that they cannot and may test the analyst, but usually the patient and analyst can reach a compromise. The unreasonable patient often cannot modulate symptoms and character traits so that they are compatible with analytic routine.

An ego defect that cannot integrate internal objects and form mental representations requires the constant presence of the nurturing or soothing person. There is no substitute for this, and these patients have not sufficiently developed the capacity for symbolization to displace their needs onto alternative objects.

Whatever the specific qualities of the infantile environment, it has been traumatic in that the child has felt abandoned. As children, they have not suffered from a total absence of object relations. Rather, they have experienced inconstant relationships, and their needs have been capriciously handled. Sometimes they have been met, and at other times they have been ignored or rejected. The external world is unpredictable, but the child's needs, because of biological rhythms, follow a predictable sequence. Inasmuch as the child does not have the security that he will be cared for, he will later form the impression either that his demands are unreasonable or that he lives in an unreasonable world.

As adults, they demand the right to be unreasonable, which represents a defense against and compensation for an unreasonable infantile environment. They require instant and total satisfaction of needs because otherwise they will not have any assurance whatsoever that gratification is forthcoming. This is the only method they have to make the world predictable.

THE PATIENT WHO HAS NOTHING TO SAY

Another extremely difficult situation that many therapists would like to avoid is one in which the patient has taken the stance that he or she has nothing to say. I assumed that this was an adolescent quality, and perhaps it is, inasmuch as adolescence is a developmental phase in which the character is still unconsolidated and fragmented and has not yet achieved synthesis and cohesion of the self-representation. Not being able to talk, that is, being incapable of free-associating in the treatment setting, often turned out to be a manifestation of not being able to allow unconscious derivatives into the sphere of awareness because various parts of the psyche were unconnected with each other. I am referring to an ego defect that has to be distinguished from repression. I am postulating a lack of a continuum between consciousness and the unconscious. When these patients state that they have nothing to say, they literally do not; they are not withdrawing, resisting, or repressing.

The following short vignette illustrates these concepts in a clinical therapeutic interaction. This nineteen-year-old patient who sought therapy because of general dissatisfaction with life and a sense of futility and not belonging would lapse into long periods of silence which he claimed he experienced as lapses or blanks. Other than ascertaining this, I did not interrupt them. We were both fairly comfortable for a while, but then he felt obligated to produce more material. As he lay on the couch, he showed signs of considerable distress. In fact, he seemed to be in tremendous pain. He would writhe and twist, his face contorted and grimacing as if he were being subjected to torture, and then he would scream and shout incoherently quite loudly. He moaned and grunted, often startling me because these agonizing outbursts would occur when I least expected them. From the defensive position in which he pulled his arms over his head and face, I at first thought he was defending himself from an anticipated blow from me.

I asked him whether he was reacting to the possibility of my hitting him, but he clarified that he was reacting to something within himself. He then described that he felt some disruptive, inchoate feeling welling up deep inside of him. Rather than being tamed as it was approaching the surface of consciousness, it would simply jump an inner gap and explode instead of being modulated by being put into words.

I thought of quantum jumps and sparks traversing a space between two electrodes, that is, of an increasing intensity of potential energy bursting into a spark. The patient spontaneously stated that he felt himself to be a Van de Graaff generator. He also recalled a science fiction movie that he had seen some years ago of a scientist on another planet who had a machine that would translate raw emotions and feelings into thoughts and words.

This patient used splitting defenses, and even his movements had an uncoordinated, fragmented quality. He was clumsy and inept with his hands, although he was intellectually superior. He was also likable, and his friends maintained a protective attitude toward him.

His treatment had many difficult moments because he was unable to modulate unconscious derivatives, that is, subject them to secondary process revision so that he could communicate his inner life by his associations. He produced either primary process outbursts or all secondary process expressions, as evidenced by his concrete thinking and the endless, monotonous, obsessive expositions of everyday events unconnected to mental processes.

He complained about his inability to make progress, and even though he blamed himself, I still felt he was covertly reproaching me. In this context, he vociferously lamented that he had nothing to say. I felt frustrated, not because of his silence but because I felt useless if I had no material to analyze. I found it interesting that he could cause me to have such uncomfortable feelings.

At first, I treated his silence as resistance and confronted him with the intention of getting him to free-associate. It was only when I began to believe that he, indeed, had nothing to say that I was able to understand my dilemma in terms of the patient's psychic discontinuity.

I finally learned that his having nothing to say was related to an inability to energize the deeper parts of his personality. At the same time, he was unable to relate to me because, at these times, I did not exist for him. I existed for others, but not him. This was depicted in a dream that was very similar to a fantasy I was having about our relationship and my nonexistence. In the dream he and I were in a dark room, but he did not know whether I was actually there because he could not see me. I had been thinking about a tree falling in the forest and the question whether it made any noise if no one were there to hear the sound.

Conceptually speaking, I felt the patient was describing a form of psychic discontinuity in which he was relatively unable to cathect his unconscious, that is, the primitive aspects of the self. As a consequence, he was unable to cathect me as well, and therefore I did not exist. He could not form and hold a mental representation of me juxtaposed with the id. In other words, in order to set the process of free association in motion, he had to initiate an energetic current between the deeper recesses of the personality and an external object—both had to be cathected. In the dream, turning on the light in the room would have illuminated both his mind and myself. At that period in treatment he could not achieve this.

Fraiberg's (1969) discussion of the lack of object constancy applies to my patient and many others with similar structural problems. Her description focused on the inability to form and hold a mental representation without the reinforcement of the actual presence of the external object. These patients demonstrate a similar phenomenon but emphasize reciprocity in that the internal world cannot cathect the external object in order to make communication between the mind and the external world possible.

This lack of acknowledgment of the therapist and the insistence that they have nothing to say makes these patients particularly difficult to treat. They often lament that they are wasting their time coming to appointments, and they frequently miss or cancel them. The therapist feels useless, and the patient strives to reinforce this feeling.

What we often fail to grasp is that, in spite of the cavalier treatment we are subjected to, we nevertheless are valued by the patient. Similarly to the transitional object, we are psychically manhandled and abused, but our presence is vital. This was impressed on me by a borderline psychotic adolescent who constantly reviled me as being useless and saw no point in continuing the therapy. He emphasized the latter because he felt strongly that he could not talk to me. During one session, my attention momentarily lagged when I looked at the blinking dots of a small digital clock, and the patient had a tantrum. He cried and screamed, paced around the room, and tore his hair. He shouted that here he was trying to open up to me (actually he was, as usual, denigrating me) and I reacted like everyone else by withdrawing and abandoning him. He impressed on me how important it was to survive his deprecations and that I be there. I became so aware of this that I felt terrible about having failed him, and I profusely apologized for my momentary inattention. He finally realized that I was truly sorry, and, although disgruntled when he left, he returned for subsequent sessions.

The therapist's survival of the patient's destructiveness and his acceptance of the role of a transitional object for the patient enables the patient to use him as a connecting bridge between unconnected parts of the psyche and as an entry into the external world. This can be a painful experience for the therapist, but he is absorbing the vulnerability and misery the patient had to endure during infancy because of being treated as nonhuman. The treatment process attempts to bring humanity into the relationship, even if the therapist has to face the inner disruption of an existential crisis and dehumanization.

COUNTERTRANSFERENCE AND THE ANALYST'S EGO-IDEAL

I first saw this patient when he was nineteen because he was having difficulties in college. He was not failing his courses, although his academic status was marginal. He just managed to get by in his quizzes, although it was clear that he was so far behind in various projects that he was not going to be able to get through the semester. The problem, however, was complex in that it involved other issues beyond academic performance. He had succeeded in antagonizing, sometimes enraging, his instructors. He had also alienated his peers and was generally considered obnoxious.

He remained with me for approximately six months, at which time he developed an intense negative transference. In the meantime, he had idealized a colleague, and I was not particularly dismayed when he decided to terminate therapy with me and see my colleague. That relationship lasted only four months because he developed a negative transference toward my colleague and now idealized me. This swinging back and forth between the two of us occurred at least four more times, causing my colleague and me to become impatient. The final straw was his wanting to see both of us at the same time.

I put my foot down, and my colleague did the same, by telling the patient he had to choose; he could not see both of us. The patient could not make such a choice, so he had to discontinue treatment, something we forced on him. Both my colleague and I had to admit that we were glad to be rid of him, although we could not really understand why.

We were trying to make the patient do something he did not have the capacity to accomplish, that is, be sufficiently integrated so that he could direct love and hate toward the same person. He was too fragmented to achieve that kind of synthesis. He seemed, however, to have sufficient organization to be able to sustain ambivalence, and in retrospect it was this appearance of cohesiveness that puzzled us.

He returned to me several years later when he was twenty-six, saying that he was stable enough to remain in analysis with one therapist. He behaved properly, indicating faith in analysis and showing me genuine respect. In spite of all this, I found myself being irritated with him, and I did not look forward to his sessions. I could not understand my reactions since he was not doing anything that was unusual or unpleasant.

I asked permission to tape-record an interview, which he generously granted. I then played the tape to both colleagues and students, and I was interested to observe that practically all the listeners felt a similar irritation toward him. Some stated that the patient was not free-associating, but they could not specify how they reached this conclusion and why this should stimulate negative feelings. Others referred to the patient's pontifical tone, but they were also puzzled about why this bothered them since they were otherwise at ease with patients who presented themselves in such a fashion.

The patient was somehow upsetting my professional stance and threatening my analytic identity. His material was infuriatingly rational, and it did not seem to offer any openings that would enable me to glimpse with him into his unconscious. I can best illustrate this by discussing the content of his discussions and referring to his pontifical tone.

He was involved in many fringe movements, such as fad diets, oriental herbs, and particularly astrology. The fact that I have referred to such activities as "fringe movements" implies that I am reacting with value judgments, an attitude which must, to some measure, be nonanalytic. He presented his position eloquently and worked hard, that is, proselytized, to convert me to his viewpoint. I sometimes felt that he was taking the extreme position of having me give up psychoanalysis in favor of astrology.

Again, these are fairly commonly encountered clinical situations, especially for clinicians who treat patients who suffer from relatively primitive fixations. Attaching themselves with grandiosity to a cause often holds together patients suffering from terrifying feelings of helplessness and vulnerability. These are psychopathological adaptations, but they are nevertheless adaptations, so why should they cause adverse countertransference reactions, not only in me but in all my colleagues and students who heard the tape-recorded interview? If it had not been for the latter, I would have classified my response as an idiosyncratic type of countertransference and would have tried to explain it solely on the basis of some peculiarity of my own.

I finally concluded that the patient's combination of rational logic and megalomaniacal devotion to systems that have no scientific foundation was the basis of my difficulty. I found myself disrupted and unable to maintain a calm, nonjudgmental attitude toward the patient.

Most of us—that is, those analysts who are willing to treat seriously emotionally disturbed patients—are comfortable with obvious craziness. We view the delusion as a necessary adaptation.

This patient's ego-ideal was able to find his paranoia acceptable because the latter was depicted in a secondary process fashion. My countertransference dilemma was the outcome of a conflict within my ego-ideal because I had not yet recognized the paranoia.

As I look at the patient's material now, it becomes obvious that he was being grandiose about his various sytems, especially astrology. He was, in fact, delusional about his powers of forecasting the future and his own unlimited abilities to determine the fate of a world which he had neatly divided according to the paranoid dichotomies of good and bad. He was omnipotently good and powerful, qualities which were demonstrated by his astrological skills, and there were external forces that were inherently evil, seeking to undermine him and to make him suffer miserably. As I present this material it seems consistent with a basically paranoid orientation, but that was not the way he described it. His discussions were calm and carried out in a well-modulated tone, indicating sensitivity and perceptiveness. He had pulled his thoughts and feelings together so that they seemed plausible on the surface.

I am reminded of certain patients whose delusional system is rationally constructed but founded on a false premise. We call these cases *paranoia vera*. I suppose my patient had qualities similar to those of this rare group of patients, but he may have been different in that there was no particular false premise serving as a foundation for a series of convictions which followed a rational sequence. All of his beliefs, if toned down, could have been true, although we would have to fill in gaps in our knowledge to be able to explore them. He was, in fact, discussing metaphysical principles without recognizing that he had gone beyond the scientific frame of reference. This must be the case with any rationally stated delusion.

My adverse countertransference reactions were manifested by an impulse to argue with him, that is, to confront the material directly and correct the reality distortions. From a professional viewpoint, this is as wrong as one can be. It is, in fact, the same thing as trying to argue a psychotic patient out of a delusion.

Some of the listeners to the tape-recorded interview complained about the patient's arrogance and his pontificating attitude. I do not believe any of us would have been affected by it if we could have seen that it was connected to his inner sense of emptiness. Instead, all of us tended to place his all-knowing attitude with his actual accomplishments, which amounted to absolutely nothing. We experienced his ignoring reality as offensive.

He had presented his material in such a fashion that we recognized neither its defensive, megalomaniac, overcompensating qualities nor the underlying helpless vulnerability he was defending himself against. As long as he succeeded in getting us into another frame of reference based on his consistency and rationality as well as his realistic limitations, we were no longer functioning as analysts. We felt guilty at having abandoned the analytic stance. Furthermore, standards that we valued, the content of our ego-ideal, were threatened.

The patient's message that I was receiving from the upper levels of his psyche was that I change my therapeutic modus operandi in favor of astrology. Reacting at only this level of communication was disruptive to me and offended my professional ego-ideal and my self-representation as a psychoanalyst. When I was able to place his admonitions in context with his severe characterological disturbance, in essence his psychosis, I was able to regain my therapeutic stance.

This patient's ability to hide his psychosis in reality, so to speak, created therapeutic impasses. Another example occurred when he accused me of not protecting him from a damaging sexual encounter that he felt would ruin him. Again this was a situation in which he was demanding that I do something beyond trying to understand how his mind worked and that I deal with him through transference interpretations. I was supposed to have taken specific action. He vociferously reprimanded me, and I resented it.

Once more he had a plausible, if not an entirely logical, argument. He spent the night with a lesbian, and now he feared that his reputation was ruined. If others found out about his tawdry sexual encounter, he would no longer be held in high esteem. He would be ridiculed and laughed at instead of being taken seriously. This struck me as strange since the patient had accomplished absolutely nothing in his life. He had never completed a course in college, finished a term paper, or concluded any project. Nevertheless, he came from a distinguished family, could trace his ancestry to some very famous persons, and belonged to a highly prestigious country club. He had responsibilities to live up to the family name, and others had high expectations of him.

On the surface, these attitudes seemed somewhat realistic—if we allow ourselves to stretch some points. Perhaps a knowledge of his encounter, in spite of our liberal sexual attitudes, might have provoked some snickers. The intensity of his response, however, and his insistence that I should have done something to stop him were totally out of proportion with the stimulus of his errant behavior. Again, I felt irritated toward him as I remained fixated on his attacks at the surface level, a fixation which, to a large extent, he forced on me. Gradually, I began to understand his response in the larger context of his psychopathology, and I was able to view once again his provocations as material.

This is another example of clothing delusional material in somewhat secondary process garb. It was true that he came from an illustrious family, and therefore it was not so strange that he felt that he should be, like Caesar's wife, above reproach. I learned subsequently that this quasi-rational attitude covered up an underlying delusion in which he believed he was the Messiah. He did not openly speak of this because it would not have been prudent to reveal himself at that moment. Nevertheless, he was the Messiah, and if others, his potential disciples, learned of his carnal indulgence, he would not be able to preserve his divine status in their eyes. That is why it was so vitally important that I protect him. Once I understood him at this level, I was able to relax and view his attacks as part of his delusion.

THE NEED TO FAIL AND THE ANALYTIC PARADOX

Severely disturbed patients have had traumatic infantile backgrounds in which they have been abandoned, rejected, or even assaulted. In treatment, they attempt to create a therapeutic ambience that replicates the traumatic infantile environment. They try to reproduce early interactions in which they have experienced maternal failure, a lack of empathy, and nongratification. The therapist is perceived as nonempathic and, in some instances, as having abandoned the patient. The latter occurs frequently enough in adolescents and is an aspect of the repetition compulsion.

As in all the examples given in this chapter, these are situations that should ideally be dealt with in a therapeutic frame of reference but which, because they touch on special sensitivities, stimulate countertransference reactions that impair the analyst's ability to maintain a therapeutic stance. The role in which the patient needs to cast the therapist runs counter to his or her therapeutic philosophy. Therapists are supposed to be empathic and accepting, not insensitive and rejecting. This is a very special instance in which analysts have to change the modus operandi of their ego-ideals. They have to understand how important it is for the patient to view them as having attributes that are antithetical to analysis.

In a way we are faced with a paradox, what I have called the "analytic paradox," by which I mean a situation in which the patient's psychopathology becomes imbricated with the therapeutic process; it is either reinforced by or clashes with the process. What I have just described is an example of clashing with the process. Analytic neutrality, however, for some patients may be experienced similarly to early rejections and abandonments, that is, archaic relationships that supplied material needs but did not relate to the child's emerging sense of aliveness. In this instance, neutrality reinforces these early traumatic situations as they are reenacted in the transference through the repetition compulsion, a reinforcement that leads to therapeutic impasses. The analyst is faced with the dilemma of changing his therapeutic style. This subject can be extensively discussed, but I will confine myself to an example in which I found myself reacting against the patient defending herself against early feelings of abandonment.

This patient is not an adolescent, but she was when I first started seeing her; she was fifteen. She remained in treatment for one and a half years and then suddenly decided to terminate. I did not believe this was a good time to stop, but she insisted, feeling she had accomplished what she wanted and leaving on good terms. She returned a year later, having for that year kept an idealized image of me. She maintained this image in her second course of treatment, which lasted for a year. She returned two years later, staying for only six months this time, but she continued idealizing me. I was mildly frustrated by the starting and stopping but passed it off as an example of adolescents' inherent difficulties anchoring themselves.

At the age of twenty-five she returned, but now her attitude toward me had completely reversed itself. She no longer idealized me; instead, she found fault with everything I did. Throughout the years she had met several of my patients and blamed me for intruding them into her life. She knew that I was not strictly to blame, but she continued reviling me. She also saw me as defensive and angry, and I imagine that to some extent I was.

I do not believe I would have had any particular reaction if she had not started manipulating her appointments. She would, for example, cancel an appointment or tell me about a trip at the last minute. She again began talking about stopping treatment, but, unlike previous occasions, she accused me of not being interested in her and wanting to get rid of her. I acknowledged to myself that there was some truth to what she said, but this was simply another source of conflict for me because I also wanted to bring the treatment of this young lady, whom I had seen on and off for a significant portion of her life, to a successful resolution.

My irritation mounted as she cavalierly canceled appointments and her unpaid bill increased. She saw nothing of value in our relationship and spent several sessions reading a book. She saw no reason why she should continue; in fact, she was going to terminate the next week. I angrily replied that she was perpetuating a pattern she had started with me many years ago and that I had reached the limits of my tolerance; if she insisted on quitting, that was up to her, and perhaps it might be best for both of us if she did. She tearfully ran out of the consultation room some minutes before the end of the session.

That afternoon I received through the mail a check paying the entire bill, indicating that she had sent it before this stormy session. At first I was relieved, but then I felt guilty. Two days later, I received a letter from her telling me how disappointed and sad she felt. She emphasized that she always thought very highly of me, but I had turned out to be just like all the other people in her life who had abandoned her. She also indicated that the date of our last session was the anniversary of her brother's suicide and her mother's death, something I was not aware of since she had never told me the exact dates of their deaths. She felt very sad about my reaction.

I was moved by her note and wrote back immediately. I took responsibility for my actions and apologized for having lost my equanimity. I told her I was also sad about what had happened, but I felt impelled to explain to her how I viewed our interaction and her participation. In essence, she had manipulated me into abandoning her as she believed her mother and brother had rejected her by dying. I had learned from previous periods of therapy that she had been raised by a series of indifferent maids, her mother never being around. During our last session she finally succeeded in provoking me into rejecting her, a repetition of the innumerable rejections of infancy.

Immediately after receiving my letter, she called for another appointment. She did not say a word about my letter and our last session but continued attacking me, although in a much milder fashion. She stated that I disappointed her but then recounted important past relationships in which she was accused of being disappointing. She was able to recognize projections. Her treatment continues, and she has now been with me for three years, the longest period of treatment she has ever sustained.

Conclusions

The crucial elements of treatment of severely disturbed patients often revolve around the transference-countertransference axis. Although this can be disruptive to both patient and therapist, the resolution of turmoil through understanding and repetition of infantile traumatic patterns can lead to significant therapeutic progress.

Patients attack the therapist in various sensitive areas. They may threaten his sense of existence and sometimes precipitate an existential crisis that the analyst will defend himself against. They may try to undermine the analyst's professional ego-ideal, trying to force him to abandon the therapeutic stance by coercing him to enter the patient's daily life or participate in a delusional system.

I have discussed several interactions based on incursions into these areas of the therapist's ego. There are other examples illustrating how the analyst's usual equilibrium can be disrupted, such as when the therapist absorbs the patient's painful excitement and is not able to contain it, but

I have to limit myself to these vignettes. The therapeutic interaction is as subtle as the two interacting minds that are participating in it.

REFERENCES

Epstein, L., and Feiner, A. H. 1979. *Countertransference*. New York: Aronson.

Fraiberg, S. 1969. Libidinal object constancy and object representation. *Psychoanalytic Study of the Child* 19:113–169.

Freud, S. 1910. The future prospects of psycho-analytic therapy. *Standard Edition* 11:139–151. London: Hogarth, 1957.

Freud, S. 1915. Instincts and their vicissitudes. *Standard Edition* 14:103–140. London: Hogarth, 1957.

Racker, H. 1968. *Transference and Countertransference*. New York: International Universities Press.

31 TRANSFERENCE/COUNTERTRANSFERENCE ISSUES IN THE TREATMENT OF AN ACTING-OUT ADOLESCENT

NATASHA L. WALLACE AND MARQUIS EARL WALLACE

The transference reaction of the patient and the countertransference of the therapist are central to psychoanalytic treatment. The concept of transference originally referred to attitudes and feelings that neurotic patients had toward whole objects (usually parents) from the oedipal phase of development. As psychoanalysis has focused on more severe forms of psychopathology and the contributions of earlier phases of development, the nature of what may be transferred has changed. At ages prior to the phallic-oedipal stage, experiences are organized differently and more primitively. When these experiences are recollected or repeated in the transference, they may be conceptualized in different ways. For example, the concept of a narcissistic transference refers to the idea that a part of the subject, as distinguished from object, is being externalized. Yet it is also possible that experiences of the environment with part-objects, that is, those serving specific needs, or even more primitive and global experiences of the environment, may also be repeated in the transference. The question presented by the case that is the subject of this chapter is whether the infant's experience of an overanxious and inadequate mother as a global object can be manifested in the transference.

The notion of countertransference has had varying meanings along various continua: from pathological to appropriate, from unconscious to conscious, from idiosyncratic to representing how the typical analyst might feel toward this patient, from a specific response to all feelings about the

0-226-24058-4/85/0012-0022$01.00

patient, and from dangerous to productive, particularly in relation to diagnostic validity. Whatever meaning and accompanying value has been placed on countertransference, there can be little debate that among psychoanalytically oriented therapists it is important and understanding it is crucial. At one point in the treatment of the case, the therapist (N. L. W.) came to doubt her own capacities, skills, and competence in dealing with the patient. This feeling so dominated the treatment that a stalemate seemed likely.

In certain cases, how and what the patient communicates to the analyst, and how the analyst responds to the patient, may be different from any other relationship in the patient's life. The psychoanalytic situation (including the analyst's basic orientation), the means of learning about the patient, and the isolation of the treatment from the rest of the patient's interpersonal world are special. The structure of treatment increases the probability that the deepest emotions and feelings will be revealed in this objectively protected atmosphere. Here the analyst will become privy to and react to aspects of the patient not revealed to anyone else. Indeed, the transference construct requires, at a minimum, that the patient must have experienced these feelings toward at least one person, other than the analyst, in childhood. Perhaps, then, only one person other than the analyst may have been in the position to respond to these attitudes. Yet, because the patient was a child, it is likely that the parent may not have known these feelings were present, or at least not in the way the therapist does.

Still, in other cases the patient feels toward and elicits from many other people the same reactions that they feel toward, expect from, and stimulate in the analyst. This more global attitude and the universal response that it causes may ultimately be the source of suffering, continuing and repeating the trauma of the patient's past. The analyst may find, in the countertransference, that he develops attitudes toward the patient that may be similar, or identical, to what others in the patient's life may feel toward the patient.

In the case to be described, each adult in this patient's world reacted to this creative, intelligent, early-adolescent girl who was seriously acting out by becoming overwhelmed. Indeed, one of the presenting complaints of her mother was, "No one can handle her." In the course of twice-weekly therapy, after one and one-half years, the transference/countertransference relationship created an intense situation, with the "overwhelmed" response reaching nearly traumatic proportions in the therapist.

The result was a therapeutic impasse which threatened to destroy the treatment and may have constituted a threat to other aspects of the patient's emotional and physical health.

Among the criticisms of the psychoanalytic method has been its circular logic and the limitations of its data-gathering method. It is alleged that whatever the analyst cannot account for as a response to the present is transference. This is then used to justify the impact of the past on the present. In the treatment of an adult, child, or adolescent, when the therapist does not have contact with the parents or significant others, verification that the patient's attitudes toward the therapist are actually being transferred from an early relationship is assumed from theory rather than proved. External sources of validity, even if available, are not used. Even if they were, one could not actually go back to the time when the attitudes and feelings were originally felt to see what the child's real feelings were. Memories undergo so great an alteration in this period that it becomes difficult to understand how early memories can survive the oedipal period intact. As a logical extension, the older child, adolescent, or adult's recollection of his childhood, or repetition in the transference, may be altered by screen memories and other ego developments after that time, further altering the content of what is recollected.

Similarly, the analyst can only rarely verify that his feelings toward the patient are appropriate diagnostic countertransference rather than the analyst's personal transference to the patient. Although material can be presented at a case conference, and others may feel the same as the analyst toward the patient, the material presented is biased by the presenter's selection of what to present.[1]

Particularly in psychoanalytically oriented psychotherapy, as distinguished from psychoanalysis, but also in the psychoanalysis of younger children, therapists have contact with adults significant to the patient. These contacts, especially in what they reveal about the patient's developmental history, often contain areas of inaccuracy and omissions owing to a variety of factors in the mental functioning of those reporting, not the least of which is their distortions of the situation at the time it originated, the change of a memory with the passage of time, and current emotional factors influencing reliability. Often this inaccuracy is not important, because working through takes place through the transference (rather than in effigy). However, in the present case, the information obtained was critical to the resolution of the therapist's countertransference.

The issue of who communicates with whom can be particularly sensitive in the treatment of an adolescent. Parents may attempt to contact the therapist even when there has been an agreement not to. Sometimes the therapist will meet with the patient and parents, together or separately, on a planned basis. In other cases parents are seen by another therapist who may obtain the history, provide counseling, or even perform therapy with one or both of the parents. As a result, there are external sources of information about the patient which may be useful.

Case Illustration

In this case, the mother was permitted to contact the therapist by phone, and the therapist would report this to the patient. On a few occasions, the therapist met with mother and patient conjointly. In addition, the parents were seen by another therapist (M. E. W.) who at times collaborated with the patient's therapist. As will be seen, this collaboration made available certain crucial information about the patient's early development which clarified the nature of the countertransference. This not only saved the treatment but led to major modifications in the patient's use of the treatment and her emotional, physical, and social well-being outside of treatment.

Carole started treatment when she was thirteen years old, stating that it was her choice to seek help because she was unable to handle her problems. She had no control over stealing and cursing at her mother, and she was not only failing at school but was consistently in trouble with authorities. There was no sector of her life that was successful or satisfactory.

Her mother complained in a similar vein. "I don't know how to handle Carole anymore. I don't know if I should send her to live with her father, because he also has given up on her. I feel overwhelmed. She treats me badly, it wears me down. I am afraid she is never going to finish school and will live a miserable life." The mother added that the public school would let Carole finish the year but would not accept her back. Shortly after the beginning of treatment, the mother did give up on Carole, who then lived in a guest house adjacent to her father's home.

In an interview with the father, he corroborated her alleged incorrigibility; he could not handle her and did not know what to do for her. Shortly after beginning treatment, she began to take drugs and to run wild with boys, and she came close to trouble with the police. On one occasion, she was physically endangered. While hitchhiking, she was picked up by a stranger, who drove her into an alley and propositioned her to perform a perverse act. She ran away terrified.

HISTORY

Carole was the result of her mother's second pregnancy; the first ended in abortion. She was described as a robust baby who was breast-fed for one month and then bottle-fed. She had colic for four months, which was hard on the mother because she could get no rest. Carole tended to "flop around" a great deal when held. She walked at nine months, at which time she also put her first words together. At eighteen months she had a habit of climbing a chain-link fence. She was "defiant as hell" and would always do the opposite of a "don't" from age eighteen months to two and one-half years.

Although the marriage was good when Carole was born, it deteriorated quickly thereafter. Her parents divorced when she was three, the father marrying the eldest daughter of the neighbor next door. When Carole continued to wet into her third year, her mother consulted an expert on the behavior of children. The expert recommended that the mother threaten to remove everything from Carole's room the next time she wet and then do so. She did this, and although the wetting stopped, this became a traumatic experience for Carole and her mother. Ten months after the divorce, the mother married this expert. The marriage was an immediate disaster. Carole became terrified of him but obeyed him, and mother turned against him. They divorced within a year.

For the next eight years, mother lived alone with Carole. From age four to eight Carole had episodes of screaming, tantrums, and throwing and breaking objects. Carole then had counseling at a clinic twice weekly. When she was discharged, they said she may need additional help as an adolescent. She did not do well in school academically but had many friends. In fifth grade, after leaving counseling, she received tutoring and was brought up to a fifth-grade level. In seventh grade she received a B/C average but began to fail at the end of eighth grade. Menarche occurred at the end of her thirteenth year, to which she had a "fine" reaction. Her first sexual experience was in her fourteenth year while she was living in the guest house near her father. During that period father's wife was pregnant with their second child and Carole became involved with drugs and flunked out of two schools.

THE TREATMENT AND THE DEVELOPMENT OF THE COUNTERTRANSFERENCE

Although Carole chose to enter treatment of her own free will, she immediately expressed no desire to cooperate verbally with the treatment.

She was silent in many sessions, sometimes even falling asleep, reading magazines, or writing letters to her friends (see Giovacchini 1973, p. 364). I felt uneasy spending the time in what seemed like an unproductive manner, and she was unable to help me understand her need to use the situation in this way.

Although I allowed this, I attempted to see what meaning I could derive from it. At a minimum, before the end of each session, I would communicate something about what I thought her behavior might be expressing about her feelings. She responded to my comments by either nodding agreement, if she was in a good mood, or telling me it was "stupid," if she was feeling unhappy. Her reactions seemed to have nothing to do with the actual content of my comments; they could not be considered confirmation. She developed and expressed an antagonistic feeling toward the therapeutic relationship, to which I reacted with a sense of bewilderment since I felt I was being particularly tolerant and accepting. She also seemed to devalue me personally in a way which made no sense. At other times, she would give me some limited hope, even if surrounded with condemnations, as when she said, "I like you, and I have nothing against you, but I don't think I am getting anything out of this." I could even find some evidence of disguised positive transference when she expressed her admiration toward items of my apparel. Similarly, at times, she would demonstrate some identification with me, which I did not find unpleasurable, when she would wear a piece of clothing similar to mine, drawing attention to the similarity, saying "isn't this like the one you have?"

Although she would have little to say during sessions, I often heard of acting out from her concerned mother weeks after the act was performed. On one occasion she stole a skirt from a department store but mentioned nothing about it until I brought it up. I said her mother wanted us to meet together because of concern over her stealing. Carole minimized the importance of the act, and said she was with a girlfriend, wanted the skirt, did not have any money on her, and so she stole it. She minimized consequences since this was her first time getting caught stealing. When I heard of the acting out, I felt that I was being drawn into some responsibility for it, and I felt guilty, frustrated, and increasingly incompetent. My interventions during this beginning phase were mainly supportive and noncritical. I was trying to establish a working alliance and to understand what was being communicated.

After seeing Carole over a year, I began assessing my capacity to help her and felt despairing and defeated. I had serious doubts about my ability to help her and her ability to be helped. I wondered if she was unable or simply unwilling to use my treatment. My guilt about accepting fees and not providing help to a patient who did not talk in sessions and acted out outside of them increased. The only positive indication I had was that Carole faithfully attended sessions, even though she remarked that she did not want to come and missed on occasion.

At this point I was asked to present an adolescent patient at a clinical seminar. At first I was apprehensive, since gains were not evident and I feared that my inadequacy as a therapist would be publicly exposed. At the same time, however, I felt strongly and strangely involved with this difficult patient. I had a desire to use any help I could receive to gain a better understanding of this young girl whom I had grown to like and feel protective toward, in spite of negative comments such as "you are not doing anything to help me and are only wasting my time and my mother's money."

During the twelve weeks of presentation, I received a great deal of support from colleagues, who assured me she was indeed a difficult patient and would require a great deal of tolerance on my part. As a result of the seminars, I began to interpret more than I had been accustomed. Although Carole was still not very talkative, I felt somewhat more comfortable interpreting more actively.

Yet when the seminar was over I became desperate once again. The patient's acting out continued. I began receiving frantic calls from the mother, who was now exploring inpatient treatment programs to attempt to control Carole, who was now living with her. Somehow, my therapeutic self-esteem had become so entangled in this case that I felt increasingly anxious and overwhelmed.

I looked for help in several ways. I sought some consultations. Several suggestions were made, including more frequent sessions, an inpatient placement, and finally referral of both parents and daughter to an expert on child management. More frequent sessions were at that time out of the question. Inpatient hospitalization or placement seemed more than was necessary. I considered referral to an expert on child management; it had some immediate appeal. Yet as I began to think of the expert on management who had cured Carole of her wetting, I became apprehensive of a repeat of a management trauma. At the same time, both parents and stepparents were overwhelmed, and everyone was ready to give up.

It was at this point that the therapist who was working with the parents reported what seemed to be new information. The mother had stated to him in a matter-of-fact way, "I had looked forward to having a child. But when they brought Carole to me, just after delivery, I was afraid to hold her. I was overwhelmed and did not know what to do. I was afraid she would break. I realize now I couldn't relate to her and did not know how to respond. While I felt I loved her, I also felt inadequate to give her what she needed." The therapist remarked that perhaps Carole was making me feel the same way the mother had felt when Carole was born. Although Carole might hope that she could find someone who could care for her and not be overwhelmed, she might fear that everyone with whom she came in contact would be as overwhelmed as her mother during her infancy.

I suddenly realized that this unfortunate girl may have been expecting that everyone in her world would be overwhelmed by her, a repetition of her early infantile experience of her overwhelmed and inadequate mother. I had become another one of these overwhelmed objects, but more intensely so in the transference. As I identified my countertransference with her mother's feelings at Carole's birth, I began to feel better. I was able to differentiate in my own mind how able I am to deal with helplessness in children and adults and how much I was not like the mother. As I refused to be overwhelmed, she began to feel more secure.

Nine months after the crisis, Carole's functioning had changed dramatically in all areas of her life. She no longer slept in the sessions. She talked about her friends at school, drugs, sexuality, and new waves of the current generation. She made excellent grades in her schoolwork. She now can interact with her mother, even argue with her, without using profanity. She is not lying or stealing; she has not run away; she has maintained a relationship with the same boyfriend for three months, which she was never capable of doing before; she sees her biological father from time to time on the weekends without incident; and she is pursuing a special talent for the performing arts.

Discussion

Carole's early relationship with her mother forged an indelible intrapsychic expectation that she was overwhelming and that mother would be overwhelmed. Derivatives of this expectation were expressed, in spite of ego controls to the contrary, in her later relations with her mother and other parental figures, except for those who used stern management, which either failed or caused her great intrapsychic distress (Giovacchini 1974).

Yet the trauma continued at an unconscious level, ready to be reawakened in the transference/countertransference regression. As described, the mother's reaction to the infant was not reported until after a year and a half of treatment. If it had been communicated earlier, I had forgotten it. The significance was not appreciated until I had been overwhelmed by my countertransference; only then could I understand the true meaning of her reaction. Until I became aware of this developmental fact, I saw my own overwhelmed feelings as another instance of failing adults in the here and now, rather than what I had become, which was the significant failing adult of her early infancy. I had been overwhelmed with concern for months, had exhausted all avenues of help, and was ready to give up the case, much as the mother had wished she had someone else to take care of her baby but at the same time wanted to hold onto her. I considered sending her to an inpatient setting for her own protection. This was to protect my own sense of well-being, just as the mother must have wished for someone to save her damaged self-esteem when she realized it might have been better for her daughter to be mothered by someone else.

Yet, when I learned of the mother's reaction to Carole as an infant, my own feelings of being overwhelmed were greatly reduced. I understood my feelings as being generated by a transference of her early experience of her mother, projected into me. It also made her symptom picture comprehensible. I was able to see her need to overwhelm all figures in her life as a repeition of the same early, traumatic, maternal deficiency and anxiety.

As I understand the situation now, the analytic relationship had generated a primitive dependency on me in which the patient repeated an early trauma with an inadequate mother. Yet this was but the last of a series of repetitions of this infantile experience. She had repeated this trauma many times during her childhood through various provocations of adults, always somehow being able to bring out whatever potential feelings of inadequacy that might be present, causing people to give up on her. This had reached a peak in her early adolescence when the controls that others could actually exert were less effective.

Conclusions

The purpose of this chapter has been to focus on how an infant's experience of the early maternal-child environment was repeated as a countertransference reaction in the therapist. Although the analyst can assume that whatever goes on in the transference and countertransference is repeating an early reaction, it is helpful, from the perspective of theory validation, to have some outside verification. This seems to have occurred here, where the outside information preceded the development of the insight. And it was the insight which saved the treatment (Harley 1970). With adolescents much of treatment becomes focused on the real relationship with the therapist. In the case discussed here, understanding of the developmental event led to interpretation and resolution of the transference/countertransference; the insight, however, was in the therapist rather than in the patient. It is also important to be reminded how much of the conduct of treatment and the patient's experience and behavior outside of treatment reflect the transference/countertransference. In this case, when the therapist's countertransference changed, the patient's behavior changed not only in treatment but outside as well (Levenson, Feiner, and Stockhamer 1975).

NOTE

1. Even if every judge agreed, interjudge reliability does not imply validity. Of course, one could make the case that when it comes to countertransference, several psychoanalysts having the same experience constitute a form of validity.

REFERENCES

Giovacchini, P. 1973. Productive procrastination: technical factors in the treatment of the adolescent. *Adolescent Psychiatry* 4:352–370.

Giovacchini, P. 1974. The difficult adolescent patient: countertransference problems. *Adolescent Psychiatry* 3:271–287.

Harley, M. 1970. On some problems of technique in the analysis of early adolescents. *Psychoanalytic Study of the Child* 25:99–121.

Levenson, E.; Feiner, A.; and Stockhamer, N. 1975. Politics of adolescent psychiatry. *Adolescent Psychiatry* 4:84–98.

32 ADOLESCENT PARANOIA: TRANSFERENCE AND COUNTERTRANSFERENCE ISSUES

W. W. MEISSNER

The transition to the adolescent phase of development is marked by significant processes that contribute to the definition of individual personality. If the latency period can be described as a period of relative instinctual quiescence, the transition to adolescence must be described as a period of recrudescence of instinctual pressures. A variety of developmental changes are thus instigated which open up areas of basic conflict that remain as residuals of earlier levels of development. This offers the opportunity for a reworking of those conflicts and their fashioning into a new and emergent sense of identity. In this chapter I emphasize that this regressive moment in the adolescent developmental process serves to reactivate and intensify the functioning of basic mechanisms of introjection and projection.

Sarnoff (1972) has described the shift in the use of projection from latency to early adolescent phases. There is a shift from projection associated with repression in the earlier phase to a use of projection associated with denial in the later phase. He particularly notes that the latter form of projection—namely, that associated with denial—is equivalent to the form of projection and displacement involved in paranoid conditions. Sarnoff's analysis makes it clear that the progression to early adolescent developments marks a definite shift more explicitly in the direction of a characteristic paranoid style of defensive projection. This shift in projection parallels a transition of the primary role of defense from fantasy and symptom formation to a role in the testing of fantasy against reality in establishing object relations. In addition, along with the partial

0-226-24058-4/85/0012-0018$01.00

dissolution and opening up of the superego to cultural influences, there is a shift from id projections to superego projections. As Sarnoff (1972) notes, "Through projection the superego is externalized. The child who attributes her formerly internalized commands to a peer or teacher stands the chance of acquiring an externalized ego ideal, with characteristics of the ego ideal of the new object. With reinternalization of the ego ideal (the projection-reinternalization is a dynamic, ongoing series of events) modifications of the superego take place" (p. 521).

The upsurge of instinctual drive intensity at the onset of adolescence obviously presents the ego with a problem. Mastery of these drives and their derivatives is one of the major developmental tasks of adolescence. As a result of these increased drive pressures, a regression in ego functioning is induced, which serves to reactivate basic unresolved conflicts from earlier developmental levels. The developing ego is thus presented with the necessity and the opportunity to rework some of these underlying conflicts in a more thoroughgoing and definitive way. There is thus the opportunity to undo earlier developmental defects and consequently remodel the psychic apparatus in more effective and positively constructive ways. Thus, adolescence opens up the opportunity for new and more meaningful identifications which can provide a major direction and organization for these remodeling processes.

The adolescent's withdrawal from the familiar objects of childhood leads to a narcissistic overvaluation of the self. The adolescent becomes increasingly aware of his inner processes. He becomes self-absorbed, self-centered, and self-concerned. This may lead to a narcissistic withdrawal and disturbance of reality testing. The adolescent often resorts to narcissistic defenses to defend against the disappointment and disillusionment of his meager position in reality. He may find it difficult to give up the gratifying parent on whom he has come to depend—especially if that parent has been overly protective and solicitous—and face his own limitations and inadequacies. He may be afraid to take responsibility for his own abilities and their consequences—as well as not wanting to be faced with the demands of adult responsibility.

With the induced narcissistic regression, the intensity of narcissistic needs is heightened. This leaves the adolescent self more susceptible to narcissistic injury and disillusionment. This provides another important source of the mobilization of introjection-projection, specifically, as narcissistic defenses. Thus, introjection and projection come into operation in specific ways to sustain the threatened sense of self and preserve its threatened integrity. The regressive activation of introjection-projection tends to intensify regressively cathexis of and attachment to parental objects.

Adolescent Paranoia

If the sense of identity requires and builds itself in relationship to a sense of communion and belonging with both significant objects and a context of belonging, as I have suggested, it is also true that an important element in the maintaining and functioning of the sense of identity is its capacity to tolerate a separation from the same significant objects. Modell (1968) has discussed this important developmental attainment in the following terms:

> That a loving parent has been internalized and become part of the self, so that one is able to love oneself, has been described as an aspect of narcissism. . . . I am suggesting that the awareness of the self as a discrete and beloved entity (the narcissistic gratification of self-love) may enable the individual to accept the fact that objects in the external world are separate and can be lost and destroyed. . . . Whether or not this assumption is correct, it is a fact that those individuals who have the capacity to accept the separateness of objects are those that have a distinct, at least in part, beloved sense of self. If one can be a loving parent to oneself, one can more readily accept the separateness of objects. This is a momentous step in psychic development. [P. 59]

The capacity to tolerate separation of significant objects is a correlative of the capacity to tolerate painful reality. It is only on this basis that a mature capacity for realistic object relations can be established and sustained. The mature sense of self, the fully enveloped sense of identity, then, is correlated with the capacity to recognize and accept the identity of others and the ability to come to terms with and acknowledge the separateness and the autonomy of those others. Where there is an intolerance for such separateness, there develops an inner need to incorporate the object within the limits of one's own self or to extend the orbit of the self to encompass that object. This incorporating or extending is accomplished through defensively toned uses of projection and introjection.

It can be quickly seen that in these terms we are dealing with an extension of the basic concerns of individuation and separation that have been an integral part of the developmental process from the beginning of the child's experience. But we need to go a step further. It is my contention here that development and maintenance of the sense of identity requires not only toleration of the separateness of objects but also active separation out from and over against such objects. I am bringing into focus, consequently, the obverse of the concerns for relatedness and belonging which I have been discussing. If the processes which underlie and build a sense of inner integrity and belonging can be seen in terms of their contribution to the process of identity formation, they must also be seen as functioning in reciprocal interaction with other processes which serve to separate the emerging identity out from and place it over against other objects and contexts—literally defining the emerging sense of identity in terms of such opposition. I am talking here substantially about the need for an enemy.

To acknowledge the need for an enemy as an integral part of personality development can be disconcerting. It is painful to reckon with the possibility that the very mechanisms which we have been at pains to define as substantially contributing to and sustaining the sense of identity are also intrinsically related to a process which serves to separate that identity out from others and to set it over against them in basic opposition. But I find myself forced to this consideration. The basic dilemma and the difficult task which are imposed on the adolescent by the exigencies of development are that he articulate a sense of himself and integrate that sense of self with a specifically defined social unit, a community which organizes itself and expresses itself in terms of specifically defined limits and internally generated and specific criteria of belonging and sharing of values.

However, as Erikson (1959) pointed out, the integration is a function of mutual recognition and acceptance. The community may feel recognized by the emerging individual who is ready to seek recognition and acceptance by the community. It can also feel rejected by those more alienated individuals who reject it, rebel against it, or simply seem not to care. If the community responds to the former with acceptance—thus promoting participation and integration—it can withhold its acceptance from the latter. This creates a paranoid impasse—a standoff of mutual rejection. The individual and the community become enemies. The paranoid process requires the individual to seek affiliation with other groupings—often countercultural subgroupings—or, failing that, to construct a more decisively pathological paranoid system.

The defining of self and the articulating of its relationship—both under conditions of mutual rejection and under conditions of acceptance—are achieved in part through a setting of the self over against other communities, other groupings, other contexts of belonging that are defined in terms of their exclusiveness from the initial social grouping and in terms of their opposition in beliefs, values, attitudes, and so forth.

Thus, the community which the adolescent shapes about himself is one that is built around a core of inherent values and attitudes but that is likewise set in opposition to other such groupings. The adolescent in our society delineates and articulates his sense of identity as participating in certain specific groupings. He envisions himself as sharing certain common affiliations with different such groupings. Thus, he envisions himself as an American citizen, or as Jewish, or as Republican, or in terms of professional affiliations as a psychiatrist, a psychologist, a carpenter, or perhaps as a truck driver.

Each of these affiliations makes a contribution which can be differentiated from others and set in opposition to them. Moreover, at certain points, when conflicts and matters of interest and advantage bring these issues to the fore, feelings and attitudes can be generated which regard the out-group specifically and concretely as the enemy of the in-group. One can observe this phenomenon with varying degrees of intensity and even pathological distortion in the social events which form the fabric of our common social experience.

The important point, however, in all of this is that such paranoid propensities make a significant contribution to the forming of in-groups which provide the context for significant adherences within which the sense of identity can articulate itself and significantly maintain contexts of belonging and sharing which serve to sustain and confirm the inner sense of individual identity. The important tasks which confront the adolescent have to do precisely with his articulating his sense of self in terms of these complex social groupings—that is, that an integral part of the forming of an identity is the acquiring of a sense of belonging to certain specified in-groups, thereby defining oneself as opposed to and separated out from other social and cultural groupings which constitute the body of the out-groupings.

The phenomenon is applicable in terms of social and cultural groupings, but it also has relevance in terms of the very personalized and individualized articulation of the sense of self as separate from and over against other selves. Thus, in a certain necessary sense, an important task of adolescent development is that the adolescent set himself apart from, separate himself from, and posit himself in opposition to his parents or other significant caretaking figures. The adolescent revolt against parental restrictions cannot be seen simply in pathological terms but must also be seen as a way of making a significant contribution to the adolescent attainment of identity. This also applies to the adolescent exigency to revolt against all forms of authority.

Thus, these considerations lead in the direction of suggesting what can be denominated as a process of "adolescent paranoia." I am suggesting that such an adolescent paranoia is based on the working out of the specifically paranoid mechanisms I have been discussing—projection, introjection, and the paranoid construction—and that it provides an essential and integral part in the process of achieving a sense of identity which is so characteristically a developmental task of the adolescent period. I am suggesting further that, even though these mechanisms are a continuation and a further expression of developmental vicissitudes, in the adolescent period they assume a specifically paranoid quality—more akin to the paranoid manifestations that we are more familiar with in the context of clinical psychopathology.

The adolescent unavoidably sees himself in some sense as the victim of parental restraints and restrictions. He must also, to some extent, see himself as the victim of social pressures and cultural constraints that require him to integrate himself with the society around him in terms of certain standards of behavior and values. It is the working of this adolescent process and its attendant persecutory anxieties that contribute significantly to the tumultuousness, the anxieties, and the rebellious turmoil that we have come to associate so explicitly with adolescent concerns. It is terribly important, however, not to lose sight of the fact that such deviant and rebellious expressions—marked by the usual accompaniments of paranoid distortions such as extreme narcissism, defensiveness, rebelliousness, hostility, and destructive potentiality—are at the same time an expression of important developmental functions which are operating in the service of establishing and consolidating a sense of identity.

Alienation and the Paranoid Process

A particular form or expression in which these processes can be identified is that of adolescent alienation. It can be readily seen that the problem of alienation can be articulated as a problem of identity—particularly identity in its extrinsic frame of reference as expressing the relatedness of the individual to this social and cultural matrix. The pathology of alienation is basically a pathology of the self. The focusing of the problem of alienation was stimulated by the social and cultural emphases of neo-Freudian theorists—particularly Horney and Fromm. However, as a result of the emergence and development of analytic ego psychology in the last few years, the relationship between man's intrapsychic life and the familial, social, and cultural contexts in which he develops and functions has undergone a profound reconsideration. In this more extended understanding of man's psychic development and structure, it has become possible to rethink neo-Freudian contributions and to integrate them meaningfully with the main body of analytic understanding.

Horney related the problem of alienation to the disparity between the idealized self and the real self. Because of the neurotic failure to measure up to the ideal, the neurotic hates himself—hates his own limitations and inadequacies. This self-hate expresses itself in relentless demands on oneself, repeated self-accusations, self-devaluation, forms of self-torment, and self-destructive behavior. In its extreme forms, such alienation can take the form of amnesia, loss of reality sense, and depersonalization. But more pervasively, alienation can take the form of a feeling of numbness and remoteness. The individual tends to become more impersonal in all his dealings. He loses a sense of responsibility for himself and for the direction of his life and activity. His continual sense of disappointment with himself and his interaction with his environment leads to a gradual disowning of his real self and a retreat into an ineffectual style of life (Horney 1950). One of the serious questions that confronts us is the extent to which this pattern of life experience is emerging as a cultural type. The line between psychopathology and cultural adaptation becomes thin and highly permeable. Alienation in its many guises may well have permeated our society to such an extent that it can no longer be regarded as deviant or as pathological in the usual sense.

The problem of alienation, therefore, carries psychiatric concern to the interface between intrapsychic dynamics and the social and cultural processes which surround the individual and inevitably influence his development and capacity to function. Alienation thus becomes a sort of middle ground on which psychiatric concern mingles with and to some extent overlaps with the concern of more social approaches to human behavior. The concept of alienation can thus be seen to carry an implicit reference to the social context which continually influences the individual and with which he is in constant interaction. Alienation is an alienation from something that is around and ouside the individual. It has been one of the most valuable insights of modern social science that patterns of deviant behavior are not merely the product of disordered intrapsychic processes or impediments of development—although these play an unquestioned and critical role—but that the organization of social structures and social processes within which the individual functions has a determinate influence on the patterns of individual adaptation.

The interrelation between social anomie and psychological alienation is complex. The cultural disparity involved in anomie has its psychological counterpart in the disorganization and inner conflicts of values within the individual. The basic question we have to face in understanding this problem is how intrapsychic and social processes influence each other in the complex process of value formation and value change. Merton (1957) has suggested that the organization of our contemporary culture with its emphasis on material wealth and competitiveness creates a certain strain toward anomie. The shift of cultural emphasis from the satisfactions involved in competitive effort to an almost exclusive concern with the outcome—in terms of measurable criteria of wealth and power—tends to create a stress on the regulatory structures and an attenuation of institutional controls. Cultural and personal values are undermined, and calculations of personal advantage and risks of punishment become the main regulatory resource. We can note that this social strain toward anomie can be paralleled by a failure of internalization processes and a regression from internalized sources of inner regulation to a more primitive and externalized reliance on external rewards and punishments, on directives and prohibitions of external authorities. The social strain toward anomie is paralleled by an inner strain toward extremes of conformity or rebellion.

The alienation syndrome has been described primarily within the adolescent and postadolescent group, but I think it has wider application than that. The elements of the syndrome include a basic sense of loneliness—the feeling that one somehow does not belong, is not a part of things, not in the mainstream of life and interests that surround one. There is a sense of estrangement and a chronic sense of frustration. The alienated person carries with him a continual sense of opposition between his own wishes and desires and the wishes and desires of those around him—with the additional feeling that his wishes, desires, and ambitions are actively being denied by others. He lives in a chronic state of disappointment—others are continually letting him down, disappointing his expectations, frustrating his designs, pressuring him to conform to their wishes and desires. His disappointment and chronic frustration produce an inner state of continual and unrelenting anger that serves to isolate him further and to put him in a condition of estrangement. Occasionally, the anger will erupt in destructive outbursts that leave him even less satisfied and further disappointed.

An important element in the syndrome is the alienated person's sense of continuing frustration. He carries within him a chronic despair—a sense of hopelessness and helplessness which he sees as unremitting. When this sense of hopelessness dominates the picture, alienation tends to take the dropout, give-up form of retreatism. The individual may resort to any number of pathological forms of behavior to alleviate his sense of inner frustration—including alcohol, drugs, or other forms of escape. Much of what we have seen over the years in the skid-row phenomenon and much of what we are seeing on the contemporary drug scene has this quality of frustrated retreatism. When the sense of frustrated rage dominates the picture, however, we are much more likely to see its manifestations in rebellious behavior of one kind or other. The sense of helplessness and the sense of smoldering rage can easily coexist in the same individual—so that the helpless victim may find himself striking out in impotent rage from time to time. A central element of the alienation syndrome is the rejection of or the conflict over social values. The alienation syndrome, as we have already noted, lies at the interface between the person and social processes.

This feature raises a problem in differential diagnosis. Psychiatrists have tended to see the clinical manifestations of the alienation syndrome more in terms of the parameters of inner psychic dysfunction and less in terms of the social parameters. Thus, the alienation syndrome is usually described in terms of some form of character pathology or in terms of its narcissistic or depressive aspects. But the associated estrangement reflects a more basic rejection of values that the society embodies and implicitly requires that adolescents accept. Their rejection of these values may leave them in a relatively valueless vacuum—or they may actively foster divergent values that they oppose to the prevailing values of the culture around them. Or there may arise an inner conflict between partially accepted values of the general culture and partially accepted values of a divergent nature. The alienation syndrome adds specifically to these other well-known clinical pictures the aspect of value conflict and a tendency to reject the accepted cultural value system of their own society.

The rebellious expression of the alienation syndrome is characterized by the formulation or acceptance of a divergent set of values. Often, this takes place in conjunction with a group of like-minded individuals who can share the same set of deviant values. It should be noted that the term "deviant" in this context does not have the connotation of better or worse but simply emphasizes that the values of the subgroup stand somehow in opposition to the general culture. Such value-oriented subgroupings are alienated from the larger social group but may be quite unified within themselves. This allows the alienated individual to achieve a compensatory sense of belonging. This compensatory aspect of group formation is a significant part of the motivation behind adolescent gangs and the youth movement in general. The value deviance can be focused and expressed in almost any aspect of behavior—clothing, hair styles, sexual mores, language, expression of values, attitudes, or beliefs. The important dimension of this value divergence is not so much the formation of new and constructive and meaningful values; rather, in the alienation syndrome the emphasis falls on the rejection and, in the rebellious extreme, on the overthrow of preexisting values. Divergent alienated groups seize on any ideology or any formulation of divergent attitudes to express their rejection. Often, in the service of frustrated and impotent rage, the objective seems to be to find the most extreme form of articulation of values that might fly in the face of the prevailing social values. Thus, rebellious groups spout the most extreme socialist and communist rhetoric—the thoughts of Chairman Mao are preferred in many quarters. There is also a need to question, challenge, and confront social institutions and practices on all levels.

Alienation is a frequent and familiar part of the picture presented by adolescents in our culture. Adolescence is a developmental period of regressive disorganization, followed, one hopes, by a progressive reorganization of the personality. This developmental progression allows the child to pass through the physical and inner psychic changes that are required for him to begin to approach his definitive role and position in adult society. But the adolescent is not really a part of that society—he is only potentially a part. He will be able to integrate himself with the adult world only by forming himself to fit adult roles and by demonstrating to the adult community that he is ready and capable of fulfilling them. Only then can the adult community recognize and receive him. During the period of adolescent development, however, he remains outside looking in. There is a sense of estrangement embedded in the adolescent experience in our culture (Berman 1970). It is an expression of what I have already described as adolescent paranoia.

Deutsch (1967) has pointed out the frequency of depressive affects in many adolescents. For many adolescents, adolescence is a traumatic period in their lives. They are confronted by the demands of reality, by performance standards, by adult competition for positions and awards that is often intense, and by an increasing realization of their own limitations. A crucial aspect of the child's capacity to adapt is related to the issue of narcissism. Promising children often come to the adolescent challenge with narcissistic dreams of accomplishment and glory—dreams that may have been fostered and prolonged by their parents. Thus, the infantile narcissism with its dreams and expectations and sense of entitlement is often prolonged into adolescence—and the inevitable disappointment becomes traumatic. An increase of narcissism is quite characteristic of adolescence anyway, but these particularly narcissistic adolescents were raised in an atmosphere of expectation generated by their parents' excessive investment in them, in the hope that they would one day compensate for their parents' own sense of disappointment and frustration.

To this basically narcissistic picture, alienated adolescents add another feature. The narcissistic investment from the mother tends to undermine the position of the father as a model for identification. The mother's disappointment is often intensified and magnified by the failure of the father to measure up to her standards. The father is thus devalued. The child who is caught up in this process must therefore devalue the father in order to share the mother's dream and to gain her approval. He too devalues and rejects the father, and this devaluation is intensified during the adolescent period. The father is seen as weak, debased, worthless, insignificant, inconsequential. At a deeper level, the adolescent boy's resentment against the father is often due to the fact that the father was too weak to protect him from an often ambivalent dependency on his mother as well as from an incestuous involvement with her. This underlying devaluation of the father often erupts in adolescence, even though it may have been there since earliest childhood. It becomes extended to the entire world of adults and adult standards and adult institutions. The adolescent rage against society, its values, and its institutions can be rooted in a rage against the devalued father and all he stands for.

Thus, the adolescent boy stands on the threshold of a world of adult standards and expectations. But it is his father's world. The devaluation of the father and the struggle against identification with the father lead to a rejection of all social commitments, all social values, all conventional roles, all responsibilities, and many of the forms of emotional relatedness with others that form the normal fabric of society. A similar problem confronts the adolescent girl. If she idealizes her father excessively, she runs the risk of devaluing and despising her mother—with an intensification of her penis envy and an impairment of a meaningful and constructive identification with her mother. She thus tends to reject and rebel against any conventional forms of feminine role or status and strives for more masculine competitiveness and forms of accomplishment. The rebellious expression of these aspects is eloquently expressed in some of the "women's lib" phenomena.

It is useful to realize that in large measure the process of alienation may serve some important developmental functions. One of the questions that the apparent increase in manifest alienation raises is the extent to which social and cultural conditions require that the forms of alienation take the patterns of expression that they do. Alienation is a feature of all adolescent development, but the reorganization of inner structures, defenses, values, and patterns of identification can be pressured into maladaptive and even pathological molds. This developmental perspective is expressed by Berman (1970) in the following terms:

> The process of identification facilitates adaptation during childhood. Its characteristics will determine how the adolescent will cope with change. When adolescence is reached, childhood identifications must undergo radical revision because of the strength of the sexual drive and the need to master it. Alienation is a mental process serving to achieve this necessary physical and psychic distance from parents and society. It is a defense against painful ideas and affects associated with the disruption of cathexis to the past relationships. The process also supports the establishment of genital primacy, new object relations, and a firm sense of self. [P. 250]

In the normal course of things, such adaptive alienation is not extreme and is resolved into new and functional adult patterns of identification and role functioning. The extremes of alienation, however, distort the growth process and make adaptive resolutions less possible and more precarious.

The problem and the paradox of alienation are acutely focused in the use of social protest and frankly revolutionary violence. Revolution and the use of violence in the service of revolution are obviously nothing new, but they took on new social implications about a decade and a half ago. The threat of violence became a familiar refrain from all sorts of disaffected and dissatisfied subcultural groups. We heard it from student revolutionaries and radicals, from black radicals and militants, and even from extremists in the women's rights movement.

The protest of students was particularly interesting in this regard. The protest of student radicals ran deep. It was a protest about and a rebellion against some important and basic values that form the essential fabric of our society. However destructive and pathological the means by which students chose to express this divergence, we miss the essential dimension if we ignore that the core issue in their dissent was a matter of values. Youth was not merely objecting to a style of life or a pattern of living in adult society; it was protesting and rebelling against the system of values that govern and guide adult society. This raised a severe problem in that adults and administrators at all levels, from the family to the larger units of social organization in educational and governmental institutions, can often see their way to discussion and debate over matters of fact, but they are usually unable to see or find their way to debate matters of value. As a result, confrontations turned out to be unsatisfactory on both sides, because the real issues were never joined.

If protest and dissent have a place in social process, what about violence? The student radicals were committed to violence. The rhetoric of student radicals proclaimed that social injustice was too deeply rooted to try to reform our social institutions. They viewed social institutions as based on the exploitation of the many in the interest of a few. They saw such institutions as unjust and evil, as controlled by a concern for nothing but money and power, and as an evil to be destroyed. They saw no possibility for reform or change from within. The only effective means for getting rid of such evil and oppressive institutions and the values that govern them was violent overthrow and destruction. They saw violent confrontation and destruction by bombings or burnings as necessary for the advancement of the cause they were promoting.

Behind this current of discontent and dissatisfaction there was a strong, ideologically colored commitment to a form of utopian idealism. Erikson (1964) has taught us that ideological commitment is a necessary ingredient in the growth of youth to maturity. But ideology can be put in the service of inner growth and the confirmation of cultural integration, or it can be put in the service of infantile needs and the dynamisms of alienation (Meissner 1978). Social idealism has served as an inspiration and a guiding dream for human social and political aspirations for centuries. But utopian ideals can represent the prolongation of infantile narcissism and wishes. Social idealism can come to embody infantile wishes to have unconditional love, protection, care, and freedom from those powerful sources representing the omnipotent parents. It may also represent the opposite and equally unrealizable wish to obtain such omnipotence for oneself.

For many of the more fanatical youth of fifteen years ago, the utopian wish had to be responded to and fulfilled immediately—without delay, planning, consideration, reflection, or questioning. They had no patience for the slow process of cultural change, they could not wait for the plodding deliberation and interaction of positions and interests that constitute the political process, they demonstrated little capacity for toleration of delay and postponement of gratification of their wishes and demands. There was a sense of urgency and immediacy to their often petulant demands. Their rejection of social values and the intensity of their rage led them to believe that the solution to their frustration was the destruction of whatever opposed their demands. The supposition was that if one destroys what one believes to be evil, good will automatically spring up in its place. In the impulsivity of their inner needs and the impetuousness of their demands, they ignored and bypassed the essential nature of social and cultural processes (Greenacre 1970).

The frustration and denial of such pressing inner demands and the deeper narcissistic expectations that so often lay beneath them led to a sense of inner disappointment and rage. Earlier we saw how the sense of powerlessness, worthlessness, meaninglessness, and social and self-estrangement can easily lead to the expression of frustrated rage. There is increasing evidence to suggest that much of the violent confrontation of the recent past was produced by a relatively small group of alienated individuals who were acting out their infantile needs and wishes in immature ways—lashing out with destructive rage without any constructive plan or purpose. There is no doubt that deeply unconscious, irrational, and infantile wishes are frequently rationalized under the guise of social idealism and that the frustration of such wishes lies at the heart of the pressure for violent social reorganization. But the analysis of inner psychodynamics does not explain away or substitute for social change. The infantile needs and behavior of a few radicals do not obliterate the need for social change nor the conditions in our society which make such change desirable or necessary.

Portrait of a Young Rebel

I would like to offer some reflections on my experience with a young man whom I treated psychotherapeutically for nearly three years. This particular patient provides a somewhat extreme example of the patterns of alienation I have been discussing. In his pathology the issues of alienation are writ large and pose a series of problems for effective psychotherapeutic intervention. The problems arise particularly in the countertransference aspects of conflicting value orientations between patient and therapist. In addition, the issue that the material of this case raises is that of the difficult interplay between the patient's distorted perceptions of the world around him and the pathological and destructive elements that persist in the social environment. The patient's paranoid perceptions are driven by inner subjective needs, but to what extent are these perceptions reflected and verified by external processes? What problems for therapy does the overlap between inner perceptions and external realities create for the psychotherapist in carrying out his professional effort?

My first contact with Jerry took place when he was brought by the police to our hospital. He had been found disrupting traffic by standing in the middle of a large highway, brandishing a crowbar, shouting at the drivers, and threatening to smash their cars with the crowbar if they tried to pass him. At the time of his arrival he was quite agitated, disorganized, somewhat confused, and delusional. He was plainly in the throes of a schizophrenic decompensation. In discussing Jerry's difficulties, I would like to look briefly at the more recent course of his illness, then go back to look at his family background and earlier history, and finally trace some of our experience during the course of approximately three years of therapy.

It turned out that Jerry's hospitalization had not been his first. His psychiatric history had started several years before when he was in the army and had to be hospitalized for a psychotic breakdown. Jerry had matriculated at a large eastern university where he spent a year that was unhappy, lonely, and only moderately successful academically. He had felt isolated from his fellow students and unable to make any substantial friendships. He decided at the end of the year to interrupt his schooling and to enlist in the army. He was assigned to a computer training program.

The army did not prove to be a hospitable environment for him. The discipline and impersonality of army life were difficult for him to accept. He again found it difficult to make friends, particularly since he looked down on the other men as intellectually and educationally inferior. He had particular difficulty adapting to the army discipline, which he found arbitrary, cold, excessively demanding, humiliating, and completely unresponsive to his personal needs and wishes. He became increasingly despondent. As an escape he had started using LSD. He began to feel that the army was trying to destroy him and ruin his mind. He became quite suspicious and began to think that the instructors in the computer program were plotting against him. He was briefly hospitalized, rather quickly recompensated, and was given a medical discharge.

He returned to college, where he again found himself isolated and having great difficulties relating to fellow students. He became heavily involved in radical student politics. He was troubled by feelings of loneliness, estrangement, feelings that people were out to get him, and feelings that people were staring at him or talking about him. Involvement in radical politics served a double purpose—it enabled him to share a common interest with other somewhat estranged and angry students and it served as a channel for the rage he felt toward the establishment. He developed his skills at haranguing groups and at organizing political activities. He finally ran for a major school office on the radical ticket. He poured all of his energy and enthusiasm into the campaign, only in the end to be defeated.

The loss was a severe narcissistic blow and proved to be one of the precipitants of his decompensation. A second important precipitant was the disruption of his relationship with his girlfriend. He had become very dependently attached to her, and they had been living and sleeping together for several months. She finally decided that he was too unstable for any serious relationship and broke it off. He was crushed, hurt, disappointed, enraged, and felt betrayed. Coming on the heels of his election loss, he felt that there was a conspiracy on the part of the school to "get" him because of his radical political views.

As the end of the school year drew near, Jerry's psychosis grew more apparent. He attended a national student conference where he became so disruptive that he had to be taken out of the meeting. He was convinced that the meeting was being controlled by the CIA and was determined to disrupt it. He interrupted the proceedings by shouting obscenities and breaking into the discussions with angry and provocative political harangues against the establishment, against then-President Nixon, against the war in Vietnam, and against the draft. He remained in this state for several more weeks, living in a commune with a group of fellow student radicals who more or less protected him.

Then one evening he decided to cross a nearby highway. He felt that the traffic was preventing his crossing the busy highway and was thereby infringing on his constitutional rights. The relentless metal machines bearing down on him, uncaringly forcing him aside without any consideration of his needs or wishes, represented the cold, uncaring, heartless, and indifferent establishment that made decisions about his life and forced him to do things he did not want to do—without consulting him in any way or taking his personal needs into account. Against this impersonal and indifferent imposition from above, he felt an intense rage and a powerful wish to strike out against it and to destroy it.

The roots of such attitudes and feelings were not difficult to find. Jerry's family had not been a very happy one. Jerry's mother was a rather affected, labile, narcissistic, demanding, and probably borderline woman. From almost the first day of her marriage she started drinking. She had been a chronic alcoholic for years and bore a number of the physical stigmata of alcoholism. His father was a trim, graying, pinstripe-suited business executive. He was pleasant and proper at all times but kept a disconcerting distance at all times. Jerry's parents did not get along at all. The marriage was torn by conflict and bitterness on the part of both parents. His father responded by a pattern of emotional and physical withdrawal. He would get up early in the morning and leave the house before mother got out of bed. He would not return home until late in the evening.

The split between the parents and father's withdrawal created other problems. Jerry was much closer to his mother. Mother also seemed to take out her frustrations and needs on him. She was perfectionistically demanding and never seemed satisfied with his performance. She easily became impatient and irritated at him and beat him in sadistic furor. He recalled episodes when his mother attacked him seemingly without reason and kept hitting him, knocking him down, and demanding that he stand up again and "take it like a man"—whereupon she knocked him down again and again. At other times, she was overly affectionate and embraced and fondled him in a manner that was physically intimate and sexually seductive.

Jerry could never figure his mother out, never knew what to expect from her. He also resented the fact that his father seemed so distant and uninvolved. He felt that his mother's problems were related to what was going on with his father. He resented the fact that his father allowed this to go on and did not protect him from his mother. In time, Jerry had two younger brothers, but he remained mother's favorite, the one whom she treated with excessive affection as well as often brutal beatings.

One of the important themes of Jerry's childhood was his continual longing for closeness with his father, a longing that was always frustrated. He hardly saw his father during the week. The family never ate together; father would come home late and the children were not allowed to disturb him while he ate dinner. By then, it was usually time for them to go to bed. If father were home, he would usually want to read the paper and was not interested in spending time with Jerry. The father also demonstrated a remarkable capacity for detachment and denial. Even in the face of Jerry's severe decompensation, he seemed incapable of recognizing or admitting that there was any problem in the family, or that he might have had any part in it. For years, he blandly denied any problems on the part of his wife, even when the evidence of her progressive alcoholism was overwhelming. This was one of the causes of Jerry's rage at him—that he could ignore the self-destructive course his mother was on and refuse to do anything about it.

Jerry was a shy and lonely child. He complained that his family lived in a remote suburban area where there were few friends he could play with, and those who were there he could not get along with. He was a fearful child with a number of childhood phobias, and he was given to severe nightmares. Nightmares were a persistent feature of his experience. His dreams were filled with scenes of bloody murder and destruction. He frequently experienced a typical incubus nightmare—feeling a heavy weight on his chest, paralyzing him, crushing him, and preventing him from breathing.

The basic difficulties in Jerry's family situation were reinforced by the pattern of the succeeding years. The father's job required frequent changes of locale. The family pattern had been one of moving every year or so, whenever father got another appointment. Jerry felt there was never any time when he could really settle in and make friends. As soon as he started to make friends, his family would move to another place. When he was old enough, his father decided to send him to preparatory school in England. The father defended his decision on the basis of Jerry's educational needs but when pressed finally admitted that he felt that Jerry's involvement with his mother was unhealthy and that he felt it was best if Jerry could escape from her. The other two brothers stayed with the family.

Jerry experienced this as an abandonment and a rejection. This feeling was reinforced by the fact that the family never visited him, that often he would not receive any presents or communications on special occasions like birthdays or holidays, that usually his father prevented him from visiting his family because of the expense. Jerry hated the school situation. He resented the harsh discipline, the intense competitiveness among the boys, the fact that they made fun of him because he was a Yank and poked fun at his mannerisms and speech, and the fact that he could not make friends. He felt lonely, isolated, hurt, abandoned, unwanted, and unloved. He reacted with angry withdrawal and rebelliousness. He was constantly fighting with the other boys and continually getting into trouble with school authorities.

He was finally sent back to the United States to complete his high school education. Father thought it would be good for him to go to the same preparatory school that he had attended. The situation in the English preparatory school was repeated, but Jerry became even more of a disciplinary problem. His marks were also very poor, and at the end of a year the school requested that he not return. He then went to live with a paternal aunt, who was a very cold, demanding, and ungiving person. She made demands on Jerry and he felt that she exploited him to do work for her that he deeply resented. He experienced all these years as a punitive exile from his family. He bitterly resented that he was forced to endure all this while his brothers could be at home. He had lost out in the sibling rivalry and had been rejected by his parents, particularly by his father.

One of the important aspects of Jerry's difficulties had to do with money. Father had always complained about money, constantly pointing out that the family was spending too much and living beyond its means. His rationalization for not visiting Jerry or for not letting Jerry come home more often had always been money. For most of his time away from home, Jerry had lived frugally, always deeply concerned yet resentful about the lack of money. Since his return to school from the army, he had lived at a bare subsistence level—spending less than a dollar a day, living commune style with fellow students, eating poorly and cheaply—but steadfastly refused to ask his father for more money. He felt that his father would only hold it against him. Money was also an issue in his illness;

father would complain about the hospital bills and insist that Jerry get out of the hospital. When Jerry got such letters, he would invariably regress noticeably and become more psychotic, until I was able to find out that he had received such a letter and we were able to discuss it.

Jerry's resentments about money were deep, especially since they were father's rationalization for so much that Jerry was bitter about. Gradually, he was able to accept the view that he had some right to help and support from father. He came to see that, even though his father complained about money, the family lived comfortably in a well-to-do suburban area, that Jerry's mother consumed large amounts of alcohol that cost a significant amount of money, and that his father could afford little indulgences like vacation trips and a sailboat. It was interesting that Jerry could displace his resentful feelings to surrogate objects and could rationalize stealing and cheating, but he had great difficulty in coming to accept even reasonable demands on his father for money.

It was clear that these experiences reinforced his deep ambivalence toward both parents. His love for his mother was contaminated by the threatening aspects of her seductiveness and overly possessive control—not to mention her sadistic punishment, which he so often felt was capricious and unmerited. He had a deep, if continually frustrated, longing for closeness to his father. But he was enraged at father's continuing indifference and cold distancing, even as he was enraged at his father's apparently blind indifference and refusal to do anything about not only his own difficulties but his mother's problems as well.

Jerry's treatment course was difficult and problematic. On his initial evaluation he was suspicious and guarded, agitated and confused, obviously psychotic. His mind was filled with ideas that he later described as "freaky"—that the world was under attack by hostile extraterrestrial forces and was threatened with chaos and destruction, with powerful forces vying with each other for control. His behavior at that point was quite paranoid.

At the beginning of his hospitalization he was quite angry, hostile, and resistive to treatment. He would break out in angry tirades, proclaiming a radical socialist philosophy and damning all the forces of the political establishment. Several times he violently disrupted patient community meetings with wild, angry, foot-stomping harangues against the doctors who were trying to subjugate and control the patients' minds and against the hospital administration, urging the patients to revolt. One of these outbursts culminated in his smashing a chair to the floor and breaking it. This behavior was quite disturbing to other patients and had to be restrained. Gradually he began to respond to high doses of phenothiazines and became less disruptive. He then entered a long period of depression and despondency that lasted for several months. His thought processes remained obviously, though moderately, disorganized for several weeks.

His psychotherapy was at first taken up by seemingly endless tirades. He fulminated against the government, against the war, against the draft, against the president, against the school administration—against any expression of or representation of authority. The tirades always had the same themes—that those who exercise power are cold, indifferent, and uncaring; and that they make decisions that affect the lives of helpless individuals without any concern or interest in what the feelings and wishes of those helpless individuals might be. These complaints were accompanied by feelings of intense rage and bitterness; it almost seemed at times as though he were going to explode. His vituperations were expressed in the most extreme and destructive terms. His rhetoric was cast in the most extreme radical and revolutionary terms. He saw no other alternatives but that the present political system and the economic structure that went with it should be destroyed. Any tactic, any device, any course of destructive action that interfered with and served to cripple or destroy the operation of this heinous system was, therefore, praiseworthy and good. Any system that so subjugated and destroyed human beings was hateful and worthy only to be destroyed. Not to work for its destruction was itself a crime. Any action taken to destroy it was an act of heroic rebellion.

Hour after hour Jerry would proclaim the rights of the downtrodden and the underprivileged—students, blacks, Puerto Ricans, women, and so forth. Every episode that suggested actions of powerful figures to take advantage of or control the lives of people became the starting point for his angry tirades. Any decision or implementation of policy in the university, any action of the government, any statement by a public official, would serve to trigger an angry outburst. There seemed to be no end to his bitterness and furious rage—and no end of subjects and targets against which he could launch it. During this period there were several student riots and strikes at the university, each of which provoked long tirades. In most of these he was actively involved. The sight of his friends being arrested and dragged off to jail was intolerable to him. When the tragic events took place at Kent State and at Jackson State, his rage was nearly psychotic.

Gradually the scope of the therapy widened. In the face of these tirades I could do nothing but wait and listen. The waiting and listening were difficult because the tirades seemed so endless and so incredibly repetitious. Little by little, however, I began to hear more of his resentments against his parents. With some encouragement from me, he began increasingly to move back and forth between his current resentments and the resentments he had felt as a child against his parents. At one crucial juncture, I pointed out to him that the language and the themes of his tirades against society and its structures were quite similar to the complaints he launched against his parents, particularly against his father. He reiterated that they were cold, indifferent, and exercised control over his life in a way that seemed to show no concern for his individual needs and wants, and that he felt himself to be helpless and victimized in the face of it.

The revelation came as a shocking and disturbing realization to him. His therapy turned much more to a problematic process of trying to disengage his infantile displacements from the real concerns that confronted him in his present experience. The realization that the intensity of his political concerns might in part reflect infantile frustrations and rage served to threaten severely his sense of political commitment. Outside of his political commitment and his idealized picture of himself as the courageous revolutionary struggling for the rights of the humiliated and downtrodden against the hateful forces of imperious subjugation, there was little with which he could sustain his sense of self-esteem and self-respect. To have that brought into question was disturbing indeed.

My therapeutic tactic was one of avoiding any questioning or confronting. I encouraged him to explore and examine his feelings and thoughts. We began to see that the intensity of his rage was often disproportionate. We recognized that it was usually triggered when he suffered some disappointment and that the frequency and intensity of his disappointment were correlated with the level of his expectations. Over and over again, he generated excessive expectations that were doomed to frustration or disappointment, which then allowed him to burst forth in frustrated rage.

One graphic event demonstrated his self-destructiveness and the consequences of his infantile rage. He became enraged about something one night and smashed his fist against the wall. He succeeded only in fracturing a metacarpal and came into my office the next day sheepishly sporting a cast on his hand. We discussed his blind anger, how his rage made him want to lash out, and how he usually ended up being destructive and self-defeating. There was a strong wish in him to be constructive, to be able to act effectively, to bring about realistic and effective changes in the evils of society he saw around him. The infantile rage made him want to lash out at the wall and destroy it rather than to find out how to work his way around it and to be able to achieve what he wanted. The dawning realization of the destructiveness of his infantile rage brought complications for him. He increasingly saw the radical activities of his fellow students as self-destructive and self-defeating; so many of them were freaking out or dropping out, and their tactics were so ineffective and were not really changing anything. He found himself increasingly alienated from them.

The difficulty was put in vivid terms. Surrendering his infantile rage and approaching the real problems of society would seem to require that he become more mature and realistic in his approach to social problems. He would have to come to terms with the means that society proposes for inner change. That might mean directing himself toward getting an education, perhaps a law degree; it meant for him the postponement of goals, of adopting a strategy of indirect action and delay, of committing himself to hard work and discipline to achieve these goals. He spoke admiringly of people like Saul Alinsky or Ralph Nader as examples of men who found more effective ways of generating change. But the threat was then that he might be "co-opted" by the system—that he might succumb to the lure of middle-class values that his parents stood for. In the face of this possibility, he could not bring himself to accept a job in any corporation, nor could he commit himself to any idea of further education. His skills permitted him employment in only relatively menial and trivial jobs, and this only compounded and intensified his rage and resentment against the system. It was extremely difficult for him to recognize or accept his own self-defeating role in this; he preferred to blame the system that put him in this position.

His relationship to me was ambivalent. He came to see me as a sympathetic and understanding person with whom he could share his concerns without any fear of retaliation of consequences. Despite his many maneuvers to get me to take a position or to oppose him, I consistently resisted this ploy and continually reinforced and supported his capacity for reaching his own conclusions and for taking responsibility for them. There was not much difficulty in recognizing the potential countertransference traps that abounded in this process. Few of the positions and arguments that Jerry assaulted me with were in any sense congruent with my own attitudes, values, orientations, and beliefs. The therapeutic interaction created a constant inner strain between my own personal commitments and values, on one hand, and the convictions and values that I felt committed to as a professional healer and therapist, on the other. On Jerry's part, throughout the therapy, he had difficulty coming to trust me. The fact was that he did trust me to a considerable degree, but it was against his principles to admit that an "establishment type" like myself could be trusted and confided in. But I became for him the father that he had longed for and had never had.

Complementarity Mode of Psychosocial Interaction

In this case we are dealing with a complex interaction of psychopathological and social variables. Jerry's problems represent a case of student activism and radicalism which had clear pathological roots in childhood experience and in the continuing sense of frustration and rejection on the part of parental figures. The argument to this point has emphasized that despite the obvious elements of displacement and projection from infantile levels of conflict and ambivalence, understanding student radicalism in exclusively these terms can be misleading. It is clear that the social context and the interactional processes involved contributed significantly to the emerging pattern of deviant behavior.

For therapists to approach such problems with a one-sided model rooted in psychopathology only would seem to reflect certain political prejudices that would tend to prejudge deviant behavior as pathological and to prejudge the social context as above reproach. As such, this model would clearly provide a vehicle for potentially unanalyzed countertransferential elements that could play a significant, if not central, role in the therapeutic interaction with such patients. From this point of view, the charge so often leveled at psychiatry of getting the patient to conform to the norms of society may be justified in some degree. The situation is obviously more complex and calls for a more complex understanding as the basis for psychotherapeutic understanding.

The dialectic of polar positions has been sketched quite effectively by Fried (1970). The psychodynamic position accounts for psychopathology on the basis of unresolved conflicts which involve intrapsychic forces—for example, impulses and defenses—in relation to significant objects. This approach does not exclude, but rather leaves open, the question of the influence of social relationships and processes. Individual differences in the ego's capacity to relate to and adapt to reality are related to individual selection rather than to systematic differentiation of social influences and patterns. The social approach does not exclude motivation but sees it as derived from social interactions and forces. The respective orientations are not only tenable but can be seen in complementary perspective.

In terms of Jerry's experience and the experience of a significant proportion of young rebels, the displacement of inner conflicts and intensely ambivalent relations with significant objects (parents) onto social structures at a university or government level is reinforced and complemented by elements of dehumanizing detachment and uncaring impersonalization, bureaucratic rigidity, authoritarian and repressive attitudes, and morally inconsistent and exploitative approaches. Jerry's projections were met and validated to a significant degree by the public situations in which he found himself impelled to protest. Thus, what can from one point of view be denominated and identified as psychopathology must to some extent from another perspective be regarded as legitimate social protest. Conversely, one might wonder whether, if social institutions did not so often operate in ways that correspond to and validate the projections of the young, the opportunities and stimulation for rebellious attitudes among its younger members would be as frequent or intense.

Therapeutic Issues

It was quite clear in my experience with Jerry that his pathology was operative in his political concerns and activity. It was not merely the striking parallels in his attitudes toward authority figures and his parents but the obvious projective distortions and the disproportionate intensity of his displaced rage—as well as the exaggerated and peremptory nature of his expectations—that reflected his pathology. It was nonetheless inescapable that university administrators and government bureaucracy responded to public issues in a manner that tended to reinforce and complement elements of Jerry's projections. The adult world seemed to react in such a way as to provoke similar responses in many of his peer group and thus provide a considerable degree of consensual validation for his often extreme views.

Therapy depends closely on clinical understanding. To presume univocally that social processes functioned normatively and provided a normal and expectable context for adaptation would have been to distort reality and to respond in terms of idealistic—if not ideological—presumptions that could not stand up to specific inquiry. I found it necessary to suspend all such suppositions in favor of open and honest inquiry. I also found it necessary to suspend my own personal ideological persuasions (not that I was in any way minded to surrender them), but in my interaction with Jerry I had to maintain my willingness to examine and question them, even as I had to acknowledge my willingness to endorse and stand by them. The basic honesty and openness required to deal with Jerry's paranoid suspiciousness and distrust demanded that I be willing to open my mind about such issues if I were to expect him to approach his own concerns with anything like an open mind.

In my own experience with Jerry and similar patients, I have found a sustained attitude of open, honest, and ruthlessly objective inquiry to be essential. One must be willing to question and hold open for investigation everything—the patient's presuppositions, attitudes, feelings, and distortions; one's own convictions, presuppositions, attitudes, and values; and the suppositions and values of the social and cultural matrix within which both the patient and the therapist move and experience reality. The inquiry must be as objective as possible, in intent if not in fact. With Jerry my tactic was at first no more than to listen to his bitter complaints and tirades. I made no objections, no attempts to correct or question his obvious distortions. I listened sympathetically and encouraged him to fill out his accounts in greater and more specific detail. From time to time—in the interests of objectivity and understanding—I wondered whether his observations were facts or whether they were his perceptions or interpretations. Little by little, the line between fact and fantasy, between real and distorted perception, between real actions and hearsay, between data and interpretation was more clearly drawn.

The inquiry was sustained at all levels. It was directed not only to his present concerns but to his past experience as well. What gradually came into focus was the insensitivity, stupidity, impersonal detachment, and even repressive hostility and destructiveness of persons and institutions that acted as the bearers of authority and power. The degree to which the respective pathologies—the indifference, repression, detachment, denial, pathological conflicts, and incapacities—of his parents played such a significant role in the patterning of Jerry's own unfortunate experience also became much clearer, as did the extent to which his own excessive expectations and the intensity of his disappointment and consequent rage caused him so much difficulty and interfered with his capacity to function more effectively.

With increasing clarity in many detailed areas of his experience, it gradually became possible to tease apart the elements and aspects of his experience that derived from infantile conflicts and projective distortions and to separate them from the more realistic and validly questionable or objectionable aspects. Jerry slowly came to see how his inner processes and resentments actually came to interfere with and distort his view of the real world and its problems. He could increasingly see such distortion as an impediment to effective action to bring about change in the world about him. He saw the futility and impotence of the destructive outbursts of his fellow student radicals.

All of this was to be counted as therapeutic progress. It would serve me well if I could report that the further course of such inquiry led to an unequivocal therapeutic success. But I cannot. After three years of sustained work, Jerry had come to the point of realizing that he was confronted with a fundamental alternative. He could yield to the demands of reality and find effective means of obtaining his ideals and objectives. But this would require discipline, hard work, hard study—and involved a risk. He might not succeed. The demanding investment might not pay off in terms of the somewhat grandiose expectations he clung to; he wanted to change the face of society to fit his somewhat utopian ideals. Reality did not offer him any assurance of success in terms that he could accept. If, however, he would cling to his infantile expectations and his rage, he could persist in his pattern of rebellious bitterness and alienation, and he could retain the omnipotent and grandiose fantasy of bringing about dramatic changes in society by means of the magic of revolutionary action. He made a clear choice. He ingested a heavy dose of mescaline, became psychotically disorganized, and was rehospitalized.

Discussion

Jerry's case is illuminating from the point of view of what contributed to its success and to its failure. Essential to its success was the combination of therapeutic alliance and a sustained objective inquiry. The transference was mixed, but with positive aspects outweighing the negative. He saw me as the concerned and available father for whom he had always yearned. Although long in coming about, the therapeutic alliance was firmly maintained through most of the therapy. It provided the emotional matrix within which an attitude of sustained, interested, honest, open, and objective inquiry could be achieved. The inquiry bore its fruits. It achieved significant therapeutic goals; but in the end, it served only to bring Jerry more fundamentally to confront the demands of reality against which he had railed from the beginning. But clearly the confrontation was different in quality and in focus. He was no longer confronting external forces of oppression and authoritarian power; he was confronting instead the inner forces of narcissistic entitlement and infantile gratification. On these rocks the treatment foundered.

There was more involved in it. My attempts to remain neutral and objective could not be sustained in the face of his efforts to bring me into a position of authoritarian intervention against which he could rebel. He had managed this with every other person and/or institution with which he was involved—why should I be the exception? He became sexually involved with another female patient of mine in what I felt was a flagrant acting out of the transference. Efforts to interpret the oedipal and preoedipal aspects were ineffective. My hand was forced. I told them both that there was no question but that their relationship was destructive to their respective therapies. Although I could not tell them what to do, I made it clear that they would be faced with a choice. They would be forced to choose between each other or therapy. I did not ask them to make the choice but merely indicated that they could not avoid such a decision. The girl made a clear choice for treatment and began to cut Jerry off. Jerry was obviously angry at her and at me. I, too, had been callously unresponsive to his needs. I had taken away from him his woman whom he felt he needed and desperately wanted. It was soon after this that he left town, and I was notified of his rehospitalization.

It is well worth bringing into focus the countertransference difficulties in dealing with such treatment problems. Jerry's tirades were in varying degrees assaults on my own middle-class values. They were a constant temptation and invitation to respond defensively and to feel that my own way of life, my profession, and my identity were being put in question in basic and anxiety-provoking ways. From a more therapeutic perspective, I could sense the distortion and self-destructiveness in so much that he said. My paternal and protective instincts told me to try to confront his distortions and show him the truth that constantly eluded him. But to do so, I would have to put myself in a position—and would implicitly put on him the demand to comply with or rebel against it. Clearly, Jerry could not tolerate a position of relative autonomy and had to find a way to polarize our relationship into one of either compliance or rebellion.

His sexual acting out served the purpose and achieved his objective. It forced me into a position which raised the threat of compliance and against which he could react with his own form of rebellion, however self-destructive and self-defeating. What is of interest here is that when he could not draw me out of my objective-neutral stance on the basis of many dimensions of my own value orientation—political, religious—he succeeded by confronting my therapeutic value system and violating it in such a way that I felt I had to take a position in the interest of preserving the therapeutic process. I think this speaks to the underlying characterological defects that remained beyond the reach of this therapy, but it also dramatically illuminates the crucial therapeutic issue.

My essential point is that Jerry's treatment—despite its failure—could not have enjoyed its success without its sustained atmosphere of inquiry. Insofar as Jerry was capable of maintaining it, the therapy progressed. It foundered at a point where the inquiry led him to the need to surrender his infantile needs. Gedo's (1972) comment offers a pertinent warning:

> Should anyone think that the destruction of our culture can leave us unscathed in some kind of therapeutic isolation, it may also be pertinent to question Hartmann's belief that these holy wars can be kept out of our consulting rooms. There may have been a time earlier in the century when an analyst could assume that persons who could benefit from the psychoanalytic procedure in other respects would prove to be analyzable because they shared our basic scientific values; I would personally doubt even this and suspect that many unexplained therapeutic failures have always been due to covert adherence to unreason, certainty, and simplicity. At any rate, times are now out of joint, and many patients whose personality structure should permit successful analysis are impossible to treat because of the content of their value systems. If these fundamental differences are not recognized, something that passes for analysis may take place without the realization that it is nothing more than a hidden argument about *Weltanschauung*. [P. 220]

Thus, the capacity to sustain objective inquiry is essential to the treatment not only of potentially analyzable patients but also of more primitive and narcissistically vulnerable patients like Jerry. But such an objective and scientific inquiry must be uncompromising if it is to be effective. In dealing with the revolutionarily minded and radical students who find their way into treatment, the inquiry must match the intensity of their rebellious feeling with a ruthless commitment to objectivity. The treatment process falters when the therapist is drawn away from such uncompromising objectivity, whether it be in the direction of unquestioning adherence to his own personal presuppositions or values or in the direction of endorsing in any degree the presuppositions or values of the patient. One must honestly and effectively leave open the possibility that the patient may choose the course of rebellion against social institutions as a result of therapeutic progress. One hopes that as a result of therapeutic progress the rebellion can be more realistically directed and realistically implemented. If, however, one loses objectivity by adhering to personal presuppositions, the therapist runs the risk of losing trust, undermining the therapeutic alliance, and becoming identified as part of the forces of constraint and repression against which the patient's paranoia is directed. If one loses objectivity by accepting or endorsing the patient's presuppositions, one runs the risk of undermining therapeutic effectiveness and eliminating the possibility of testing the patient's perceptions and attitudes in realistic terms.

Conclusions

The direction of my argument and my experience with Jerry and similar patients is that one cannot attain or sustain the objectives of scientific and objective inquiry without supporting it by a theory of psychological and social complementarity. It is only by seeing personal pathology and social process in their overlapping and intermeshing functions that one can maintain an unprejudiced set of mind that will support the therapeutic inquiry. The therapist must be as able and willing to recognize the pathological and destructive aspects of the social environment as he is able and willing to recognize and acknowledge the pathological aspects of the patient's psychic functioning.

REFERENCES

Berman, S. 1970. Alienation: an essential process of the psychology of adolescence. *Journal of the Academy of Child Psychiatry* 9:233–250.

Deutsch, H. 1967. *Selected Problems of Adolescence*. New York: International Universities Press.

Erikson, E. H. 1959. *Identity and the Life Cycle*. New York: International Universities Press.

Erikson, E. H. 1964. *Insight and Responsibility*. New York: Norton.

Fried, M. 1970. Social problems and psychopathology. In H. Wechsler, L. Solomon, and B. M. Kramer, eds. *Social Psychology and Mental Health*. New York: Holt, Rinehart & Winston.

Gedo, J. E. 1972. The dream of reason produces monsters. *Journal of the American Psychoanalytic Association* 20:199–223.

Greenacre, P. 1970. Youth, growth and violence. *Psychoanalytic Study of the Child* 25:340–359.

Horney, K. 1950. *Neurosis and Human Growth*. New York: Norton.

Meissner, W. W. 1978. *The Paranoid Process*. New York: Aronson.

Merton, R. K. 1957. *Social Theory and Social Structure*. New York: Free Press.

Modell, A. H. 1968. *Object Love and Reality*. New York: International Universities Press.

Sarnoff, C. A. 1972. The vicissitudes of projection during an analysis encompassing late latency to early adolescence. *International Journal of Psycho-Analysis* 53:515–522.

33 THE FAMILY MEETING AS A DARKROOM: COUNTERTRANSFERENCE ISSUES WITH SEVERELY DISTURBED ADOLESCENTS

DAVID B. FEINSILVER

In my work with severely disturbed adolescents and young adults at Chestnut Lodge over several years, I have consistently noted the following phenomenon: Shortly after beginning psychotherapy with a new patient, always a very exciting and puzzling experience, I would have an initial "getting acquainted" meeting with the patient's family, usually including the patient. Not trying to structure the meeting in any particular way, I would immediately note that the family members seemed to be under pressure to pursue an agenda of their own with seemingly irrelevant or inconsequential matters. Soon, however, it would become apparent that the family members were enacting, unconsciously, something related to the genesis of the patient's pathology. In fact, it seemed to me that the family were staging a play in answer to the question, "What do you think caused your child's illness?" Moreover, it would seem to me that previously hidden central aspects of the basic transference-countertransference situation in the psychotherapy were suddenly emerging into the spotlight, much like the image emerging in the darkroom on previously exposed sensitized paper as it lies in the developing tray.

A particular clear and concise example will perhaps convey more clearly my observation. When I met with the parents of a severely regressed assaultive paranoid young man who was confined to a seclusion room, the mother immediately began besieging me with questions about the status of her son's cough. This took me completely by surprise because I

0-226-24058-4/85/0012-0021$01.00

had been seeing the son regularly and had not noticed such a symptom. I found out later from our staff that the son had indeed been showing symptoms of a minor cold, and this was mentioned by the staff in an effort to pass on what they thought was relatively inconsequential news. Almost before I could attempt to answer the mother's questions, she launched into an associative monologue about her own mother's death of lung cancer around the time of the patient's birth. The presenting symptom of this cancer was a hacking cough which had gone unnoticed for many years. Our patient's mother, from the time of her son's birth, always had the strange fear that her son would someday develop this illness, a concern which then pervaded her fears about him at every step of his development. This genetic perspective suddenly helped me understand the vague countertransference feeling that my efforts to engage him would somehow be controlling and annihilating him. I was becoming identified with this overprotective symbiotically involved mother.

In the following case material, I would like to show how this phenomenon of dramatic re-creation by the family of the genetic origins of the patient's illness helped to clarify a particularly confusing primitive transference-countertransference situation.

I will be using the term countertransference in the sense of Kernberg's (1965) definition of "totalistic countertransference," meaning the totality of the therapist's feelings in response to the patient. In work with severely disturbed patients, I believe, it is only through such an overinclusive definition that one can properly contain what is being generated by the patient (Feinsilver 1980, 1983).

Initial Presentation of the Case

When I first saw Marilyn, I knew only the barest outline of her case. She was a nineteen-year-old girl who had been in and out of various forms of treatment, inpatient and outpatient, since age ten. Throughout her early years, she was not seen as ill by her family, although she was reported repeatedly by school authorities to be having problems which required attention. After a premature menarche at age ten, she became a disruptive influence in the classroom, and her illness could no longer be ignored. She began behaving in an inappropriately, sexually provocative way, was called a "flake" by her classmates, and was scapegoated. She responded well at that time, at least symptomatically, to a treatment which combined supportive psychotherapy and medication. Marilyn was the oldest daughter of parents who had fought consistently throughout their married years, using sex and sexual affairs as ammunition in their battles. The patient's first hospitalization was precipitated by the parents' announcing their intention to separate when Marilyn was sixteen years old. Marilyn was described on admission as in an agitated, psychotic state, hypomanic with grandiose and sexual content. Over the next two years, up to her admission to our hospital, her treatments followed a recurrent pattern, with Marilyn at first showing rather rapid symptomatic response to hospitalization and medication, which included various phenothiazines and lithium. Father, however, would then be reluctant to follow through on recommendations for long-term treatment, choosing instead to try to keep her at home while she attended some special school. Marilyn, however, would soon have to be hospitalized again in an acutely agitated psychotic state. Marilyn had been diagnosed at different times as chronic schizophrenic, schizoaffective schizophrenic, or borderline schizophrenic.

When I approached Marilyn for our initial session in the living room of her unit, the room was dimly lighted and she was standing in a particularly shady corner. I was struck as I approached her by an impression of ambiguity that was highlighted by the dim shadows—an ambiguity which would persist almost hauntingly in our interactions for some time. She seemed, fleetingly, like a genuinely attractive young woman; then, at another instant, from a different angle, like a gross caricature of a garish prostitute; and then, at another instant, as I got closer still, like bizarre, severely disturbed "human wreckage."

As I introduced myself, she stammered back blankly. I was just about to conclude that she must be hallucinating or autistically withdrawn when she responded in a surprisingly normal-sounding way, asking what I wanted to know about her. I was further startled when I hesitantly asked her, as I might normally ask a private patient in my office, if she could, "Tell me a little bit about what brought you to the hospital." She then responded in a clear, coherent way, giving me a very reasonable, affect-laden, factual account of her past. She recounted the theme of being a "misfit" and did so with a surprising amount of feeling that was easy for me to empathically share with her. She spoke with great poignancy about how she saw herself coming to Chestnut Lodge as a last resort, after repeatedly experiencing herself in situation after situation as failing to find the love she craved. She confessed in an embarrassed way that she could not control herself sexually for this reason and often got into trouble because of it. She kept finding herself rejected, with the feeling that she must be like the "Boston Strangler"—whose identity nobody knew but for whose surfacing everybody anxiously waited. She began to sob in a way that seemed easy to empathize with—in fact, a very unusual occurrence on a first meeting with most of the patients who come to our hospital. She elaborated on how she had first started experiencing this feeling of shameful rejection while growing up in her family whenever her parents fought, feeling vaguely ashamed and guilty about their difficulties and particularly for their ultimate separation. She then described how this was part of a bad, ugly sense of herself that was somehow reinforced when she became a woman "too soon."

This initial hour ended with my having confusing, contradictory impressions. On the one hand, I felt that I had encountered a normal engaging young woman who could give me a readily understandable account of why she felt so bad; on the other hand, this did not fit with the severity of her illness as manifested by the lifelong history of repeated breakdowns and hospitalizations. There was certainly no hint of a schizophrenic, "there but not there," wall-like atmosphere (Pao 1979). Was Marilyn really as ill as reflected in her history, or as well as reflected in her presentation to me, or some combination of these presentations that needed to be further clarified?

The details of Marilyn's history, as they were gathered from past records and social worker's interviews with the family, elaborated further details but did not really clarify the diagnostic dilemma or the confusing ambiguity about who Marilyn really was as she related to me in our initial psychotherapy hours. Mother, a severely disturbed child herself, with an inadequate mother and an overly seductive father, seems to have re-created the same situation for Marilyn. She describes herself as totally inadequate as a mother and having to turn over much of the responsibility for Marilyn's rearing to the father. As if to emphasize the roots in her own past, her mother described Marilyn's development as faulty from the moment of conception, denying penetration by father during the sexual act. Mother was always very fearful for her developing infant, being particularly concerned about dirt and being afraid to be alone with her. She also admitted frequently taking out her frustrations on Marilyn and hitting her, especially when she refused to eat. In addition to the father's taking over much of the mother's caretaking activities, he has always been noted by observers to be behaving in an overly seductive manner toward Marilyn. They have often been described as behaving like husband and wife.

Father is a successful professional and apparently the psychologically stronger of the two (relatively). He, too, had an inadequate mother but was spared much of the ill effect by the presence in the home of an overcontrolling grandmother who took over his parenting. Father's own father was unavailable because of his involvement in running his business. Thus, father, too, seemed, in many ways, to be re-creating his own parenting with Marilyn by trying to be the parent figure who takes over for the inadequate original ones. Marilyn's developmental landmarks were said to be normal, but by the time she reached nursery school she was undeniably recognized by her teachers to be withdrawn, shy, and performing badly, although basically having superior endowment. Recommendations to pursue treatment were repeatedly unheeded, until severe disruptions began at age ten after Marilyn's premature menarche.

Reflecting the initial confusion in our diagnostic impression, the planning by our treatment team wavered between two extremes, first considering Marilyn to be more capable than she was and then to be sicker. In brief, this initial phase, lasting about six months, up to the time we had our introductory family meeting, went as follows: Because Marilyn seemed in good reality contact and had been off medication for several months, we decided to see how far we could go trying to maintain and mobilize her healthy functioning. We tried to actively support her wishes to finally obtain her high school diploma by arranging for her participation in a special program, as well as encouraging her active involvement in hospital activities. But within a few months Marilyn began to regress. In her individual therapy, I had tried to maintain a supportive focus on her daily concerns, minimizing the focus on transference. Things seemed to go well for a while as we walked and talked informally around the grounds for our sessions, but shortly after we began to meet in my office, Marilyn began to show increased agitation on leaving our sessions, particularly on weekends. Just prior to a long holiday weekend, Marilyn suddenly became agitated and deluded, obviously psychotic, making references to sex and sexual attack. Though she then showed rapid symptomatic response to lithium, she was unable to maintain a coherent reality-oriented conversation with me and seemed sufficiently concerned about my attacking her and her attacking me that we both agreed that, in order to help her feel more controlled and comfortable, we would begin meeting for hours with her regularly restrained in a cold wet sheet pack (see Feinsilver [1980] for further details of this procedure).

Although Marilyn was able to be sufficiently organized to continue doing well in her preparations for her high school diploma and to participate in hospital activities, she remained relatively disorganized in our hours and tended to remain withdrawn and quiet or locked in psychotic fantasies. A central delusional belief (although probably not taken as total reality), was about herself being Marilyn Monroe and my being either Joe DiMaggio or Arthur Miller. She also spoke about fears of my rotting or dying and, sometimes, of my somehow killing her or of killing herself. Of particular interest were recurrent vague stories about incestuous experiences with her father or an uncle, which, although reported as actual historical events, had vague fantasy qualities that made them sound dubious. What was most curious, however, was that, despite knowing that these stories were delusions, I found it difficult in listening to them not to get caught up in feeling that these traumas had actually befallen Marilyn.

Family Meeting

As I approached the meeting room, my concerns about the traumatic incestuous experiences between father and daughter seemed to be substantiated—though as it turned out, incorrectly. The social worker who arranged the meeting rushed up to me, took me aside, and told me that I had just missed "the most amazing display of inappropriate hugging and kissing between a father and daughter" that she had ever seen. But this proved to be a mere diversionary fleeting prologue and disappeared by the time I entered the room. We were barely finished with the formal introductions when daughter, assisted by father, began making a presentation to mother of a small birthday gift. After a few stereotyped birthday exchanges, mother retreated into the background, not to be involved again until the end of the meeting, and father took over control of the discussion. It was as if the family were dramatically re-creating the history of how Marilyn was given over to father, as a present to mother, to relieve mother of the responsibility of her parenting role.

We seemed to be entering act 2 as the father took over, entirely dominating the proceedings. He began grilling me much as a parent concerned about his child's performance might grill a teacher. He asked about why his daughter was not doing better, participating in more activities, and progressing in her therapy. The father seemed to be anxiously pursuing this line of questioning without waiting for a response, more out of an interest in registering a complaint than in having a real discussion. Soon Marilyn began to respond instead, cutting him off, defensively arguing about how well she was doing in her special tutoring program and other activities around the hospital. Father then quickly cut her off and the two of them went back and forth in an argumentative exchange that had the quality of a dance they must have done many times. As I observed this, it seemed to me that father was saying, "Why are you such a failure?" and Marilyn was saying, "I am not really failing, I am really doing okay," a theme that seemed to have echoes of her past history as well as the course of treatment with me. I recalled the recurring theme of her performing poorly in school as well as in her successive treatment efforts. I recalled how it was only as a result of Marilyn's blatant failures that she seemed able to get her father's attention in the first place, either to get herself into treatment or subsequently for him to rescue her from it.

At this point I interrupted and asked whether the idea of Marilyn's failing, not doing as well as expected, was perhaps a familiar theme. This led to the father's talking directly to me for the first time, saying, "Of course, this has always been my complaint about Marilyn." He then went on to elaborate in a complaining tone about how he has always worried about her wasting time and efforts.

At this point, Marilyn also began to speak to me directly for the first time, saying that of course she felt she was often wasting her time. What else could she do? She also felt she was being sent off by her parents to one place or another—school, treatment, friends. They all felt like places she was being sent away to. When she then began to elaborate about how she always felt there was some bad shameful thing that was causing this rejection and abandonment by her parents, I thought immediately about the incestuous theme. I began to question further about what this bad and shameful thing might be. Marilyn's response was striking in many ways—in its absence of any direct or indirect reference to sexuality, in its striking clarity of describing simply an experience of parental rejection and abandonment, and in its poignant affect. She described in detail, with a great deal of feeling, the sense of shameful abandonment she experienced as her father first brought her to the lodge. She described how this was similar to when her father took her to her first psychiatrist. She elaborated on how her sense of shame was associated with the feeling that she was not living up to his expectations in some way. Father always complained of her not being a "mensch," but she felt unclear about this. It seemed unfair to her and she felt that somebody—father, mother, or somebody—should make this up to her in some way.

At this point, it seemed clear that father and daughter were dramatizing a story of mutual abandonment. Marilyn seemed to be saying that failing was her way of registering her complaint that father was unfairly imposing expectations that she could not fulfill. This left her feeling rejected and abandoned. Father, in turn, seemed to be saying that his daughter was indeed always failing his expectations for her and in this way rejecting and abandoning him. This was strikingly reminiscent of the way I had felt Marilyn had failed me after showing such promise in our initial engagement and comfortable informal beginning. I was reminded of her increasing vague separation anxiety after our hours just prior to her complete disorganization. I was further reminded of how Marilyn's concerns about attacking, and being sexually attacked by, me surrounded her separation anxiety. It suddenly seemed clear to me how Marilyn's incestuous concerns were indeed a mere opening prologue to the more central basic issue of mutual rejection and abandonment between father and daughter. In brief, the blame and counterblame interaction between father and daughter seemed to be a personification of the way I might have felt about Marilyn dashing my expectations—that is, if I were clearer about why I felt so confused about why I thought of her first as so normal and later as so sick. My confusion mirrored her fragmentation as we both labored to ward off these aggressive wishes.

In the meeting, her father then continued demonstrating exactly how he might have gone about further cementing this rejection and abandonment in his daughter. He began jumping in and cutting her off with blame-establishing questions of the double bind variety such as, "When are you going to stop this fooling around and accept your illness?" "When are you going to stop wasting time and begin working with your doctors to get well?" All this was, of course, said with the clear implication and expectation that Marilyn was such a bad person that she would never and could never do differently. It was also striking to me, at this time, how much father's specific complaints of Marilyn being somebody who "just fooled around" and "wasted time—was a complete waste" recalled for me the fragmented, devalued self-images that had struck me as disconnectedly present since our first meeting—the "garish prostitute" and the "human wreckage." Of course, such complaints by the father also implied an expectation of his daughter's being capable of doing and being otherwise. This was a normal image which he also had his reasons for seeing in Marilyn, and she had her reasons for trying to live up to it. I was reminded of the disconnected images that I had experienced in our initial encounter, and here it seemed as if I could almost see how those disconnected images were being hammered into place.

Therapeutic Interaction

Although Marilyn continued for some time in her relatively fragmented state in our hours, remaining restrained in a cold wet sheet pack, shortly after this family meeting I was able to begin applying in a useful (though not dramatic) way my clearer sense of what our confusing interchanges were about. The following hour occurred a few months later and will serve as an example:

I began to note in the nursing reports that Marilyn was becoming increasingly sexually provocative on the unit, particularly on weekends and at other times at separation from me after sessions. In the hours, Marilyn would frequently become sexually abusive for no apparent reason. One day, just before a long weekend, I entered her room for an hour and she, lying in her cold wet sheet pack, stared away from me and remained totally silent. After about ten minutes, she began writhing in the pack in an unmistakably sexual rhythm. She ignored my efforts to engage her verbally, but instead just kept writhing in a way that started to make me feel quite uncomfortable and annoyed with her—ordinarily she would at least give me some sort of verbal response. In addition, her writhing itself was making me very angry. I had always found her blatant sexuality quite disgusting and obnoxious. Much to my surprise, however, I found myself becoming sexually aroused with her for the first time. I then noted an interesting chain of fantasies and associations centering around my angry feelings. I wished she were a different person; I wished we were in a different place; I wished it were a different time. Then it struck me. This must be how father made her feel. In short, I was being victimized just as Marilyn must have been. This must be what she experienced as rejection and abandonment at the hands of her father and was at the core of what was making her feel like such a rage-filled misfit, sexually stimulated and frustrated by incestuous fantasies.

I then offered Marilyn a speculative, interpretative comment, saying that I thought she was doing to me probably what she felt I was doing to her, an experience she had repeatedly with her father, namely, being forced into a situation of expectation and promise, creating a sense of sexual stimulation and excitement, only to find herself repeatedly rejected and abandoned. She began talking in the hour for the first time, although in a monologue way, as if not really addressing me. She began retelling the story of how her father brought her to Chestnut Lodge, as she had done with so much feeling in the family meeting. She then focused on an aspect she had not spoken of before, about how father first took her for a few hours to an amusement park before bringing her to the hospital. Her voice then trailed off as she focused in detail on a scene in the parking lot where she said they met a little puppy who wanted to be picked up and held. At that point, I broke in and asked her if she wasn't talking about feeling very rejected and wanting to be picked up and held like the puppy dog. Without waiting for an answer, I suggested further that, although I did not expect her to acknowledge or respond to this, I suspected that she might very well be feeling something like that right now, then and there with me, around the forthcoming weekend separation. She did not answer directly but tried instead to start writhing again as if to block everything out. She stopped quickly, however, this time apparently no longer able to get into it. It was near the end of the hour, and she remained silent. When I then said it was time to stop and started to get up to walk out the door, she stopped me and said in a very pointed way that seemed to be her way of acknowledging and responding to my remarks, "Have a nice weekend, Dr. Feinsilver."

Discussion

I will give a brief survey of the family interaction literature and then take up what seemed to be the essential elements of the "darkroom phenomenon," first from the perspective of the therapist and then from the perspective of the family.

The family interaction of severely disturbed patients has been of considerable interest to researchers and clinicians for many years, focusing on specific patterns of communication (Bateson, Jackson, Haley, and Weakland 1956; Lidz, Fleck, and Cornelison 1965; Palazolli 1978; Walsh 1979; Wynne, Ryckoff, Day, and Hirsch 1958); studies of verbal communication (Feinsilver 1970; Mischler 1968; Morris and Wynne 1965; Wild, Singer, Rosman, Ricci, and Lidz 1965; Wynne and Singer 1963); role relations (Ackerman 1956; Bowen 1960; Lidz et al. 1965); symbiosis (Searles 1965; Summers and Walsh 1977, 1979); specific traumatic events (Walsh 1978); sharing of unconscious mechanisms (Reiss 1981); and maintaining specific part-object relationships (Zinner and Shapiro 1972).

To my knowledge, very few writers link these observations about family interaction with the emergence of the patient's transference relationship in individual psychotherapy. In his article in which he covers many clinically useful aspects of the relationship between family therapy and individual therapy, Searles (1965) touches on the issue in general. He describes various ways in which one can see in the family interaction manifestations of the patient's inner objects. He cautions against the pitfall of believing the patient's complaint that the source of his difficulties lies only in these family interactions. Searles argues for the possibility of combining the benefits of dealing with the interpersonal problems in the family work with the intrapsychic problems in the individual therapy, but he does not focus on the re-creation of a specific transference-countertransference situation. Shapiro, Shapiro, Zinner, and Berkowitz (1977) point out how, for the borderline patient, conjoint family therapy can be very useful in helping the individual therapist clarify, for the patient, emerging transference patterns both in the family meetings as well as in the individual therapy. They focus on the effect of strengthening the patient's reality-oriented ego and the alliance. Shapiro (1978) focuses similarly on combining individual therapy with conjoint family therapy as a place for resolving the here-and-now reality resistance of the transference manifestations in the actual family interaction that otherwise could present formidable resistances to the individual work. Of particular interest for this chapter is Shapiro's observation that adolescents seem to have a need to confront their parents with the historical truth about the origins of their illness. He cites Freud's Dora case and states, "Patients such as Dora therefore may legitimately insist that the genetic meaning of their sickness find recognition within an assessment . . . of the historical truth of their family experience. . . ." It is also interesting to note that, in a list of purposes for combining the family meeting with other forms of therapy for the various individuals, Stierlin (1980) does not even mention a diagnostic purpose. All these articles, however, focus on the therapeutic benefit of the family meeting for the patient and do not take up the clarifying effect on the therapist, particularly with regard to his countertransference.

Let us consider why this countertransference clarification phenomenon has not been previously recognized—although, I suspect, it has been probably noted and passed over by observers for some time. I believe the answer lies in the special circumstances of a therapist in an ongoing therapeutic relationship with the patient being introduced into the ongoing family situation. Let us consider this first from my perspective—exclusive therapist for the patient—and then from the perspective of the family in meeting the therapist of the designated patient.

I approached these families as the therapist who has already become exposed to the patient's transference with its effect on my own countertransference processes (largely unconscious at this point in the therapy). I came to the family meeting with Marilyn, for instance, having experienced an initial engagement and subsequent disintegration only dimly aware of the unconscious impact on me. However, I recognized immediately, as familiar from my own experience of Marilyn's transference, her father's complaint about her failing him, and her self-destructive retaliatory response of failing as a way of dealing with abandonment and rejection. In fact, this is the negative aspect of the transference-countertransference interaction that had been ejected from the dyad as part of a dual effort to maintain the positive idealized relatedness between us and my projectively identifying blame on the family. Marilyn is probably activating this interaction with her father as a way of displacing it out of the therapy, as I am similarly projectively looking for it there as part of my complementary displacement. My tendency to hear Marilyn's memory-fantasy of incest as an actual trauma for which to place blame on the family is an example of how this kind of projection was taking place all the time. Thus, my previous experience with Marilyn's unfolding transference sensitizes me and serves in the family meeting as an unconscious searchlight—ready to stop when it passes over what it recognizes.

Other observers with different experiences with the patient and family would see the same interaction completely differently. For instance, the social worker in this case, having developed a strong alliance with the father and encouraging him to speak about his concerns, tended to see Marilyn's reaction to her father's questions as unfortunate responses to the father's realistic concern about his daughter's progress. As another example of this in the introductory vignette, it is easy to see how the mother, asking about her son's cough, might be seen as involved in a reasonable motherly concern or an annoying irrelevance and easily dismissed. Similarly, it is easy to see how a researcher or a clinician, with other tasks or frames of reference and no need to project any particular aspect of his ongoing relationship with the patient, might come to rest his searchlight on any one of a number of interesting aspects of the interaction that would miss the connection with the transference.

Now from the side of the family, how can it be that the members invariably present the relevant transference to the sensitized observer? (I have not yet met with a family where this has not occurred.) The most obvious answer is that the family, just like individual patients, cannot avoid enacting its family transference because it does so all the time. This is undoubtedly true and part of the answer, but I believe there is another major factor that must be taken into account that relates to how the particular interaction seems to focus on the designated patient, seemingly "confessing" the story of what the family has done to the child. I believe that it has to do with the introduction of the family to the therapist who they all hope will cure the patient's problem—much like an initial interview with an individual patient, or a first dream in psychotherapy. Under these circumstances, the patient seems to be presenting to the healer, in unconscious terms, his major unfulfilled wishes, along with their history in condensed terms, and his hopes and expectations for the future. Often much of this will be verbalized by the family members with specific comments, such as, "Doctor, I hope you will finally be able to do something for X's problems" or "Doctor, I think you should know about this important event that happened to X as a child" or know "about this bad thing that happened between us." Often such topics become explicit matters to speak about, but I believe that if no explicit agenda is preset to focus the family's conscious attention and predetermine the family's interaction, they will unconsciously tend to join to find a way of expressing their deepest concerns, in unconscious behavior terms, as they approach the healing person by whom they wish the problem to be cured.

If one then adds to this setting the situation of the patient's bringing to the family the specific intolerable aspect of the transference that he is needing to eject from the therapeutic relationship, one can easily see how this will feed into the always present family dynamics in a way that will tend to re-create the ways in which all the family members originally dealt with this conflict. This may also then feed into the patient's search for truth noted by Shapiro—or, indeed, may be responsible for it.

Conclusions

The net effect of the family meeting for the therapist of the severely disturbed patient is to provide an opportunity to see in live action the shadowy, largely unconscious, primitive part-object transference-countertransference relatedness that he perceives only dimly in his interaction with his patient. For the therapist, it is as if he were photographing his interactions with the patient in the dark and then having the opportunity, in the family meeting, to bring out these images in bold relief and clarity.

NOTE

The author wishes to acknowledge the assistance of Muriel S. Levine, M.S.W., in the clinical work as well as for comments on the manuscript.

REFERENCES

Ackerman, N. W. 1956. Interlocking pathology in family relationships. In *Changing Concepts of Psychoanalytic Medicine*. In S. Reda and G. Daniels, eds. New York: Grune & Stratton.

Bateson, G.; Jackson, D. D.; Haley, J.; and Weakland, J. H. 1956. Toward a theory of schizophrenia. *Behavioral Science* 1:251–264.

Bowen, M. 1960. A family concept of schizophrenia. In D. Jackson, ed. *The Etiology of Schizophrenia*. New York: Basic.

Feinsilver, D. 1970. Communication in families of schizophrenia patients. *Archives of General Psychiatry* 22:143–148.

Feinsilver, D. 1980. Transitional relatedness and containment in the treatment of a chronic schizophrenic patient. *International Review of Psychoanalysis* 7:309–318.

Feinsilver, D. 1983. Reality, transitional relatedness and containment in the borderline. *Contemporary Psychoanalysis* 19:537–569.

Kernberg, O. 1965. Notes on countertransference. *Journal of American Psychoanalysis* 13:38–56.

Lidz, T.; Fleck, S.; and Cornelison, A. R. 1965. *Schizophrenia and the Family*. New York: International Universities Press.

Mischler, E. G. 1968. *Interaction in Families: Family Process of Schizophrenia*. New York: Wiley.

Morris, G. O., and Wynne, L. C. 1965. Schizophrenia offspring and parental styles of communication: a predictive study utilizing excerpts of family therapy recordings. *Psychiatry* 28:19–44.

Palazolli, M. S. 1978. *Paradox and Counter-Paradox*. New York: Aronson.

Pao, P. 1979. *Schizophrenia Disorders*. New York: International Universities Press.

Reiss, D. 1981. *The Family's Construction of Reality*. Cambridge, Mass.: Harvard University Press.

Searles, H. 1965. The contributions of family treatment to the psychotherapy of schizophrenia. *Collected Papers on Schizophrenia and Related Subjects*. New York: International University Press.

Shapiro, E. R.; Shapiro, R. L.; Zinner, J.; and Berkowitz, D. H. 1977. The borderline ego and the working alliance: indications for family and individual treatment in adolescence. *International Journal of Psycho-Analysis* 58:77–87.

Shapiro, R. L. 1978. The adolescent, the therapist and the family: the management of internal resistances to psychoanalytic therapy of adolescents. *Journal of Adolescence* 1:3–10.

Stierlin, H. 1980. *The First Interview with the Family*. New York: Brunner/Mazel.

Summers, F., and Walsh, F. 1977. The nature of the symbiotic bond between mother and schizophrenic. *American Journal of Orthopsychiatry* 47:484–494.

Summers, F., and Walsh, F. 1979. Symbiosis and confirmation between father and schizophrenic. *American Journal of Orthopsychiatry* 49:136–148.

Walsh, F. 1979. Breaching of family generation boundaries by schizophrenics, disturbed non-schizophrenics and normals. *International Journal of Family Therapy* 1:254–275.

Walsh, F. 1978. Concurrent grandparent death and birth of schizophrenic offspring. *Family Process* 17:457–463.

Wild, C. S.; Singer, W.; Rosman, B.; Ricci, J.; and Lidz, T. 1965. Measuring disordered styles of thinking in the parents of schizophrenic patients on the object sorting test. Parts I and II. In T. Lidz, S. Fleck, and H. Cornelison, eds. *Schizophrenia and the Family*. New York: International Universities Press.

Wynne, L. C.; Ryckoff, I. M.; Day, J.; and Hirsch, S. I. 1958. Pseudomutuality in the family relations of schizophrenics. *Psychiatry* 21:205–220.

Wynne, L. C., and Singer, M. 1963. Thought disorder and family relations of schizophrenia. II. A classification of forms of thinking. *Archives of General Psychiatry* 9:199–206.

Zinner, J., and Shapiro, R. 1972. Projective identification as a mode of perception and behavior in families of adolescents. *International Journal of Psycho-Analysis* 53:523–530.

34 COUNTERTRANSFERENCE ISSUES IN PSYCHOTHERAPY WITH ADOLESCENTS[1]

STEPHEN L. ZASLOW

Countertransference Issues in Psychotherapy with Adolescents

Psychotherapy should be—and is—a process congenial to many adolescents who are stuck or blocked in moving forward, who are too fearful to try out new roles and relationships, or who are too inflexible or unlucky to mature in the process. The primary task of the adolescent's therapist is to foster the adolescent's emerging personal identity, that is, to help him define himself in the many spheres of life. "Countertransference" is the term I use along with Epstein and Feiner (1979) to refer to "the therapist's contribution to the therapeutic situation." They see countertransference "as a normal, natural interpersonal event" involving a therapist "who is a genuine coparticipant in an ongoing process . . . rather than as an idiosyncratic phenomenon." It is expected and accepted that countertransference is normal, natural, inevitable, and informative. Because of the centrality of the transference-countertransference drama in psychotherapy, and because this chapter demonstrates therapeutic uses of countertransference, I will outline some concepts from the literature which have influenced my work.

Freud (1910) first articulated the concept of "counter-transference," noting that it developed in the physician "as a result of the patient's influence on his unconscious feelings." This recognition demanded "innovations in technique," namely, that the analysis begin with self-anal-

0-226-24058-4/85/0012-0014$01.00

ysis and that the analyst should "continually carry it deeper" while "making observations on his patients." Freud (1912) was well aware of the interactive implications of transference, for he insisted the analyst "must turn his own unconscious like a receptive organ towards the transmitting unconscious of the patient. He must adjust himself to the patient as a telephone receiver is adjusted to the transmitting microphone. Just as the receiver converts back into sound waves the electric oscillations in the telephone line which were set up by sound waves, so the doctor's unconscious is able, from the derivatives of the unconscious which are communicated to him, to reconstruct that unconscious, which has determined the patient's free associations."

Epstein and Feiner (1979) show how Freud's writings wove two strands of an ambivalent view of countertransference: as a hindrance to be analyzed out and as an asset which the physician can use to aid his patient. In considering the analyst's emotional response as one of the most important tools in analytic work, Heimann (1950) expanded the view of countertransference to include all the therapist's feelings toward his patient. She assumed that the analyst's unconscious understands the patient, an understanding that becomes conscious within a countertransference context and which she viewed as "the patient's creation" and "part of the patient's personality." She recommended that the analyst apply evenly hovering attention to his own responses, thereby using countertransference as an ally. Such an approach was a welcome antidote to anxious and guilt-ridden self-scrutiny, as were the ideas of those who stressed the processes of induction within the bipersonal field (Langs 1976), Grinberg's (1962) work on "projective identification and projective counter-identification," and Klauber's (1981) attention to the "secret loving and secret hating" that goes on in analytic therapy.

Winnicott's (1949) paper, "Hate in the Countertransference," was a refreshingly direct statement that analysts could and should hate on occasion. Indeed, the analyst's hate could be just the "objective" feedback the patient needed, if the patient was asking to be hated. "If the patient seeks objective or justified hate, he must be able to reach it, else he cannot feel he can reach objective love." Little (1951) also grappled with the analyst's need to contain, process, and use the tension and impulses generated by very disturbed patients. Each of these authors admitted the analyst's need to react, even primitively and spontaneously at times, for the needs of both the patient and the analyst—who sometimes has to "detoxify" his feelings to continue to function constructively. With primitive patients, then, countertransference feelings may have to do much of the work. Little also suggested the analyst accept, admit, and—when possible—explain his mistakes, for patients' paranoid anxieties can be relieved by experiencing the analyst as a human (i.e., limited) being.

Racker (1968) wrote about countertransference phenomena, which he accepted as natural and normal. When the analyst finds himself in the emotional position of a child to his patients, Racker called this a "countertransference neurosis." Countertransference identifications are either "concordant" (i.e., empathic with the patient's thoughts and feelings) or "complementary" (i.e., a negative reaction to the patient's projections). Epstein (1977), Tauber (1978), Wolstein (1981), and others have examined the inevitable intimacies of the doctor-patient relationship.

The following clinical examples are selected to shed some light on the process of identity formation in adolescence and how issues for the adolescent often intertwine with significant professional issues for the therapist. In addition, they reveal some typical issues of opening, middle, and end phases of treatment and indicate how I process my inner experiences and use them in the treatment of patients. The therapist's expectations can interact with the patient's expectations to produce a stalemate, as I will discuss.

Winnicott (1971) concludes that "psychotherapy takes place in the overlap of two areas of playing: that of the patient and that of the therapist. Psychotherapy has to do with two people playing together. The corollary of this is that where playing is not possible the work of the therapist is directed towards bringing the patient from a state of not being able to play into a state of being able to play." The idea of therapy of play reminds us, too, of Blos's (1962) conceptualization of adolescence as "the second individuation process," wherein peer groups permit teenagers opportunities to try out new roles, without the necessity of permanent commitment either to the group or to the new roles. Psychotherapy involves much of this.

We approach the initial meeting with the adolescent with these frames of reference. Meeting the adolescent as a human being comes first, and an important aspect of this involves understanding his life space before he officially becomes a patient. "Man does not live by reality alone, even less by psychic reality," wrote Klauber (1981). So we must attune ourselves to the multiple realities of the adolescent's life and psyche from the beginning of the therapeutic relationship. If the adolescent is not eager to begin, it might be wise to supply him with the data, as we know it, about the referral—for instance, as his mother provided it in the phone contact—rather than inquire directly about his perceptions and motivations. This gratifies his need for information and context. It affords him the opportunity to correct data, define issues, and develop his relationship with the therapist.

When the teenager still remains silent, we need to pay special attention to affects: his and ours. Is he expressing via silent containment and control uncertainty or bewildering confusion, panic, shame or dread, challenge or implacable coldness? Do we feel curious or eager to guide, testy, repelled, or drawn in? Early in our careers as therapists we are apt to overvalue therapy, perhaps to overcompensate for "the feeling of therapeutic inadequacy [that] might be called the depressive position of the newly qualified analyst" (Klauber 1981). We lean toward needing our patients to need us, subtly coercing them to become patients and to need therapy. Concurrently we may idealize adolescents, overvaluing their strengths—their presumed autonomy, willfullness, and liveliness. Then we project our helpless irritation into them and accusingly sense in their silence a challenge, rejection, or resistance to therapy. Thus the therapist's concern with his new identity as a therapist can impose an attitude of his own and make it more difficult for the silent teenager to express his own conflicts about being in the patient's chair.

Case Report

Ellen's mother urged me to see Ellen as soon as possible but insisted on seeing me alone to brief me first, while father and Ellen waited outside. She efficiently compressed life history, psychiatric history, and present illness into fifteen minutes. Ellen, an eighteen-year-old learning-disabled only child, had identified with her parents' values for academic success and achievement and made it her ambition to graduate from college and become an architect. By dint of extreme hard work and exclusive focus on academics, she graduated from high school. She had few friends, fewer personal interests. During periods of threatened or actual failure, she concealed difficulties from her parents, until either she prevailed or the school brought them to her parents' attention.

Several consultations with other therapists had been failures, mother warned, because therapists had ignored her advice about the goals she had set for Ellen and the therapist. For example, in the senior year of high school, Ellen was agitated and insomniac and afraid she would fail her examinations. Mother wanted to help her over the hump so she would graduate. The therapist, however, insisted on psychological tests. Ellen took these but became so resistant that thereafter she would not see the therapist. Mother stressed that therapists tried to do too much, that Ellen could not even admit a problem. So, she advised, I should proceed slowly.

Yet the current predicament concerned her gravely. Ellen was failing several college courses. She had not gone to school for a week. She had cut off all contact with peers. She stayed in her room studying or pacing. She barely sat through dinner, snapped when spoken to, and offered nothing spontaneous. Perhaps she talked to herself, as well, and thought people were against her.

By the end of mother's mini-session, I felt irritation about being pressed into what seemed to be an impossible situation. I recognized my sense of helplessness.

As Ellen slowly responded to my greeting, I felt that she looked at me only out of polite obligation. Her dress was drab, clean, and slightly askew; her complexion pasty; and her hair mousy and shapeless. She walked into the office like a weak automaton and sat flaccidly and still. Her speech was faint, and affect was vacant. She offered no comment when I shared some of mother's recitation. She had no purpose in being here and did not wish to discuss anything. She did permit me to question her. She said she had no problems, was feeling OK, and was only interested in finishing school. She would not comment on other interests, friends, or family. I spoke of her polite and quiet manner, her apparent self-control, and of my suspicion that she was straining to contain herself despite great stress. She smiled ruefully and agreed that she tried to stay in control, but the stress was not so great. I felt a bit of contact and asked, Was the stress sadness within? "A bit," she said, then looked in the distance and withdrew. I felt I was losing her, that I could not hold her attention. Perhaps this reflected her inner life, I silently wondered. After a while I said I did not know what was happening to her, but perhaps she was feeling a loss, a void. I wondered aloud whether she had lost something dear to her—an ideal, a goal, a cherished wish—and that life might seem meaningless without it. "Not exactly meaningless," she said—which answered my concern about suicide. But she could say no more. Again I felt contact followed by disconnection.

In a brief conference with the parents I predicted that Ellen's condition might soon change, perhaps for the worse, and they might have to consider hospitalization and perhaps medication. We set another appointment. That night Ellen became violent. She also called mother "Mommy" for the first time in a year and asked to be hospitalized. She was hospitalized.

I believe that many factors contributed to Ellen's being able to ask for help rather than withdrawing. I used my countertransference responses toward her mother—such as feeling the pressure of urgency yet being constrained, helpless, and angry—and my responses to Ellen. The latter consisted of feeling accepted and then shut out, generally feeling sad. This enabled me to predict how Ellen would react. I believe I helped her to get in touch with inner feelings of helplessness and express her neediness without challenging the control that she and mother sought to retain. She was able to reach out powerfully to "Mommy" but still managed to maintain some distance by going to the hospital.

Case Report

In the middle phases of therapy, and in the middle phases of a therapist's life, certain countertransference orientations emerge regularly. One is the therapist's satisfaction in being successful with his patients, and the adolescent who is doing well gratifies him through affirming his therapeutic endeavors. The adolescent may be fixated on childish goals and adaptive patterns and unable to mature because of character pathology. We may believe, however, that we have initiated a thoughtful therapeutic strategy and established a working alliance. Particularly with a compliant obsessional, we may have organized a quietly successful obsessional therapy, where affects are accepted, interpersonal maneuvers recognized, and dreams and symptoms understood. The patient may have functioned better and better in numerous areas of living. But somewhere along the way, perhaps a year or two, a stalemate may be recognized and may be related to the therapist's too easy acceptance of the situation. In the following instance, Roy's transference clarified my countertransference, and our mutual insight led to mutual change.

Roy, a bright sixteen-year-old, whose two-year course of therapy seemed to be progressing well from a technical viewpoint, complained of continuing depression despite personal awareness and school and social success. He was dissatisfied with therapy specifically because it was "boring." After discussion and reflection, I had to agree: therapy had indeed become depressingly boring. I openly suspected that I contributed in no small measure. Initially Roy shouldered the blame: it felt boring because of his "neurosis, depression, masochism." I insisted that I, too, must play a role. He then homed in on my oversolicitousness and seriousness—which replicated in large measure his experiences with anxiously concerned parents. Previously he had engaged and confronted his parents on these issues with little satisfaction. They said that was right, that was the way they were, and he would have to get used to it. I shared with him my perceptions of him which had led me to react as I had—his timidity, fragility, and perfectionism. I also validated his perceptiveness about oversolicitousness and seriousness being character traits of mine, not all generated by him. I resolved to change, to "lighten up," to see if *I* could change the tone of therapy. In sessions I labeled and laughed at absurdities without exploring or belaboring. As I changed, he changed. Therapy became fun and playful—no longer obsessional, though we still worked at clarifying. He exclaimed he no longer felt like a patient, a "weirdo," the outsider he had always pictured and felt himself to be. He saw himself as just another teenager with sensitivities and problems.

Roy's confrontation helped free me. My self-examination indicated that I linked him with people in my life toward whom I had been protective and from whom I expected little. My smug self-satisfaction with Roy's "neat" therapy could not be denied as he deflated me by stating it was "boring." The therapist-as-parent role which initially provided a sense of trust, confidence, and security for this anxious, insecure, and dependent lad later served to reinforce dependence and feelings of inferiority and unworthiness. We had bogged down into obsessional boredom. Roy's transference and courage in complaining were effective in reaching and changing me. This provided a structural and stylistic change in the treatment. A new interpersonal partnership replaced an outgrown professional-type alliance.

Case Report

In six months of my work with seventeen-year-old William, we observed some working through of anxiety related to feeling and expressing closeness to males (so-called homosexual anxiety or panic) as termination approached. As William achieved some success through his own efforts, he grew more anxious, because success meant giving up his role of child-victim and its not-so-secret gratifications of disparaging and provoking his father. We considered his fears of my narcissistically feeding on his dependency, of my exploiting him to aggrandize myself. As we analyzed his macho rebellion against male authorities, he differentiated between his father, his employer, and myself. He was then able to feel affection for men in a limited way, when permitted to feel respect and identification with strength. He could then view himself as a potentially autonomous and independent person.

William, then a high school senior, and I were in our fourth year of work. As a child, he had had five years of individual and family therapy with a competent therapist because of school failure, impulsive and provocative behavior, poor judgment, extreme fearfulness, and social isolation. Having significant learning disabilities and a physical defect, he was the most impaired of a series of sons of an intact, close, and intrusive family. Of average intelligence, William used denial, projection, regression, and acting-out defenses.

One night a brother came into his bedroom as he was trying to sleep. William started a violent fight, revealing how terrified and angry he was at being intruded on. He was also fearful of and sensitive to his father's intrusions but not particularly sensitive to those of his mother. I suggested he had "a chip on his shoulder," refusing to let father care about him. He rejected my interpretation, but his relationship with his father became more relaxed. He began to understand that his father was revealing his own fearfulness rather than persecuting him. He nearly had several automobile accidents. I suggested he was trying to get father and me to worry about him and to treat him as an incompetent. He denied this, too, but he drove better.

In mid fall he announced he would be moving out of state at the end of the school year. "Don't be disappointed. This is the last year I'll see you. Don't take it the wrong way." "You mean I shouldn't feel rejected and possessive of you?" "Exactly," he said, deadly serious. He shared his pleasure in his grades and his accomplishments at work. Now he could let his mother be happy for him, but he resented his father's solicitous bragging about him. He also continued to have nightmares and insomnia.

I wanted more from him, some real acknowledgment. Our time together was growing short, and we were not resolving the problem of homosexual panic. I was tempted to press him to admit his dependency, attachment, and fondness for therapy and for me. I thought better of the idea, lest I replicate the intrusive and narcissistic demands which infuriated him in his parents. Instead, I said I thought he was afraid that I would be angry at him when he moved away if he did not miss me enough. He was puzzled. He said, "You don't treat me like that, you let me have my own thoughts and reactions. My father treats me like that. I have to put on a big show for him and I hate that. You're not like that. You're low key." I told him that men can like each other and share friendly feelings without being "wimpy, faggy, or mushy." He didn't think so! Nonetheless, the nightmares disappeared by the next session, and he continued waking refreshed instead of irritable. He dreamed of his father as a successful executive, then as his employer. For the first time ever, he planned a trip and took it. Abandoning the helpless, dependent, furious child-victim identity, he began to feel adult competence. Acknowledging respect, if not affection, for me permitted identification with strength and care and replaced oppositional rebellious orientations. My rare use of direct confrontation and not making demands permitted William to feel in control of our relationship and to sustain a sense of trust.

Bonime (1962) differentiated the patient's healthy reluctance to terminate from resistance to termination. Although he wrote about adult patients, his ideas are valid for adolescents. I place the healthy reluctance to relinquish a meaningful relationship first, as he does, both because I believe it needs reemphasis, and because I believe that when it is not mutually given its due, the holding on to pathology cannot be given up. Bonime (1962) stated:

> Not all reluctance to terminate is pathological. Genuine affection, gratitude, and enjoyment of the relationship has grown to some degree out of the camaraderie and personal growth experienced in the jointly undertaken long-term activity. There have been significant changes wrought in the patient's way of living, and life is more valuable than it was at the start. The meaningfulness of the friendly, communicative contact with the analyst is even greater in the case of a lonely patient, still unmarried, and without enough nonpathological time behind him to have cultivated enduring intimacies. Some have no family, or no potential in the family as it is presently constituted, for emotionally rewarding experience. The factor of healthy warmth towards the analyst, a prizing of the contact, must be considered. . . . For the analyst to mistake for pathology this fondness, which is based upon a hard-won capacity for affection and intimacy, will produce at termination the same kind of hurt, and, more serious, the same emotional confusion. What is more, the opportunity for resolving such a therapeutic mistake may not occur if analysis is terminated. The healthy reluctance to relinquish a meaningful rela-

tionship must be recognized, respected and welcomed, and placed for the patient in the perspective of his increased prospects for greater and more fulfilling intimacies than are realized with the analyst.

Resistance to termination can signify clinging to the treatment and unwillingness to make commitments to progressive changes as well as a refusal to assume full personal responsibility for mature adaptations. For example, a competitive patient may refuse to terminate because that would give the therapist credit for therapeutic success and the patient would be deprived of the satisfaction of torturing someone in his life.

As a young therapist I was overwhelmed to the point of tears and wordlessness when a six-year-old autistic lad, on leaving our last session, knelt and kissed the base of the office doorframe. Since then I have not faced so poignant a parting, but I have become more comfortable with intense and tender affection.

Conclusions

Therapists integrate and treasure experience with past patients as they look forward to new interchanges. By stimulating countertransference feelings, patients heighten the therapists' sensitivities so that they can appropriately respond to their needs.

NOTE

1. This is an expanded version of a talk presented at the joint meeting of the American Society for Adolescent Psychiatry and the American Academy of Psychoanalysis, New York City, May 1983.

REFERENCES

Blos, P. 1962. *On Adolescence*. Glencoe, Ill.: Free Press

Bonime, W. 1962. *The Clinical Use of Dreams*. New York: Basic.

Epstein, L. 1977. The therapeutic function of hate in the countertransference. *Contemporary Psychoanalysis* 13:213–234.

Epstein, L., and Feiner, A. H., eds. 1979. *Countertransference: The Therapist's Contribution to the Therapeutic Situation*. New York: Aronson.

Freud, S. 1910. The future aspects of psycho-analytic therapy. *Standard Edition* 11:144–145. London: Hogarth, 1964.

Freud, S. 1912. Recommendations to physicians practising psycho-analysis. *Standard Edition* 12:115–116. London: Hogarth, 1964.

Grinberg, L. 1962. On a specific aspect of countertransference to the patient's projective identification. *International Journal of Psycho-Analysis* 43:436–440.

Heimann, P. 1950. On countertransference. *International Journal of Psycho-Analysis* 31:81–84.

Klauber, J. 1981. *Difficulties in the Analytic Encounter*. New York: Aronson.

Langs, R. 1976. *The Bipersonal Field*. New York: Aronson.

Little, M. 1951. Countertransference and the patient's response to it. *International Journal of Psycho-Analysis* 32:32–40.

Racker, H. 1968. *Transference and Counter-Transference*. London: Hogarth.

Tauber, E. S. 1978. Countertransference reexamined. *Contemporary Psychoanalysis* 14:38–47.

Winnicott, D. W. 1949. Hate in the countertransference. *International Journal of Psycho-Analysis* 30:69–75.

Winnicott, D. W. 1971. *Playing and Reality*. New York: Basic.

Wolstein, B. 1981. The psychic reality of psychoanalytic inquiry. *Contemporary Psychoanalysis* 17:399–412.

THE AUTHORS

ELISSA BENEDEK is Clinical Assistant Professor of Psychiatry, University of Michigan, and Director of Training, Forensic Center, Ypsilanti State Hospital, Ypsilanti, Michigan.

IRVING H. BERKOVITZ is Clinical Associate Professor of Psychiatry, University of California at Los Angeles Center for the Health Sciences.

IRVING N. BERLIN is Professor of Psychiatry and Pediatrics and Director, Division of Child and Adolescent Psychiatry and the Children's Psychiatric Center, University of New Mexico School of Medicine, Albuquerque.

NORMAN R. BERNSTEIN is Professor of Psychiatry, Abraham Lincoln Medical School, University of Illinois, Chicago.

CHARLES A. BURCH is a staff member, Sinai Hospital of Detroit.

SUE S. CAHNERS is Director of Social Service, Shriners' Burns Institute, Boston.

BARRY S. CARLTON is Assistant Professor of Psychiatry and Associate Director of Adolescent Psychiatry, Northwestern University School of Medicine, Chicago.

JONATHAN COHEN is Lecturer, Department of Human Development, and Adjunct Associate Professor in psychology and education, Teacher's College, Columbia University, New York.

REBECCA S. COHEN is Director, Clinical Social Work, Department of Psychiatry, Michael Reese Medical Center, and Assistant Professor of Psychiatry, Pritzker School of Medicine, University of Chicago.

MARY DAVIS is Assistant Professor of Child Psychiatry, Division of Child Psychiatry, Medical College of Wisconsin, Milwaukee.

MAIRIN B. DOHERTY is Assistant Professor of Psychiatry and Pediatrics and Director, Child Inpatient Services, University of Massachusetts Medical Center, Worcester.

WILLIAM ELLIS is Assistant Professor of Child Psychiatry, Child Study Center, Yale University, New Haven, Connecticut.

AARON H. ESMAN is Professor of Clinical Psychiatry, Cornell University Medical College, Faculty Member, New York Psychoanalytic Institute, and a Senior Editor of this volume.

DAVID B. FEINSILVER is Staff Psychiatrist, Chestnut Lodge, Rockville, Maryland.

SHERMAN C. FEINSTEIN is Clinical Professor of Psychiatry, Pritzker School of Medicine, University of Chicago, Director, Child Psychiatry Research, Michael Reese Medical Center, and Coordinating Editor of this volume.

ROBERT M. GALATZER-LEVY is Lecturer in Psychiatry, Pritzker School of Medicine, University of Chicago, and Faculty Member, Chicago Institute for Psychoanalysis. He is a Special Editor of this volume.

BENJAMIN GARBER is Clinical Assistant Professor, Pritzker School of Medicine, University of Chicago (Michael Reese Hospital), and Training and Supervising Analyst, Chicago Institute for Psychoanalysis.

PETER L. GIOVACCHINI is Clinical Professor of Psychiatry, Abraham Lincoln College of Medicine, University of Illinois, Chicago. He is a Special Editor of this volume.

MEYER S. GUNTHER is Clinical Associate Professor, Departments of Rehabilitation Medicine and Psychiatry, Northwestern University Medical

School, and Training and Supervising Analyst, Chicago Institute for Psychoanalysis.

ROSA A. HAGIN is Professor of Psychological and Educational Services, Fordham University, New York.

CLARICE J. KESTENBAUM is Clinical Professor of Psychiatry, Columbia University College of Physicians and Surgeons, and Director of Training, Division of Child Psychiatry, New York State Psychiatric Institute.

BONNIE E. LITOWITZ is Adjunct Associate Professor, Departments of Communicative Disorders and Linguistics, Northwestern University, Evanston, Illinois.

JOHN G. LOONEY is Staff Child Psychiatrist, Timberlawn Psychiatric Center, Research Psychiatrist, Timberlawn Psychiatric Research Foundation, Dallas, and a Senior Editor of this volume.

RITA L. LOVE is Psychiatric Social Worker, Mental Health Service, Northwestern University, Evanston, Illinois.

DENNIS L. MC CAUGHAN is a faculty member, Teacher Education Program, Chicago Institute for Psychoanalysis and Chicago School of Professional Psychology.

ROBERT MARTIN is Professor of Psychiatry and Associate Head, Department of Psychiatry, University of Manitoba Faculty of Medicine, Winnipeg, Canada.

JOHN E. MEEKS is Associate Clinical Professor of Psychiatry, George Washington University Medical School, Washington, D.C., and Medical Director, Psychiatric Institute of Montgomery County, Rockville, Maryland.

W. W. MEISSNER is Clinical Professor of Psychiatry, Harvard University Medical School and Supervising and Training Analyst, Boston Psychoanalytic Institute.

NICHOLAS MEYER is an author and director who lives in California.

DEREK MILLER is Professor of Psychiatry and Director of Adolescent Psychiatry, Northwestern University School of Medicine, Chicago.

SOL NICHTERN is Assistant Clinical Professor of Psychiatry, New York Medical College, and Director of Psychiatric Services, Jewish Child Care Association, New York.

KAMBIZ PAHLAVAN is Clinical Instructor in Psychiatry, Harvard Medical School, Boston.

HARRY PROSEN is Professor and Head, Department of Psychiatry, University of Manitoba Faculty of Medicine, Winnipeg, Canada.

IRVING H. RAFFE is Social Worker, Division of Child Psychiatry, Medical College of Wisconsin, Milwaukee.

PERIHAN ARAL ROSENTHAL is Associate Professor of Psychiatry and Pediatrics and Director of Child Outpatient Service, University of Massachusetts Medical Center, Worcester.

JACQUELYN SANDERS is Senior Lecturer, Department of Education, and Director, Sonia Shankman Orthogenic School, University of Chicago.

JOHN SCHOWALTER is Professor of Psychiatry and Pediatrics, Child Study Center, Yale University, New Haven, Connecticut.

ALLAN Z. SCHWARTZBERG is Associate Clinical Professor of Psychiatry, Georgetown University School of Medicine, and a Senior Editor of this volume.

THEODORE SHAPIRO is Professor of Psychiatry and Psychiatry in Pediatrics and Director of Child and Adolescent Psychiatry, Cornell University Medical College, New York.

ARCHIE A. SILVER is Professor of Psychiatry, Division of Child and Adolescent Psychiatry, Department of Psychiatry and Behavioral Medicine, University of South Florida, Tampa.

ARTHUR D. SOROSKY is Associate Clinical Professor of Psychiatry, University of California at Los Angeles, and a Senior Editor of this volume.

FREDERICK J. STODDARD is Assistant Clinical Professor of Psychiatry, Harvard Medical School, Clinical Associate in Psychiatry, Massachusetts General Hospital, and Director of Psychiatry, Shriners' Burns Institute, Boston.

MAX SUGAR is Clinical Professor of Psychiatry, Louisiana State University, Director Children's Unit, Coliseum Medical Center, New Orleans, and a Senior Editor of this volume.

JOHN TOEWS is Associate Professor of Psychiatry, University of Manitoba Faculty of Medicine, Winnipeg, Canada.

MARQUIS EARL WALLACE is Associate Professor, University of Southern California, and Research Clinical Associate, Southern California Psychoanalytic Institute, Los Angeles.

NATASHA L. WALLACE is a member, Department of Psychoanalysis, California Graduate Institute, Los Angeles.

SIDNEY WEISSMAN is Director, Residency Training and Education, Department of Psychiatry, Michael Reese Medical Center, and Assistant Professor of Psychiatry, Pritzker School of Medicine, University of Chicago.

HELEN A. WIDEN is Psychotherapist, Mental Health Service, Northwestern University, Evanston, Illinois.

STEPHEN L. ZASLOW is Associate Clinical Professor of Psychology, Adelphi University, and faculty member, Long Island Institute of Psychoanalysis.

CONTENTS OF VOLUMES I–XI

NAME INDEX

SUBJECT INDEX